The Estimation of the Time Since Death in the Early Postmortem Period

The Estimation of the Time Since Death in the Early Postmortem Period

Second Edition

Claus Henssge MD
Professor of Forensic Medicine,
Acting Head of Institute of Forensic Medicine,
University of Essen, Germany

Bernard Knight CBE, MD BCh, MRCP, FRCPath,
DMJ(Path), Barrister
Emeritus Professor of Forensic Pathology,
University of Wales College of Medicine, Cardiff, UK

Thomas Krompecher MD
Associate Professor, Institute of Legal Medicine,
University of Lausanne, Switzerland

Burkhard Madea MD
Professor of Forensic Medicine,
Head of Institute of Forensic Medicine,
Rheinische Friedrich-Wilhelms-University,
Bonn, Germany

Leonard Nokes MD, BCh, MSc, PhD
Department of Medical Engineering,
University of Wales, Cardiff, UK

Edited by Bernard Knight

A member of the Hodder Headline Group
LONDON

First published in Great Britain by Edward Arnold 1995
This second edition published in 2002 by Arnold,
a member of the Hodder Headline Group,
338 Euston Road, London NW1 3BH

http://www.arnoldpublishers.com

Distributed in the USA by
Oxford University Press Inc.,
198 Madison Avenue, New York, NY10016
Oxford is a registered trademark of Oxford University Press

British Library Cataloguing in Publication Data
A catalogue record for this book is available from the British Library

Library of Congress Cataloging-in-Publication Data
A catalog record for this book is available from the Library of Congress

ISBN 0 340 71960 5

1 2 3 4 5 6 7 8 9 10

Commissioning Editor: Serena Bureau
Production Editor: Jasmine Brown
Production Controller: Iain McWilliams
Project Manager: Tim Wale
Cover Design: Terry Griffiths

Typeset in 10/12 Minion by Phoenix Photosetting, Chatham, Kent
Printed in Italy by Giunti

What do you think about this book? Or any other Arnold title?
Please send your comments to feedback.arnold@hodder.co.uk

Preface to Second Edition

The text of this Second Edition has been thoroughly overhauled, and although there has been relatively little original research published in the field of death-time estimation in the years since the book first appeared, a number of changes and additions have been made. A new section on the use of gastric contents has been added, and Professors Henssge and Madea have refined some of their original work on temperature and other methods.

It is hoped that this new edition will continue to be the only work in the English language to provide up-to-date data and references on this important subject.

Bernard Knight, Editor
June 2002

Contents

Contents

General introduction

BERNARD KNIGHT

The importance of estimating the time since death must have been appreciated for centuries, probably millennia. Even in the most unsophisticated societies, when homicides took place the community would inevitably have correlated the location and movements of the prime suspects with the apparent time of death – however crude that comparison might have been – to test what would later become the defence of alibi.

Little has changed from those early days, except that their data acquisition equipment was merely the back of a hand to test the coolness of the corpse's skin, and their eyes and nose to evaluate decomposition. We now have multichannel thermometry with thermocouples sensitive to a fraction of a degree, enzyme methods, vitreous chemistry, muscular reactivity and several other avenues for collecting data. Regrettably, the accuracy of estimating the postmortem interval has by no means kept pace with the enormous strides made in technological sophistication.

It is obvious why an accurate estimate of the time of death is of such importance in many criminal cases, but there are other reasons why it may be required. For example, the coroner, medical examiner or other equivalent authority needs to know the date of death for registration purposes. Indeed, the legal basis of the English coroner's jurisdiction is to 'enquire where, when and by what means, a person came to his death'. Where a body is found, without witnesses to the death, the death may have occurred in the early morning or the previous evening, with a consequent change of the registrable date of death at midnight. This may have other implications in civil law, in that matters of attaining majority of inheritance may hinge upon that date. Where two deaths, especially of spouses or siblings, occur close together, the order of death – and hence survivorship – may have profound effects upon the transfer of estate and property. Other matters may revolve around insurance and contracts and culpability for delayed death following an accident or assault. Admittedly, these aspects are much rarer than the usual criminal connotations, but are nonetheless important on the occasions when they do arise.

It is not only the defence of alibi that has such relevance to the estimation of the postmortem interval in criminal deaths. In the earliest stage of many criminal investigations, before any suspect is questioned or charged, a knowledge of the approximate time of death is vital if the investigating officers are to direct their enquiries in the appropriate direction. The relationship of the time of death to other events, to persons in the vicinity and to those who could not have been in the vicinity, will automatically channel investigative efforts along certain lines. When several suspects are being considered, the best estimate of the time of death forms a primary screening procedure to eliminate some putative killers, who could not have had access to the deceased at the material time, and may strengthen suspicion against others whose movements coincided with the estimated time. There is thus a heavy responsibility upon the doctor who offers an opinion as to the probable time of death – if he or she is significantly in error, the investigation may be dislocated at its earliest and perhaps most vulnerable stage.

The onus is therefore upon the doctor to provide a *range* of times within which he/she thinks the death occurred, which is as accurate as is justified in the circumstances. Even more importantly, it must not be so unreasonably precise as to exclude incorrectly the true time of death, as this may provide a false alibi for one or more suspects.

When a suspect is charged and becomes the accused, the estimate of the time of death may come under intense scrutiny and robust challenge by the defending lawyers, if a defence of alibi is to be run. The opinion of the doctor may be dissected minutely, criticized and denied by one or more expert forensic witnesses of equal or perhaps much greater experience. It is therefore vital for the doctor to justify the accuracy of measurements, the correctness of calculations, and the logic of method. What the doctor puts into his or her report at the time of examination must be of sufficient resilience to survive intense cross-examination in the court room many months later. It is useless for the doctor to offer the investigators a firm opinion, but fail to adhere to this when in the witness-box. The editor has been present in a court room when a High Court Judge stopped a murder trial and discharged the accused, because two doctors failed to agree on the *day*, let alone the *hour*, of the death of the victim.

To offer an unreasonably accurate time of death is worse than providing such a wide range of times that the police derive no help from it. In the latter situation, they at least then know that they have to use other methods in their investigation, but to mislead them by some outrageously precise time runs the risk of their excluding the true culprit, as well as falsely implicating an innocent party.

Unfortunately, it is often the least experienced medical witness who tends to offer the most accurate estimate, not having seen enough cases to appreciate the many pitfalls and fallacies in the process. Certainly, with all the methods available up to the present time, the opinion of any doctor who offers a *single* time of death, instead of a range – or one who includes any fraction of an hour, instead of a whole hour – must be viewed with considerable scepticism.

Temperature-based methods I

BERNARD KNIGHT AND LEONARD NOKES

TEMPERATURE MEASURING SCALES

Fahrenheit

This scale was devised in about 1714 by the German instrument-maker Gabriel Fahrenheit (1686–1736). He used a mixture of ammonium chloride and ice for his zero, and his own body temperature for the 100-degree mark. On this scale, the freezing point of water was 32 and its boiling point 212.

Centigrade

This scale is divided into 100 degrees, with the freezing point of water as zero and its boiling point at 100. It is often misnamed 'Celsius', after Anders Celsius (1701–1744), a Swedish astronomer, who proposed a 100-degree scale in 1742. However, he placed the freezing point of water at 100 and the boiling point at zero; it was reversed 8 years later by his pupil Martin Stromer.

Reaumur

This scale was devised in France in 1731 by Rene Reaumur (1683–1757). He used an alcohol thermometer, using the freezing point of water as zero, then graduating the stem into degrees, each of which contained one-thousandth of the volume of the bulb and stem up to the zero mark. Arbitrarily, the boiling point of water lay at 80 degrees on his scale.

Early work on temperature and time of death

BERNARD KNIGHT

Although the general principle that corpses cool progressively after death has been appreciated since time immemorial, the first attempts to place the phenomenon on a scientific footing appeared towards the middle of the nineteenth century, as far as writings in English are concerned.

In 1839, a book was published in London by Dr John Davey, which was entitled *Researches, Physiological and Anatomical*, in which Chapter 13 dealt with 'Observations on the Temperature of the Human Body after Death'. In this, the author described his experiments in thermometry conducted on the bodies of eight British soldiers in Malta in 1828, and subsequently on ten others after his return to the cooler climate of the British Isles. Considering that he was such a pioneer in this field, as well as the primitive facilities of his day, Davey's methodology and his insight into the results were remarkably modern. In Malta, the bodies were placed, soon after death, on a wooden table in a large room and covered only with a sheet, so ensuring relatively uniform environmental conditions. Davey recorded the ambient temperature in all cases. No details of his thermometer are given, other than it had a (presumably mercury) bulb and was calibrated in degrees Fahrenheit. Unlike many workers who followed him, Davey did not confine his measurements to only one body site, but recorded the temperatures in various places within the tissues. No skin, mouth, axillary or rectal temperatures were taken, and it seems obvious that the measurements were recorded during the course of autopsies. They were taken between 3 and 29 hours after death, and most were later than 12 hours postmortem. Davey made no attempt to estimate the time of death from his data – much of the discussion in relation to the Malta bodies concerned the very high temperatures discovered in some corpses, which reached 108° and even 113°F some hours after death. He decided that the hot climate and the common infective causes of death contributed to this phenomenon, but also began the long-running speculation about postmortem production of heat in the organs and tissues. However, Davey rejected this hypothesis after some discussion. Following his return to England, Davey decided to continue his measurements in a more temperate climate, and conducted similar tests on soldiers dying in Chatham General Hospital in Kent. In his preamble to this section, Davey offered the first mention of the forensic use of body temperature:

'It may often be a question, how long a body has been dead. By attention to its temperature, particularly of the deep-seated parts, taking into consideration the circumstances affecting temperature, probably in most instances an answer may be given approximating to the truth and which may be of considerable use in evidence'.

Davey's final comments are worth recording, as although in hindsight the first part has proved over-optimistic, his last caution is as true today as when first written, over 150 years ago:

'These observations may enable the enquirer, instituting similar trials and reasoning analogically, to arrive at a tolerably positive conclusion, in doubtful cases of death, as to the time which may have elapsed between the fatal event and the postmortem examination. *Much judgement, however, and nice discrimination may be requisite on the part of the medical man in appreciating the circumstances likely to modify temperature, so as to enable him, when called on for his opinion, to give one which will be satisfactory to the legal officers and to himself, on reflection*'.

Soon after Davey, there were some brief records published in America, in the journal *The Medical Examiner* of Philadelphia, though this has no medicolegal connection with the modern office of *Medical Examiner*, being a general clinical publication. In June 1845, it published an abstract from an article in the *Western Journal of Medicine and Surgery* for June and October 1844 by Dr Bennett Dowler of New Orleans, concerning his temperature measurements of a variety of corpses. This was followed in August, September and October 1845, by letters from Dr Dowler with further information. His main interest was again the 'postmortem caloricity' noted by John Davey – the frequent marked rise in body temperature after death. Dowler took temperatures at different sites, both on the body surface and internally, and also measured them at intervals. His records are a mixture of Fahrenheit and Reaumur, but he does not describe his thermometer. However, he seems to have had not the slightest interest in using his data for medicolegal purposes.

Dowler's publications stimulated another letter to the Philadelphia *Medical Examiner* in January 1846, this time from a Dr Benjamin Hensley, who gave an address in Marietta, Ohio. He said that he used the thermometer mentioned by Dr Dowler, which was composed of a large glass cylinder with a bulb at one extremity, the large cylinder enclosing a smaller one, which was graduated in degrees Reaumur. The boiling and freezing points were found to be correct to within less than half a degree on the scale.

Hensley took many temperatures from various sites, including the skin, axilla, rectum, vagina antecubital fossae, muscle and under internal organs. He repeated these at varying intervals and built up quite a mass of data, though he seems to have made no real use of it. He also took the temperature of the 'dead-house' and in some cases, measured the body temperature several hours *before* death, presumably in those of his patients whom he knew were going to die.

After these rather futile beginnings, as far as post-mortem interval is concerned, there was gap of some 17 years before the subject was tackled again. In 1863, a substantial paper was published in London, which is often cited as if it was the very first in the field, in spite of it quoting Davey, Dowler and Hensley. However, it was the first English-language paper to concentrate on the forensic aspects of the topic. It was a long article by Taylor and Wilkes[1] from Guy's Hospital, published in the Reports of that institution.

Alfred Swaine Taylor was a Lecturer in Medical Jurisprudence at Guy's, and was the author of the famous book *Taylor's Principles and Practice of Medical Jurisprudence*, which was first published in 1865 and was for a century the premier textbook of forensic medicine in the English language. The article had a typically lengthy title for that era, being called 'On the Cooling of the Human Body after Death – Inferences Respecting the Time of Death: Observations of Temperature made in 100 Cases'. The 30-page paper is largely anecdotal and discursive and, although very interesting, is rather disappointing from the scientific aspect. It begins with several pages devoted to putrefaction, a subject hardly relevant to the title.

Taylor and Wilkes' experimental results are marked by several major faults, which cannot be blamed on the facilities available in the middle of the nineteenth century. First, almost all the hundreds of temperature measurements were made 'by placing the naked bulb of a good thermometer uncovered on the skin of the abdomen'. This is highly unsatisfactory, as the thermometer readings must have varied with air temperature, stray draughts, humidity and also with the inconstant area of contact of the curved bulb with the abdomen – to say nothing of the variable relationship of any such small area of skin with the deep tissue temperature.

The other error, which is admitted in the paper, was that for the first 27 cases of the series of 100, the authors omitted to record when the bodies were brought from the hospital wards to the 'dead-house', so it was quite unknown for how long there was a different environmental temperature.

All but four of the hundreds of measurements were taken on the skin surface, and the results were grouped into four ranges: 2–3, 4–6, 6–8 and 12 or more hours after death. As the variation of temperature within each group was very wide, and also because the size of each group varied from 29 to 76 people, the statistical value of the results is very limited. As with previous authors, Taylor and Wilkes made no effort to derive any formula from their data, to assist in calculating the time of death.

Amongst the generalizations and numerous anecdotal cases, there is some interesting observation and speculation. Like previous writers, Taylor and Wilkes noted that there is sometimes a postmortem rise in temperature, and they discuss possible mechanisms for this. These include, of course, the frequent infections that were a common cause of death. They also noted, though without giving it a name, the temperature 'plateau' that still gives rise to controversy and which was to become so important in later research. Other aspects discussed were the effect of environmental temperature, clothing and the effect of immersion in hastening cooling. The first concept of a heat gradient from the interior to the surface is discussed, as well as the obvious fact that the interior of the body can remain warm after the skin is cold.

Two other phenomena were quoted from other authors, which have passed into forensic mythology and still appear, without any scientific foundation, in some textbooks today – though to be fair to Taylor and Wilkes, they were partly dismissive of the claims. The first was quoted from Dr W. B. Richardson, who also wrote in 1863, though the reference is not offered.

He stated that 'a loss of blood, as in cases of death from haemorrhage, whether the blood is effused externally or internally or even temporarily withdrawn from the heart as in syncope, is a cause of rapid cooling of the body'. Taylor and Wilkes point out that 'the sudden cold of collapse is here confounded with the slow and progressive cooling of the dead body'. To Richardson's claim that 'if the body is left dead from direct and absolute loss of blood, cooling to the temperature of the surrounding medium is completed in regard to the external surface in two hours', they comment that 'this may lead to a serious error and implicate an innocent person in a charge of murder'.

The second myth is quoted from Nysten, though again no reference is provided. Nysten claimed that 'the bodies of persons who have died from asphyxia by hanging or suffocation or from the inhalation of carbonic acid gas, do not cool until from 2–48 hours after death and that sometimes, even three days have elapsed before the body has become completely cold'. Taylor and Wilkes disparage this statement by saying 'Too much importance must not be attached to this statement, since it is quite certain that in some cases of fatal asphyxia, the body has cooled just as rapidly as in death from other causes'. However, this justifiable criticism is contradicted elsewhere in the paper, when the authors are describing the death of the Prince of Conde, Duke of Bourbon, who was found hanging by his cravat from a window shutter. Here they say 'As in asphyxia from hanging, the warmth of the body is preserved longer than under common circumstances'. They also make the unfounded assertion that 'Where death has taken place suddenly, as from accident or acute disease or apoplexy, a body has sometimes been found to retain its heat for a long period'.

To summarize, although the article of Taylor and Wilkes has been acclaimed as the earliest paper on postmortem temperatures, it is in fact neither the earliest nor particularly erudite though it has great interest in other ways, such as a record of a hundred common causes of death in mid-nineteenth century London and a series of Victorian anecdotes, which throw a fascinating light on both patients and doctors of that era.

The next important contribution to the literature came three years later, and was of a different scientific calibre altogether. It was written in 1868 by Harry Rainy,[2] Professor of Medical Jurisprudence at the University of Glasgow, who wrote with a clarity of thought and the use of mathematics that at least equals many modern papers on the subject. Rainy acknowl-edges the publications of previous authors and credits the collection of his own data to Dr Joseph Coates of Glasgow Royal Infirmary. They measured abdominal skin and rectal temperatures on a hundred bodies, but sensibly discarded all the surface readings in favour of those from the rectum. They also rejected 54 cases because the temperature of the mortuary was not constant during their experiments. Four, and sometimes five, serial temperatures were measured on each body, between limits of 30 minutes to 63 hours after death. Rainy then calculated the 'ratio of cooling per hour' for each measurement, by expressing the proportion which the excess of temperature above the ambient at the end of an hour, bore to the excess at its commencement, the latter being taken as unity. Rainy was the first to mention Newton's law of cooling, but rightly declared that it was not absolutely correct when applied to dead bodies. 'Bodies recently dead are not found to cool in conformity with this law', he states, and goes on to recount that some actually rise after death, again quoting Davey, Dowler, Taylor and Wilkes in this respect. 'We scarcely hesitate to ascribe this rise in temperature in these cases to physiological processes which are continued after the action of the heart ceases'. Rainy comments on the 'plateau', though again does not name it as such. He says 'It follows that the cooling may be retarded in the earlier stages by the continuance of obscure vital processes … these processes must be kept in view in estimating the time which has elapsed since death'.

Like Fiddes and Patten,[3] Marshall and Hoare,[4] the present author[5,6] and others in the twentieth century, Rainy[2] states categorically that more than one temperature reading is needed to determine the time since death.

It will be obvious that it is important to ascertain, not merely the relative temperature of the body and the surrounding medium when the body is found, but also the rate at which the process of cooling is going on during that period. This requires two observations at an interval of an hour, or if possible, two or three hours.

He goes on to state another truth which is still disregarded by many pathologists and police surgeons even today '… having obtained these data, though we cannot exactly calculate the period which has elapsed since death, we can almost always determine a minimum and a maximum of time within which that period will be included'. This is a statutory warning, from well over a century ago, for doctors not to be so rash as to volunteer a single time of death, but rather to give a preferred range within which they consider that death occurred.

Rainy was the first to offer a formula for calculating the central point of that range of time since death.

'Let the excess of temperature of the rectum at the first observation be t, and at one hour later $t - n$: and let the excess of temperature of the body at death be $n + D$, where D = the rectal temperature at death minus environmental temperature. Further, let $t/t1 = R$ and because t is greater than n and consequently will be greater than unity, then:

$$\frac{\log D - \log t1}{\log R} = x \qquad (2.1)$$

which is the number of hours that have elapsed since death. The number of hours, x, determined by this calculation will in almost every case be *less* than the actual time which has elapsed since death. This arises from the fact that in the early stages, the cooling proceeds more slowly than the assumed (Newton's) law and that the calculation furnishes us with a minimum time.'

Here, Rainy is acknowledging the plateau: he goes on to say

'It is more difficult to fix a maximum time with precision, but a careful comparison of recorded cases will show that in all cases in which the temperature of the rectum is found to be below 85°F, the time elapsed since death has been less than the minimum multiplied by 1.5.'

Rainy then offers the delightful comment, still often appropriate in respect of the mathematical ability of many doctors, that 'Persons unacquainted with logarithms may make the necessary observations when the body is found – and the proper inferences may be deduced by competent parties afterwards!'

This article was the first that can truly be recognized as a proper scientific contribution to the subject and, in spite of its relatively early date, the style and content compare favourably with many modern publications.

Interest increased in the topic, both in English and Continental journals. In 1870, Goodhard[7] published a report, though he contributed little that was useful.

Wilkie Burman,[8] a medical officer at a mental asylum in Wiltshire, published papers in 1874 and 1880, describing his experiments with a special thermometer which he had designed. This was bent at right-angles so that the bulb could be left in the axilla whilst the mercury level was read. Burman first reviews the writings of Hensley and Dowler (who he calls 'Fowler') and of Taylor, upon whose failure to record the time of removal to the mortuary he seizes. In his own experiments, all of which were carried out on skin temperatures, he found no plateau – again showing that the delay in the fall of core temperature must be due to the interval needed for the establishment of a heat gradient. Burman tested a number of cases from a 'lunatic asylum' in Yorkshire and pointed out that 'his results were of greater value than those of Taylor and Wilkes', because his special thermometer could be read without disturbing its position in the axilla, and also because all his estimations began either at the moment of death or even before death took place. Burman's article was the first to exhibit a graph of results, which indicates an almost linear fall over the first 12 hours, with no trace of a plateau. He calculated that the mean drop in temperature was 1.6°F per hour. One of his deaths showed a slight postmortem temperature increase and, in common with the material of many of the early writers, the temperatures at death are often markedly elevated, presumably due to infective disease.

Burman stated that cooling was much faster in the immediate postmortem period, as there was no plateau in skin measurements. The mean rate of cooling for hyperthermic bodies was 4.4°F per hour. As a recommendation for calculating the time since death, he advocates dividing the observed drop in temperature in degrees Fahrenheit by his factor of 1.6, which is really the same rule-of-thumb method recommended right up to the present day by some authors. In fact he suggested, in 1880, that the factor be rounded down to 'one and a half' – exactly the figure given in standard books for so many years. To give credit to Burman, he adds all the usual cautions and advocates modifying the result according to environment, clothing, etc.

The first author writing in English to move to the Centigrade system was Womack[9] in 1887. Womack used a special mercury thermometer with a flattened bulb of very thin glass, which he strapped to the abdominal wall with white adhesive tape. This obviously gave better results than Taylor and Wilkes, method, as it reduced cooling of the bulb by draughts and convection. However, Womack claimed that the thermometer could be read to an accuracy of 'better than a fortieth of a degree', which seems unrealistic even by today's standards and, for 1887, it seems unlikely that comparably exact calibration could have been available.

Womack used sophisticated mathematics, including calculus, to apply Newtonian theory to his 118 cases, and illustrated his article with several graphs. These he referred to as 'woodcuts', as they were white on a black background – perhaps an early precursor of our 'reverse video'!

Once again, Womack found no initial plateau, due to his choice of the skin as a measuring site. Although Womack's paper is an impressive piece of mathematics, it is marred in retrospect by the unrealistic accuracy with which he computed his time of death. In his first illustrative case, he apologizes for estimating the time of death as minutes to 5 o'clock, whereas it was really 5 minutes past 5 ... yet the first temperature reading was not taken until half past twelve. In his second example, Womack again calculates to within a few minutes of the true time, more than 5 hours after the death, from two skin temperatures taken 30 minutes apart. Over his series of 118 cases, he recorded an accuracy of better than 25 minutes from the true time for 57 deaths – an impossible result given the method used.

One of the best-known of the 'modern' publications in the field of temperature and time-of-death is that of De Saram et al.,[10] who carried out their research in Sri Lanka (at that time Ceylon). This appeared in 1955, and began a new era of investigation in the subject. Some of the interest stemmed possibly from the rather macabre fact that the work was carried out on victims of judicial execution, but the intrinsic worth of the research is undoubted, even though the algorithm produced has never enjoyed widespread use in practice.

De Saram and his collaborators worked in a tropical country where the ambient temperature was high, so that their results were not readily applicable to temperate climates. They investigated the cooling rates of 41 executed criminals under strictly observed conditions, by taking hourly rectal temperatures beginning usually an hour after execution.

They noted a 'lag period' or plateau of about 45 minutes, and added this to their estimates of time since death arrived at from their calculations. De Saram et al. recommended using a formula which incorporated all the known variables, rather than the use of a general calculation followed by further modifications according to local circumstances. His actual submission is that: 'The time of death (should) be estimated, not, as at present, by a generalised formula where the influence of modifying factors are assessed, so as to say, empirically, but by the use of a formula which itself embodies the influence of these factors'.

De Saram et al. included the humidity of the environment, which in Ceylon varied between 70 and 90% saturation, considering that this was a potent factor in altering the cooling rate. The presence of thick cotton overalls on the bodies was dismissed as having little influence, as five of the bodies from a different prison were measured unclothed.

The De Saram formula combined heat losses from convection, radiation and conduction and the mathematical principles of his methods are discussed in a later chapter of this review. His discussion from first principles is an excellent review of the whole problem, and well repays study even from this distance of 47 years.

In 1956, Lyle and Cleveland[11] entered the scene with new technology in the form of a six-channel thermocouple device which continuously recorded temperatures at a number of sites, these being plotted on a strip chart every minute. These were from the skin of the chest, forehead, rectum, liver, brain and thigh muscle. Valuable data were acquired, demonstrating that the rate of heat loss was widely different at different sites, but that extrinsic variables had less effect on brain than on rectal temperature. They also pointed out the well-known fact that time of death could not be determined satisfactorily after 24 hours or where the difference in environmental and body temperature was only a few degrees. Lyle and Cleveland did not derive any practical formula from their work, and the main legacy of this research is some of the actual data from the recordings.

Karl Sellier[12] from the Bonn Institute, published a paper of considerable mathematical complexity in 1948, based on the concept of the infinite cylinder. Most of his work was pure mathematics and heat mechanics, and was a very useful dissection of the theoretical basis of the problems, discussed further in Chapter 3 of this book. Sellier was obviously very much influenced by the work of De Saram, to whom he refers constantly. He states that the experimental material in his own Institute was not usable because the environmental temperature was too variable and the bodies did not stay long enough, so he used the data of De Saram for his manipulations.

He made the interesting assertion that the retardation of cooling in fat bodies was not due to the insulating effect of the 'fatty pads', as he called them, but to the fact that the excess adipose tissue increased the radius of his cylinder.

Also in 1958, the seminal paper of Fiddes and Patten[3] appeared which, like that of De Saram et al.[10] is still held up as one of the models of theorizing about the use of temperature in time-of-death estimation. Fiddes and Patten pinned their hopes on assessing the rate of fall of the temperature, by using two or more temperature measurements. They also developed the concept of 'virtual cooling time', this being the time taken to cool through 85% of the difference between normal body temperature (not defined, but assumed to be 37°C) and the environmental temperature. This is discussed in more detail in Chapter 3.

Fiddes and Patten devised a 'percentage cooling rate', in which the fall in temperature from 'normal' is expressed as a percentage of the difference in temperature between 37°C and the ambient. This is calculated for two or more points separated in time, and the postmortem interval calculated by applying the data to a standard graph offered by the authors from 100 known cases. The method can be applied only if the ambient temperature remains constant throughout the whole investigation and if the initial body temperature is assumed to be 37°C (or some other fixed assumption). The merits and disadvantages of Fiddes and Patten's method are discussed further in Chapter 3. It might also be noted that when James and Knight[13] used the Fiddes and Patten double-measurement method in their research into errors, they found it to give no added accuracy compared with a simple single-exponential method.

Professor T. K. Marshall of Belfast is one of the most prolific writers of recent years (up to the 1970s) and, with several collaborators, produced a doctorate thesis and six other publications on temperature and time since death. The best known paper is that by Marshall and Hoare,[4] published in 1962. The paper showed that a dead body did not cool according to Newtonian principles during the first 12 hours after death. These authors suggested that the deviation from Newton's law is due to postmortem metabolism and the development of temperature gradients in the surface layers of the body, resulting in a sigmoid rather than single exponential cooling curve.

However, after about 12 hours, the curve approximates to an exponential expression and is then amenable to use for postmortem interval calculation, as the rate of heat loss is then directly proportional to the excess of temperature of the body over its surroundings.

The rate of cooling per degree of temperature difference (the 'cooling factor') was then said by Marshall to be proportional to the ratio of the effective radiating surface of the corpse to its mass (the 'size factor').

Marshall and Hoare[4] devised a formula, discussed later in this chapter, which expressed two exponential terms: first, the cooling proportional to the excess of the temperature excess of the body over its environment; and second, the influence of modifying factors.

By reference to many experimental results, which provided 'standard cooling curves', the use of this formula was held to provide satisfactory results. Their data have been reworked several times by others, though with conflicting results. The recent computer and nomogram methods of Henssge et al.[14] described at length in later chapters of this book, are substantially based on Marshall and Hoare material. In the many other papers by Marshall, with and without collaborators, the basic theory has been discussed and refined. Perhaps one of the most useful comments of this prolific author is contained in the very last sentence of an article in the *Journal of Forensic Sciences*[15]: 'It would seem that the timing of death by means of temperature can never be more than an approximation'.

Body temperature at the time of death

LEONARD NOKES

It is very difficult to specify a 'normal' body temperature, as this value can vary considerably between individuals. Rectal temperatures in a group of healthy subjects can vary between 34.2 and 37.6°C, with a mean of 36.9°C. Rectal temperature is often referred to as 'deep central temperature', similar in value to that of the brain, heart, lungs and abdominal organs. As reported by Mead and Bonmarito[16] in 1949, variations in rectal temperature can be obtained depending on the location of the measuring instrument. If it is near a large vein, the heat within that region is dissipated more readily than an avascular area. Vital organs such as liver and other abdominal viscera produce about 70% of the total body heat while at rest. During exercise, the main heat-producing components are the skin and muscles.

The temperature differences between the major internal organ areas, skeletal masses and the skin led to the concept of a 'mean body temperature (Tb)'. At a comfortable room temperature (24–25°C), two-thirds of the body mass is considered to be at a core temperature, represented by the rectal thermal reading (Tr). One-third of the body mass is assumed at a shell temperature, represented by the skin thermal reading (Ts). The 'mean body temperature', therefore, can be represented by:

$$Tb = 0.67Tr + 0.33Ts$$

This relationship is, however, subject to errors, as the proportion of body mass at core and shell temperatures changes as a function of environmental temperatures. Isotherms demonstrate that in cold climates the core temperature is reduced, which results in a lower 'mean body temperature'. The rectal temperature may increase slightly due to peripheral vasoconstriction resulting from direct thermal stimulation or increased sympathetic activity.

Many factors influence body temperature. Most individuals show a diurnal rhythm in which the body temperature fluctuates by ±0.5°C around the person's normal mean temperature (Fig. 2.1). These cyclic patterns persist regardless of activity or disease states, but they are less well established in small children and may be reversed in adults who change their working patterns or rapidly cross international time zones. Other factors which influence body temperatures are:

- Emotional stress of pleasure or displeasure.
- Febrile disease states (fever) and non-febrile disease states (hyperthyroidism).
- Exposure to a severe cold environment.
- Metabolic disorders, including hypothyroidism.
- Peripheral circulatory disorders.

Age also affects body temperatures; children tend to have higher rectal and oral temperatures (37.5–38°C) than adults. Newborn and premature infants have body temperatures that are highly dependent on their thermal environment because they do not have well-developed thermoregulatory systems. Most women show body temperature changes related to the menstrual cycle.

The thermoregulatory system has three major components, as shown in Fig. 2.2. Sensory thermore-

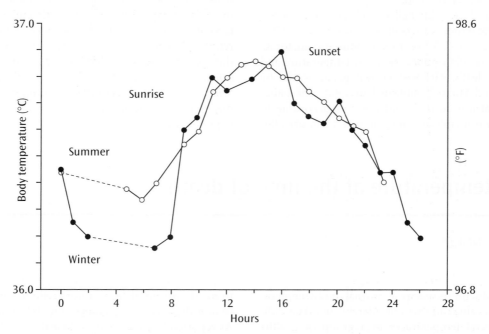

Figure 2.1 *Circadian rhythm in body temperature. Body temperature is lowest in early morning, gradually increases during the day, and reaches a maximum in mid-afternoon, during peak activity (from Selkurt[17]).*

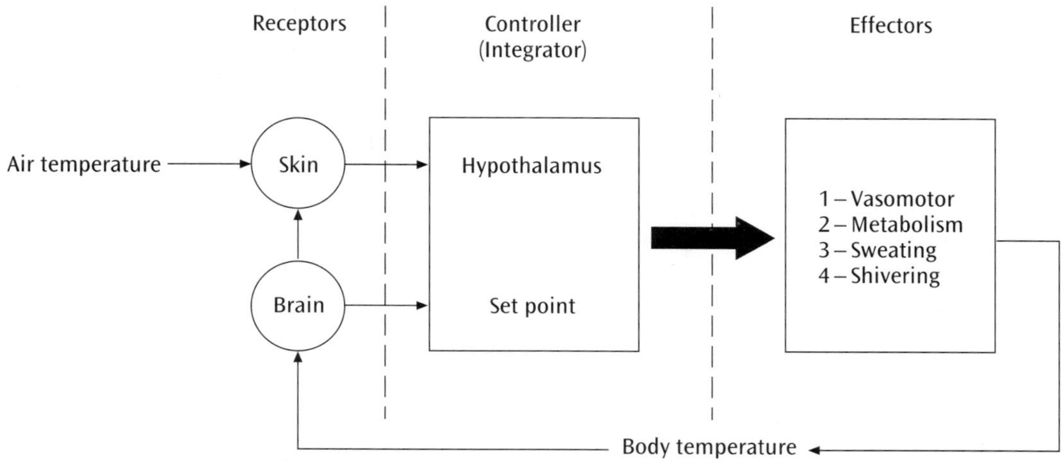

Figure 2.2 *Basic components of the thermoregulatory system, showing receptors (skin and central receptors), hypothalamic controller (or integrator) with central set point, and effector systems regulating heat production, conservation and loss (from Selkurt[17]).*

ceptors supply skin and deep temperature information to the central integrator, which compares this information with a standard reference value. On the basis of any difference, the integrator sends information to effector systems which control heat production or loss.

Conditions that prevent heat loss or heat production and which lead to thermoregulatory imbalance are numerous. These disorders can cause the following heat illnesses:

- Skin disorders such as sunburn.
- Fainting resulting from combined effects of extensive peripheral vasodilatation and cerebral ischaemia.

- Heat stroke, which is primarily a result of an inability to sweat, causing brain temperature to rise to a critical level (41°C).
- Heat exhaustion, which is a malfunction related to water and electrolyte metabolism.

Sedatives and tranquillizers suppress temperature regulation and cause vasodilatation, leading to fainting. Cold disorders influence the ability to tolerate cold by involving peripheral circulation or cardiac defects. In some individuals, cold induces haemagglutination, which reduces cutaneous blood flow and heat transfer. This makes the individual more susceptible to frostbite and increases their hypersensitivity to a cold environment.

The cooling of a corpse

LEONARD NOKES

The cooling of a human corpse and the factors which affect cooling are well described in a paper by Joseph and Schiekele[18] in 1970. This section mainly reports their analysis of how the body cools and its various cooling parameters.

THE COOLING OF A PHYSICAL OBJECT

The heat flow from an object is described by:

$$\text{Flow} = \frac{K \times \text{difference in energy level}}{\text{resistance}} \qquad (2.2)$$

where K = constant of proportionality. The flow of heat along an object is described by:

$$\text{Flow per unit area} = \frac{C \times \text{difference in temperature}}{\text{insulation thickness}} \quad (2.3)$$

where C is the thermal conductivity of the material. Consider a solid cylinder of uniform temperature, Tc, placed in a cooler environmental temperature, Te. Heat will flow from the surface to the environment. A temperature gradient between the surface and the region just below it will be established. The gradient will work its way inward, slowly at first, building to a maximum rate, and then slowing again as the temperature at the centre reaches that of the environment. The whole process takes the appearance of the well-observed sigmoid curve.

The shape of the cooling curve is not the same throughout the body. Figure 2.3 shows the cooling curves at the surface, midpoint of the radius and at the centre of the body. The use of rectal temperatures as a measure of mean body temperature is not strictly accurate. A thermometer placed in the rectum records the temperature of the tissues in the immediate vicinity of the rectum. The time taken for a corpse to cool is a function of the size and shape of the body and the insulation surrounding it. By assuming the body to be an infinitely long cylinder, Joseph and Schiekele[18] and Sellier[12] concluded that the major factors influencing the cooling time were the radius and insulation of the body. This is the basis of Marshall's 'size factor', which states that the larger the body, the greater the volume which must be cooled, relative to the surface through which cooling takes place.

1. The heat lost from the core of a body encounters a series of barriers to the flow:
2. The resistance offered by the more peripheral tissues.
3. The resistance of the clothing or covering.
4. The resistance at the outer surface of any body covering.
5. Of the air drifting by and picking up heat.

By using the analogy of an electrical circuit, we can assume that the individual resistances are in series and can be added together to give an overall value of resistance. The total resistance can be

$$\text{Total resistance} = \frac{Tc - Te}{\text{heat flow}} \quad (2.4; \text{ from eqn } 2.2)$$

The usual unit of resistance to heat loss is the Clo. One Clo is considered to be the insulation provided by ¼ inch (6 mm) thickness of still air. The Clo measures the resistance to the conduction of heat through a material and to both the convection and radiation losses at the body surface. Some relevant Clo values are shown in Table 2.1 (first presented in Joseph and Schiekele's paper[18]).

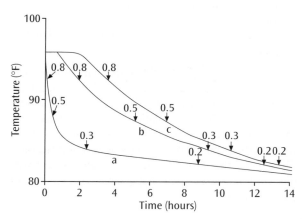

Figure 2.3 *Observed course of cooling at surface (a), midpoint of radius (b) and centre (c).*

Table 2.1 *Clo values for barriers to heat loss from the body core*

Resistance	Range of insulation offered	Clo units
Shell tissues	0.2–0.8	Usual value 0.3
Clothing	0–4	
Body support (bed, ground, etc.)	Variable; about 8 for a 2″ (5 cm) mattress	
Ambient air	Very still	1.0
	Closed room	0.8
	5 mph wind	0.4
	10 mph wind	0.3
	High wind	0.2

In addition to the series resistance to convection and radiation losses from the body surface, clothing and air, there are two more possible resistances in parallel with these. The first is evaporation loss due to drying out of tissue, whilst the second resistance is due to 'explicit radiation'. Explicit radiation may be associated with the presence of external heat or cold near the body. A resistance diagram including values for a typical indoor situation is shown in Fig. 2.4.

To quantify the various resistances in the cooling body, Joseph and Schiekele investigated the heating and subsequent cooling effect of a rubber cylinder. The data from a thermocouple placed in the long axis of the cylinder are shown in Fig. 2.5. These results reflect the influence that various conditions have on the cooling of the cylinder. Note in particular the high rate of cooling and the shape of the curve for the cylin-

der in 'still' water. The curve may be called 'compound', representing a non-uniform cooling pattern. The increase in the conductivity of the water after some hours is counterbalanced by the reduced convection currents in the water compared with air. The cylinder is then additionally insulated by a thin layer of still warm water near the surface.

Compound cooling curves shown in Fig. 2.5 (d, e and f) illustrate the effect of getting into bed. At first, the body is chilled, and only when the bedding has absorbed some heat does it begin to insulate and to slow down heat flow.

Due to the complex shape of the curve and the corresponding model needed to describe it, it is advisable not to move the corpse during the determination of its time since death using temperature measurements.

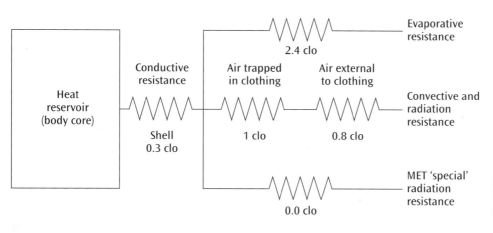

Figure 2.4 *Resistance to heat flow from the body core.*

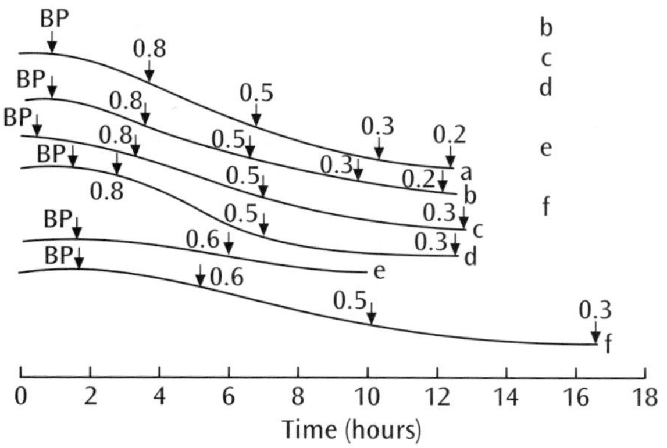

Curve	Temp drop from centre to air	Conditions of run
a	25.5	Cylinder standing upright
b	18	On concrete
c	16.5	In water
d	20.5	On cushion and uncovered
e	17	On cushion covered with double blanket
f	17	Upright 1.5 clo insulation

Figure 2.5 *Course of cooling at the centre of a test cylinder under various conditions.*

The temperature plateau

LEONARD NOKES

The shape of the cooling curve of a human corpse is of great importance as it is inevitably the basis on which all postmortem temperature investigations are made. Many investigators have presented cooling curves derived from different environmental conditions and varying body temperature measurement sites.

In general, it is reported that the body cools in a manner adequately described mathematically by the double exponential sigmoid formula (Fig. 2.6). However, some investigations present cooling curves which can be represented by a single exponential or a straight-line formula. The accuracy of these models is examined later in the chapter. Generally, the more complex the cooling model, the more difficult it is to apply. Simple models are usually as good as the more complex over the region of the cooling curve that approximates a straight line or a single exponential (Fig. 2.6). The regions which cause concern are those at the start of the cooling and at the end, as the body temperature approaches that of the environment. It is in these regions that the simple models break down,

and where the more complex versions may be of some assistance in determining the time since death.

Most models fail to take into account a phenomenon described as the 'plateau'. In 1880, Burman[8] stated that 'Whilst admitting the undoubted rise in axilla temperature that does, in some instances, take place after apparent death' he interestingly adds 'that death does not take place until the body commences to cool down'! The reference in his paper to other workers in this field undoubtedly supports the fact that it was not uncommon to observe a postmortem temperature rise and a *delay* in cooling, i.e. a 'plateau'.

In 1955, De Saram *et al.*[10] presented cooling data that supported the existence of a plateau, though it should be pointed out that the conditions under which they obtained these data were markedly different from those of other investigators, in that the environmental temperatures were approximately 85°F. Other workers in temperature conditions similar to those of Britain have reported the existence of a plateau.[4,19,20] Shapiro was one of the first investigators to analyse in detail the postmortem plateau. He points out observations made by Fiddes and Patten[3] and other co-workers, that any temperature-based technique used to determine the postmortem period must include provisions for the possible existence of a plateau. Hutchins[20] reported that, in 20 patients, after death there was a postmortem rise in rectal temperature, with temperatures returning to the premortem level over a 3-hour period. He does not disclose the environmental temperature, but states that all bodies were usually unclothed, wrapped in a shroud and on a metal stretcher in a postmortem room. He concluded that the initial rise in postmortem rectal temperature may be caused by the continuing metabolic activity of body tissue and of bacteria in the intestine after the cessation of heat dispersal by circulation and respiration.

For the plateau to exist, certain factors must have been present, involving either the production of heat, or the prevention of heat loss after death. If the body is well insulated by heavy clothing, this would present the mechanism by which the body loses heat to its surroundings; namely, evaporation, conduction, convection and radiation. Cooling by radiation, convection

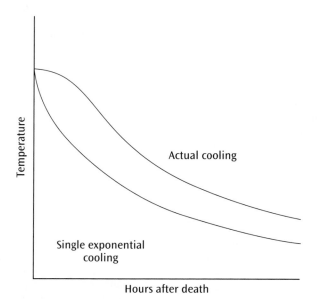

Figure 2.6 *Graph of actual body cooling and single exponential cooling.*

and conduction are dependent on the temperature of the body surface. Evaporation of moisture from a dead body is little understood; De Saram et al.[10] suggested that a reduction of moisture evaporation after death would be expected due to respiratory and circulatory failure.

Shapiro[19] and Brown and Marshall[21] postulated that the postmortem plateau is due to the delay in establishment of temperature gradients which involves heat loss from the centre (core) of the body by conduction to the surface and further heat loss to the atmosphere by radiation and convection. Fiddes and Patten[3] were of the opinion that metabolic processes do not necessarily cease at the moment of death but continue for a short period after clinical death, producing heat; indeed, some constitute an additional factor contributing to the maintenance of the plateau. The cessation of blood circulation will cause the oxygen tension in the tissues to fall rapidly, resulting in no further aerobic activity. Anaerobic metabolism in muscles may, however, attain a high level, with the production of lactic acid from glycogen. Nearly all the muscle glycogen is broken down during the first few hours after death. Evolution of heat from other autolytic processes will occur, but the amount produced would be less than that caused by glycogen breakdown. Nokes et al.[22], in 1985, speculated that glycogenolysis is responsible for maintaining a temperature equilibrium in the human corpse shortly after death. Lundquist[23] claimed the initial rate of cooling to be 0.5°C/hour, rising to 1°C/hour during the maximum rate of cooling. For a 70-kg body this represents a heat loss of 35 kcal/hour and 70 kcal/hour, respectively.

Lundquist also stated that the breakdown of muscle glycogen to lactic acid, and hence internal heat generation, is approximately 140 kcal for a human body, released over a period of several hours. For a plateau to be maintained, heat loss must equal heat gained. From Lundquist's data it would appear that this could be the case, provided that the body is well insulated and the environmental temperature is relatively high.

Several literature sources have presented cooling curves of dead bodies that do not exhibit a temperature plateau.[11, 24] The occurrence of a plateau appears to be dependent upon four factors:

- the position on the body of temperature measurement;
- the environmental temperature;
- surface insulation; and
- the size of body.

An obese body wearing heavy clothing and lying in a place with a relatively high environmental temperature would be more likely to produce a cooling plateau than would a thin, naked body under similar conditions. The existence of a plateau greatly affects the calculations for time since death as nearly all theories describing cooling of human bodies need to be adjusted to take the cooling delay into account.

To conclude, it is important that environmental temperature, clothing and size of body be taken into account when analysing early postmortem periods of up to 6 hours. If the case under investigation appears to be a likely candidate for exhibiting a delay in cooling, it is advisable to add 1–2 hours to the estimated postmortem period.

Single exponential models

LEONARD NOKES

One of the earliest investigators to develop a model to fit his clinical observations was Rainy[2] in 1868, who reported data from 100 cases over a finite postmortem time period. The temperatures were recorded at the umbilicus and rectum but, in presenting his data, Rainy disregarded the umbilical temperatures. He reduced his sample size to 46 cases in which the temperature of the 'dead room' remained constant. This, he states, was done with the view of eliminating as far as possible all the circumstances which might complicate the law of cooling. He correctly noted that Newton's law of cooling could not be applied in the true sense to a cooling human corpse. Newton postulated that the rate of cooling is proportional to the difference of temperature between the surface of a hot body and surrounding cool medium. Rainy noted that the rate of cooling of a corpse varied, due to:

- the increase in body temperature after death, possibly up to 4 hours' duration; and
- the general shape of the cooling curve (later described as 'sigmoid').

In developing his model, Rainy assumed the rectal temperature at the time of death to be 100°F; he also stated that the accuracy of the model should be accepted with caution. The calculated postmortem period gives a time that should lie between a maximum and minimum period. The derived formula relies upon two rectal temperatures, taken at least 1 hour apart and is described as:

$$x = \frac{\log D - \log t'}{\log r} \qquad (2.5)$$

where x = number of hours after death, D = rectal temperature at death minus the environmental temperature, t = rectal temperature minus the environmental temperature, t' = rectal temperature 1 hour later minus the environmental temperature, and $r = t/t'$.

It is interesting to note that Rainy's formula is one that has appeared numerous times in the literature since the turn of the century, albeit in various formats. From his equation, the minimum postmortem time is calculated in the early stages of cooling (if rectal temperature 85°F). The maximum time is calculated by multiplying by 1.5 × calculated time (if rectal temperature 85°F).

The next paper to describe a model derived from postmortem data was that of Womack,[9] in 1887. This paper, although 100 years old, is an example to all modern-day research workers in its objectives, analysis, discussion and conclusion. A criticism is that temperature measurements were taken on the abdominal surface. However, in his development of a model, Womack assumes Newtonian principles of cooling, which assume surface heat loss, and although its practicality in determining the postmortem period may be less than ideal, his model, on theoretical grounds, is perfectly correct. He also presents other workers' data and, on analysis of the 'woodcuts' (graphs), reiterates the point that the rate of cooling is greater in the early postmortem period (see Fig. 2.6). Due to lack of data from previous investigations, Womack decided to take temperature measurements from various corpses in order to develop a model of cooling. He dealt with the cooling problem in two parts: first, to determine the

temperature of the body when brought into the mortuary; and second, to find at what time previous to this did the excess of temperature over that of the hospital ward where the corpse lay correspond to a normal abdominal temperature of 36.2°C. A graph of a set of typical temperature measurements from a corpse is shown in Fig. 2.7. The principal difficulties pointed out by Womack were:

- The unknown temperature at death.
- The development of rigor mortis and postmortem rise in temperature.
- The varying temperature of the atmosphere.
- The varying locality of the body.
- The varying condition of the body.

Womack concludes by stating that, of 118 corpses, 57 exhibited an error between actual and calculated time of death of 25 minutes. Of the remainder, 33 cases exhibited an error of 40 minutes, 12 cases 60 minutes, and 16 cases greater than 60 minutes. The later corpses, Womack states, had abnormally high temperatures at death.

In 1980, Kuehn and co-workers[25] reported a case involving an 8-year-old girl found frozen, and the use of Newton's laws of cooling to determine the postmortem period. Experiments on dogs under similar conditions indicated that Newton's simple model had to be abandoned and a new approach developed. The

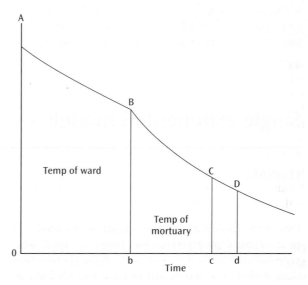

Figure 2.7 *Reprint from Womack's paper of a graph showing a set of typical abdominal temperature measurements from a corpse.*

alternative model incorporated a three-stage response in which the skin, muscle mass and body-core heat-flow characteristics could be taken into account. By trial and error, which involved determining various constants experimentally, the new model was applied to the victim. The calculated postmortem time was found to be in close agreement with that obtained in evidence presented at the trial of the suspected killer. The authors concluded that the success of the technique in this particular case was primarily due to the extensive documentation of the circumstances, particularly the environmental temperature, history and the thermal condition of the body prior to sudden death. Caution was expressed regarding use of the technique in cases which involve a gradual loss of consciousness associated with hypothermia.

An alternative use of a single exponential model in determining the postmortem period was the application of Newtonian cooling to temperature measurements taken from the trachea after death[26]. The technique involved taking two temperature measurements 1 hour apart, and hence determining the time constant which enabled the postmortem period to be calculated. Prior knowledge of original trachea temperature was required, which was assumed to be 37°C. The authors stated that various factors could affect trachea temperature; these included metabolic activity, increased breathing and climatic conditions.

A change of 1°C could yield an additional error of up to 30% on the estimated postmortem time. The technique, however, did have some advantages over other methods. No knowledge was required of the environmental temperatures, clothing or the surface area of the corpse.

Double exponential models

LEONARD NOKES

Since the time that the first investigators in the nineteenth century began to plot temperature measurements from cooling corpses, it became apparent that the body cooled sigmoidally (see Fig. 2.6). Investigators including Rainy[2] in 1868 and Womack[9] in 1887, commented on the changes in rate of cooling seen just after death, and as the temperature of the body approached that of the environment. In the 1960s, numerous publications by Marshall and co-workers analysed the cooling curve of dead bodies and postulated that the best mathematical expression to describe the data was that of a double exponential model. To understand Marshall's approach, it is necessary to start with the single exponential equation. The next few pages will be of interest to the numerically minded, and can be avoided if desired without any loss to the theme of this review.

DEVELOPMENT OF DOUBLE EXPONENTIAL MODEL

The Newtonian law of cooling can be represented by:

$$q = hA \, (Ts - Tf) \qquad (2.6)$$

where q = the heat transfer rate from the surface of the body; h = the heat transfer coefficient from the surface to the environment; A = the surface area; Ts = the surface area of the body; and Tf = the temperature of the environment.

If we make an assumption that the human body is thermally thin and has a physical size, density (d), specific heat (s) and thermal conductivity (k), eqn 2.6 can be rewritten as:

$$-MS \, \frac{dtb}{dt} = hA \, (Tb - Tf) \qquad (2.7)$$

where M = the mass of the body; S = the specific heat of the body; and dtb/dt = the rate of change of the body temperature (with respect to time) after death.

Assuming that the environmental temperature does not change with time, integrating eqn 2.7 gives:

$$\frac{Tb - Tf}{Tbo - Tf} = \frac{\exp \, (-hA \, t)}{(MS)} \qquad (2.8)$$

where Tbo = initial body temperature at the time of death; hA/MS = cooling factor (Z).

Many investigators have usually implied that eqn 2.7 is Newton's law of cooling, but this is incorrect, as only eqn 2.6 is the true statement of Newton's law of cooling. Eqn 2.6 will reduce to eqn 2.7 only under limiting cases of a thermally thin body – which the human body is certainly not, as the rectum is at a very different temperature from the skin.

The sigmoidal curve has appeared many times in the literature concerning heat conduction. In 1959, Corslaw and Jeager[27] showed that the sigmoidal curve can be described by an equation having an infinite series of exponential terms. The observed human cooling curve can therefore be expressed as:

$$\frac{Tr - Tf}{Tbo - Tf} = \sum_{n=1}^{n=\infty} An \exp(-\alpha nt) \qquad (2.9)$$

where Tr = the temperature at some radial position, r, inside the body at a time, t, after death; An and n = functions of radial position, r, overall body diameter, body density, specific heat, thermal conductivity and surface area heat transfer coefficient between the body surface and the surrounding environment.

A paper by Brown and Marshall[21] in 1974, concluded that Eqn 2.9 could be reduced to:

$$\frac{Tr - Tf}{Tbo - Tf} a_1 \exp(-\alpha_1 t) + a_2 \exp(-\alpha_2 t) \qquad (2.10)$$

as an additional exponential term is redundant after the first 3 hours after death. The same conclusion was reached by Marshall and Hoare[4] 12 years earlier, as their cooling formula also contained two exponential terms:

$$Tr - Tf = B \exp(-Zt) + \frac{C}{Z - p} \exp(-pt) \qquad (2.11)$$

B, C, Z and p are constants of the corpse under investigation, and it is assumed that $Z > 0$, $p > 0$, and $p \neq z$.

The first term expresses simple exponential cooling, whilst the second term takes into account the changes in the cooling factor, Z. In order to evaluate the constants in Marshall and Hoare's formula, knowledge of the height and weight of the body is required, as is the environmental temperature history and the corpse core temperature at the instant of death.

The constants a_1, a_2, α_1, α_2 in Brown and Marshall's equation (eqn 2.10) are determined experimentally by taking two sets of temperature measurements a finite period apart and at least 12 hours after the suspected time of death. To determine a_1 and a_2 requires further information about the size of the body. Evaluation of the 'size factor' involves the ratio of the surface area exposed to cooling and the body mass (A/M).

In 1985, Nokes et al.[22] further developed the double exponential cooling model postulated by Brown and Marshall. The resulting formula, based on taking four sets of temperatures 15 minutes apart, enabled the postmortem period to be determined without recourse to:

- Calculation of ambiguous constants.
- No allowance for size or clothing of the body under investigation.
- Calculated postmortem period dependent only on actual data taken from corpse.

The disadvantages involved the need for accurate temperature measurement of at least 0.1°C and the assumptions of a constant environmental temperature and original body temperature.

Other models of body cooling

LEONARD NOKES

In 1955, De Saram et al.[10] reported from Ceylon (now Sri Lanka) a number of cases perhaps unique in the investigation of postmortem cooling. Rectal temperatures were obtained from 41 corpses whose time of death was accurately known. These unfortunate individuals had been executed by hanging, which enabled temperature measurements to be made minutes after the point of death.

In formulating a model to represent their temperature data, De Saram et al. examined the heat losses from dead bodies by conduction, convention and radiation. They suggested that the relationship between the rate of cooling of the rectum $-d\theta/dt$ (the negative sign implies a decrease in rate of rectal cooling with time) and the temperature difference θ between the rectum and a constant environment, might be expressed as:

$$\frac{-d\theta}{dt} = b\theta + \alpha \qquad (2.12)$$

where a and b are constants for a particular body under investigation, which can be obtained by plotting the rectal temperature drop against time. Eqn 2.12 has a solution of the form:

$$\alpha + b\theta = K \exp(-bt) \qquad (2.13)$$

where K is constant.

The validity of the model was examined by comparing the experimental data and the calculated temperature measurements from eqn 2.13. De Saram *et al.* noted an error of less than 1°F between actual and calculated points. This is not surprising, having used the original experimental data to develop the model. It would be pertinent to try the model on other sets of temperature data from cooling corpses.

Dividing both sides of Eqn, 2.13 by b, it can be shown that the postmortem period can be calculated from:

$$t_1 - t_0 = \frac{\log(\theta_0 - p) - \log(\theta_1 + p)}{\log(\theta_1 - p) - \log(\theta_2 + p)}(t_2 - t_1) \qquad (2.14)$$

where θ_0 is the original body temperature minus the environmental temperature, two temperature measurements taken some time t_1 and t_2 apart. Since there is no practical way to calculate p, eqn 2.14 reduces to:

$$t_1 - t_0 = \frac{\log\theta_0 - \log\theta_1}{\log\theta_1 - \log\theta_2}(t_2 - t_1) \qquad (2.15)$$

On examination, this is no different from the single exponential model and does not take into account the plateau often seen in warm climates, such as Sri Lanka.

One of the most complex mathematical analyses of the cooling of a human corpse was carried out by Sellier[12] in 1948. In order to model cooling curves, different geometrical dimensions, heat transfer coefficients and ambient temperatures had to be considered. Sellier stated that eqn 2.16 represents the heat balance of an infinitely long cylinder with radial heat flow:

$$\frac{d^2\theta}{dt} = a\left[\frac{d^2\theta}{dr^2} + \frac{1}{r}\frac{d\theta}{dr}\right] \qquad (2.16)$$

where a = thermal diffusivity; t = time; r = some radial position inside the cylinder; and θ = temperature of cylinder minus surrounding temperature.

The general solution to eqn 2.16 is:

$$\theta = \sum_{n=1}^{n=\infty} D_K \exp(-n^2) K \exp(at) J_0(n_K - r) \qquad (2.17)$$

The various constants in eqn 2.17 are determined by the boundary conditions of the object under cooling. Various parameters of eqn 2.17 were investigated, including the heat flow at the surface (function of r) and the thermal conductivity (function of a). The most important parameter which influences the cooling curve was found to be the radius of the cylinder. The establishment of the temperature gradients and hence the slow rate of initial cooling is strongly influenced by the radius of the object.

One of the simplest and most often-quoted means of determining the postmortem period is based on the percentage method devised by Fiddes and Patten in 1958.[3] These authors measured the difference in temperature between the rectum and the environment for over 100 corpses and analysed the varying rates of cooling. Due to the decrease in cooling rates when the rectal temperature approaches that of the environment, they developed the concept of 'virtual cooling time'. This assumed that the time taken to reach a 15% difference between the rectal and environmental temperatures represented 100% virtual cooling time. Calculating the time since death involved taking two sets of temperature measurements a few hours apart. The percentage reduction of the temperature difference between the rectum and the environment at both times is plotted on the graph shown in Fig. 2.8. The estimated postmortem period is calculated as a

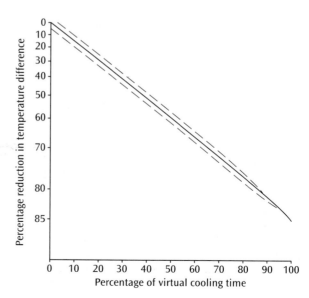

Figure 2.8 *The percentage reduction in temperature difference between rectum and environment against percentage of virtual cooling time.*[1]

percentage of the virtual cooling time obtained from Fig. 2.8.

The negative aspects of the Fiddes and Patten method include the upper and lower limits expressed on the graph in Fig. 2.8. When the limits are incorporated into the postmortem calculations, they can lead to large errors. The decision as to which side of the average line a body is likely to lie, depends on the size and the clothing of the corpse. Well-clothed subjects of good nutrition fall above the line, whilst thin, poorly clad individuals fall below the line. The exact point on the graph for these two examples is not quite clear. Finally, the method is based on a single exponential model of cooling which, as previously explained, fails to take into account the changes in the rate of cooling often seen in the early postmortem period.

An interesting, though somewhat confusing, paper was that presented by Botezatu[28] in 1977. He analysed various biochemical components of blood and pericardial fluid, together with measurements of rectal temperature of corpses who had died under various circumstances. The indices measured included total nitrogen, albumin fractions, electrolytes (Na^+ and K^+) and the enzymes aldolase, aspartate and alanine-aminotransferase, with deaths having occurred from trauma, asphyxia, electric shock and sudden cardiovascular failure. Over 14 000 blood and pericardial fluid analyses were carried out at various environmental temperatures ranging from 10 to 23°C. For clarity, an example is given of how the postmortem period is estimated using Botezatu's approach. In cases of death due to head trauma and in an environmental temperature of between 10 and 15°C, total nitrogen was estimated in blood from the right side of the heart and from a femoral vein blood sample. Serum potassium from both sites was also measured, as was the rectal temperature over a finite postmortem period. These sets of data were then substituted into five separate formulae designed to show the relationship between time of death and the individual indices. All appear to represent parabolic equations. The constants for these five formulae change depending upon the mode of death and the sites from which the samples were taken for biochemical analysis. The time of death is calculated by averaging the results obtained from the five formulae. Botezatu claims that, for death due to head trauma, the error between actual and calculated postmortem interval is within 0.05 hour.

For death due to drowning, samples are obtained from 'vessels in the region of the death spots', and 'measurements of general protein' are also included in the calculations. We leave the reader to ponder on these statements.

The final section of the paper further complicates matters by stating that once the values from various equations for a particular mode of death are established, a graphical solution is used to determine the time since death. No reference is made to this graph in the earlier sections.

The methodology is interesting, but Botezatu fails to explain why he selected the various indices and their relationship to modes of death and environment. The wide variabilities make it highly impractical without recourse to expensive and complex equipment.

Using similar analogies suggested by previous investigators, Hiraiwa et al.,[29] in 1980, derived a cooling model of the human corpse from the concept of the infinite cylinder. To address certain points raised by previous researchers, the following were investigated:

- The accurate position of the rectum inside the body.
- The effect of the radius of the cylinder.
- The possibility of estimating the postmortem period.
- The behaviour of the rectal temperature when there is some fluctuation in the ambient temperature.

In an attempt to answer some of these questions, a mathematical expression was developed based on work presented by Joseph and Schiekele.[18] The differential equation for an infinitely long cylinder incorporating the theory of heat transmission is given in eqn 2.16.

A solution to eqn 2.16 can be obtained by assuming certain boundary conditions. In order to investigate the effects of the environment on the model, eqn 2.16 was replaced by:

$$2a \frac{d^2\theta}{dr^2} = \frac{d\theta}{dt} \qquad (2.18)$$

which assumed that the fluctuation in ambient temperature be represented by:

$$\frac{d\theta}{dr} = 0 \text{ at } r = 0 \qquad (2.19)$$

The final model assumed a solution to eqn 2.16 using a finite difference technique.

The validity of this cooling model involved accurate measurement of the rectal position using computed tomography and the use of data obtained by De Saram *et al.* from corpses as reported in their paper in 1955. Constant updating of various parameters, including the heat thermal diffusivity, was also undertaken. The size of the corpse was included in the post-mortem calculations by the measurement of the hip circumference.

Hiraiwa *et al.*[29] claimed errors of less than 1 hour using their technique, but several assumptions were made in calculating the postmortem period:

- The environmental temperature remained virtually constant over the postmortem period (no more than 2°C variation).
- Rectal temperature at time of death was 37.64°C.
- Failure to take into account the possible existence of a temperature plateau.

The report of Hiraiwa *et al.*, however, introduced the concept of developing a dedicated computer to determine the postmortem period.

In order to avoid the use of body-size parameters when estimating the time since death, Green and Wright[30] developed the time-dependent Z equation (TDZE) method. This technique is relatively simple to use and relies on three sets of data, including two rectal temperatures taken 1 hour apart and an ambient temperature. By completing some simple arithmetic and with the aid of a graph (Fig. 2.9), the time of death can be estimated.

The theory is based on the observation that the rate of cooling (Z) varies as the body cools. By analysing the changes in the rate of cooling, and assuming that the body cools in a manner adequately described by a double exponential mode, a reference curve was constructed. The postmortem period is estimated using the formula:

$$T = -F \times A/G \qquad (2.20)$$

where $G = (\theta R1 - \theta R2)/(tR2 - tR1)$; A < ($\theta R1 + \theta R2)/2 - Te$; $\theta R2$ = the rectal temperature (second reading); $\theta R1$ = the rectal temperature (first reading); $tR2 - tR1$ = the time between measurements.

To find F requires the calculation of a constant termed the reduced θR:

$$\theta R = (\theta R1 - (\theta bo - \theta R2)/2)\theta bo - Te \qquad (2.21)$$

where θbo = original body temperature, and Te = environmental temperature.

The value of F is obtained from the graph shown in

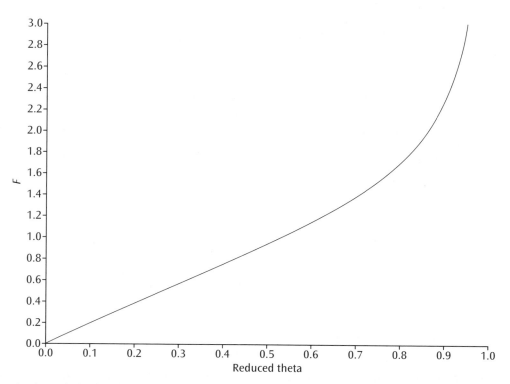

Figure 2.9 *The theoretical reference curve relating reduced theta with the numerical function* F.

Fig. 2.9, which shows the generalized relationship between the reducing temperature and F.

Green and Wright compared their method with other techniques for estimating the postmortem interval, and concluded that the minimum error using their logarithm occurred in the early cooling period, and that this was acceptable due to the comparatively short period since death compared with percentage errors over a longer time period.

Problems which may arise from using Green and Wright's method are similar to those inherent in other techniques using the double exponential model, that is:

- The assumption that the body temperature at the time of death is 37°C, which need not be the case.
- The assumption that the environmental temperature remains constant over the cooling period.

Large errors can be introduced by the use of ambiguous constants, and great care is therefore required to implement the technique correctly.

In 2001, Al-Alousi et al.[31,32] reported their findings on the cooling of 117 cases, both clothed and unclothed. Measurements included brain, liver and rectal temperatures using microwave thermography. Average cooling curves were constructed relating temperature ratio with time after death. The graphs are shown in Fig. 2.10. The temperature ratio is defined as:

$$\frac{Tbt - Tet}{Tbo - Tet} \tag{2.22}$$

where Tbt = the temperature at any body site measured at a given time; Tbo = the temperature of any body site at the moment of death; Tet = the temperature of the environment measured at time t.

Equation (2.22) was used in preference to simple temperature measurements in order to compensate for the fluctuation of the environmental temperature.

Knowledge of original body temperature at various sites at the time of death is very important, as this can lead to large errors. Al-Alousi et al.[31,32] acknowledged this point, and suggested figures shown in Table 2.2 as possible values. We find it slightly perplexing that the liver – a site of energy metabolism and hence a major

Table 2.2 Average values for body site temperatures at time of death[30]

Body site	Average temperature (°C)	Standard deviation (°C)
Brain (naked)	26.5	3.7
Brain (covered)	27.7	3.7
Liver (naked)	27.5	3.1
Liver (covered)	32.7	2.9
Rectum (naked)	36.6	2.0
Rectum (covered)	32.2	4.8

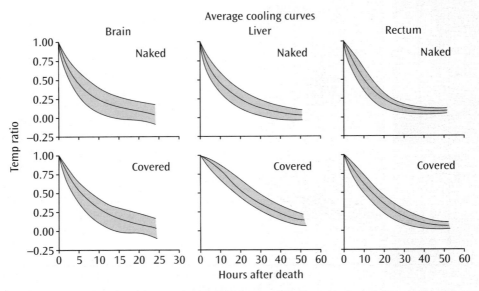

Figure 2.10 Average cooling curves for three sites in naked and covered bodies. The shaded areas indicate the range of error corresponding to ± 1 standard deviation.

heat-producing organ – has a lower value than the rectum. Our own investigations have shown repeatedly that the liver temperatures are higher than those of the rectum, even after death.

On examination of the cooling curves shown in Fig. 2.10, it can be seen that the one standard deviation area can introduce large errors in the calculated post-mortem period. The authors in their conclusions state that: 'Estimation of the time of death using this method gives accurate confidence limits and is of major value in forensic investigation. However, it is insufficiently precise to be used in evidence'.

Temperature measurement

LEONARD NOKES

The simplicity of the mercury-in-glass thermometer (Fig. 2.11) and the convenience of a direct-reading temperature scale have enabled the measurement of body cooling to be made with some degree of accuracy. By adopting a careful experimental technique, it is possible to estimate the temperature between the range 0 to 100°C with an accuracy of 0.5°C.

Possible sources of error in mercury thermometers include:

- The variation in diameter of the capillary bore.
- The variation in the fundamental interval from 0 to 100°C.
- The influence of the variation in the external pressure on the bulb due to alterations in atmospheric pressure.
- The effect of the internal pressure on the volume of the bulb, due to the height of the column of mercury above the centre of the bulb.
- Changes in the zero or 'ice point' reading.

The composition of the glass is very important, as some glasses can show very large thermal hysteresis. The best results are obtained with pure potassium glass containing a large percentage of silicon and calcium and small amounts of sodium and potassium oxides.

Calibration involves the removal of strains set up in the glass during manufacture. This is resolved by annealing the thermometer at a higher temperature than its working range. The bore is then calibrated and the fundamental range is obtained from the ice (0°C) to steam (100°C) points. Comparison with other standard mercury or electrical thermometers can be made at a number of temperature points.

Adaptations of the standard mercury thermometer, when used to measure temperature of cooling corpses, have involved the construction of a right-angled instrument. The bulb is kept in the corpse's axilla, and the shaft lies across the chest. This enabled the read-

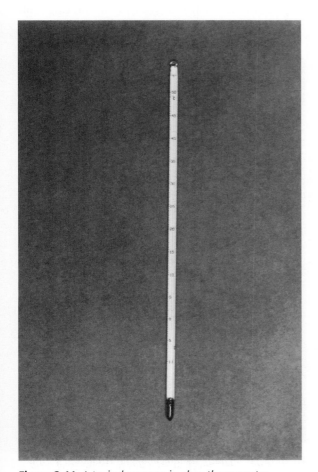

Figure 2.11 *A typical mercury-in-glass thermometer.*

ings to be made without disturbing the corpse or removing the thermometer. In 1887, Womack[9] flattened the bulb and used a thermometer made of very thin glass, which was strapped to the abdomen of the corpse by adhesive tape. Womack stated that 'the thermometers could be read to one fortieth of a degree C and estimated to less than this'.

Some of the first investigators to use electrical instrumentation to measure temperature from corpses were De Saram *et al.*[10] in 1955 and Lyle and Cleveland[11] in 1956. The principle of thermocouples is shown diagrammatically in Figs 2.12 and 2.13. If two dissimilar metals are joined together and one junction is heated to a temperature t_1, the other remaining at a temperature t_0, then a current will flow in the circuit. The electromagnetic force (EMF) developed may be

used as a measure of the temperature difference between the two junctions. In order to measure the EMF, the circuit shown in Fig. 2.13 is usually employed. Here the couple, which has been indicated as a platinum against an alloy of rhodium and platinum, is opened at the cold junction t_0 to where it is connected to a measuring system such as a potentiometer or a millivoltmeter. Thermocouple accuracy is normally in the range of +0.1 to +0.2°C. This degree of accuracy requires relatively expensive equipment and precise laboratory calibration. Many recent methods to determine the postmortem period require temperatures to be measured to at least 0.1°C.

Sources of error include the presence of stray EMFs and differences in the thermoelectric properties of the circuit. Instability and drift can also occur when the output voltage and the thermoelectric power change over a period of time.

Many recent time-of-death studies have used thermocouples to measure the cooling of dead bodies. This has the advantage of displaying and storing cooling data. Figure 2.14 shows a simple hand-held ther-

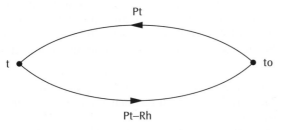

Figure 2.12 *Principle of thermocouples. Pt, platinum; Pt–Rh, platinum–rhodium alloy; to, cold junction temperature.*

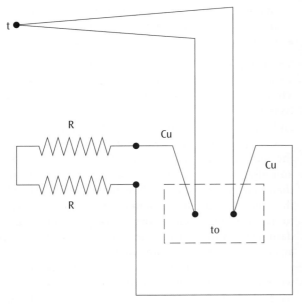

Figure 2.13 *Practical thermocouple circuit. Cu, copper; R, resistor.*

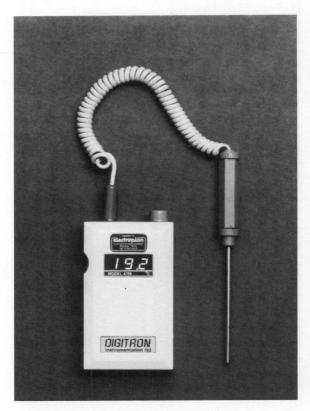

Figure 2.14 *A typical hand-held digital readout thermocouple temperature device.*

mocouple device which is typical of that used by many to record body temperatures.

Lyle and Cleveland,[11] in 1956, and Nokes et al.[26] in 1986, recorded the cooling curve of individual corpses directly onto paper in real time. Green and Wright[30] stored temperature measurements on a data-logger. The advent of relatively cheap computers now enables easy storage and rapid analysis of data, and techniques which 100 years ago could not have been employed without some difficulty can now be carried out with relative ease.

Other methods used to record body temperature after death include the use of the hot-wire principle described by Kuroda et al.[33] in 1982. The apparatus shown in Fig. 2.15 was used by Kuroda to estimate the thermal conductivity of the human skin. A heat source (chromel wire) and a thermocouple were placed in a polytetrafluoroethylene tube held between two pieces of excised skin. The temperature distribution within the assembly was made uniform by being kept in an incubator for 1 hour at approximately 31°C. Heat was then applied via the chromel wire and the temperature recorded. Figure 2.16 is a graph showing the relationship between temperature and log time. From the slope of the graph and various end-condition estimations, the average thermal conductivity of skin was found to be 0.30 kcal/mh°C.

Body heat can be recorded optically and is often measured by thermal devices used, for example, by the

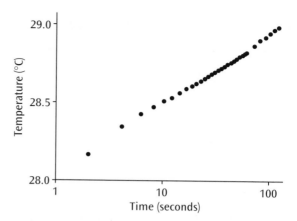

Figure 2.16 *The relationship between temperature and log time recorded using the equipment shown in* Fig. 2.15.

fire service to detect trapped victims. An alternative non-invasive thermography method is that described by Al-Alousi et al.[31,32] The thermal radiation from the human body consists mainly of three wave types, of which microwave is one. The amount of microwave emitted is relatively small and requires considerable amplification in order to record the levels. The measurement of thermal radiation does enable heat generated deep in the body to be recorded non-invasively, but this advantage may not be sufficient to detract from the cheaper, more accurate methods such as thermometers and thermocouples.

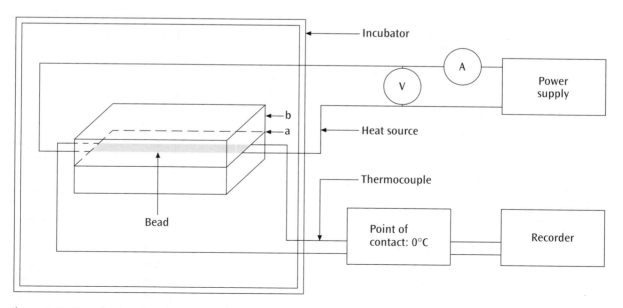

Figure 2.15 *Hot-wire technique to measure skin conductivity. a, surface; b, subcutaneous.*

Temperature probe sites

LEONARD NOKES

The earliest investigators into postmortem cooling recorded temperature measurements from external points on the body. The axilla was a popular site because of its relative ease of access and the minimum amount of disturbance to the thermometer readings from changes in environmental temperature. The external abdominal temperature was also recorded by some. Burman[8] in 1880, quoted Taylor as stating that:

'Fallacious results may arise from the customary method of judging of the degree of coldness of the body by the mere and unaided sense of touch. The dead human skin is a good conductor of heat and thus the surface may appear cold (though it be not really so) to a moderately warm hand; and that, moreover, the condition of the hand itself may lead to an erroneous impression, for instance, if the two hands be different temperatures, a recently dead body may appear cold to one and warm to the other'.

Taylor rightly urges that 'in all observations of the temperature of the dead body, a thermometer should, if possible, be employed, and be applied, not only to the exterior surface of the body, but also to the interior parts'. Even after this sound advice, Burman (to his later regret) recorded data from the external surface of the abdomen. It was felt that this was justified because the skin over the abdomen was thin and thus enabled the temperature recording of the 'most important heat-producing viscera'.

One of the earliest records of analysing rectal cooling of corpses was carried out by Rainy[2] in 1869. He investigated 100 bodies in order to develop an equation to determine the postmortem period. Some 80 years later, in 1949, Mead and Bonmarito[16] published a paper that questioned the reliability of rectal temperatures as an index of internal body temperature during life. A flexible catheter with an array of thermocouple tips along its length was passed up the rectum of several volunteers to a depth of 8 inches (20 cm). The temperatures near the tip of the catheter were, in almost all cases, lower than the temperature recorded simultaneously at intermediate points along the catheter. Radiography showed that the tip of the catheter in a majority of instances lay near the posterior wall of the pelvis, and that cooled blood from the surface of the body passing through the pelvic wall veins was responsible for the recorded drop in temperature at the catheter tip. These authors concluded that an index of deep body temperature was meaningless unless measurements were taken at a constant position and beyond the direct influence of the temperature of blood in the large pelvic vessels. Numerous investigators have since provided an analysis of rectal temperature readings, but few have modified their experimental protocol in order to avoid the problems highlighted by Mead and Bonmarito.

Multisite temperature recordings of cooling bodies were reported by Lyle and Cleveland[11] in 1956. Figure 2.17 shows the cooling curves from various sites from a corpse over a 25-hour period. These authors also presented a comparison between rectal and brain postmortem cooling (Fig. 2.18). It is interesting to note that, although they declined to draw any conclusions from their data, they did suggest that the brain was likely to be less affected by factors that could affect the cooling of other body structures.

Simonsen et al.[24] in 1977, also concluded, after examining the multisite cooling curves of 20 cases, that the brain temperature in association with an evaluation of the development of the signs of death, was the most reliable means of estimating the postmortem interval. Figure 2.19 is a graph of the various cooling curves from multitemperature sites on a corpse analysed by Simonsen et al.

It is interesting to note that, with reference to Figs 2.18 and 2.19, the brain appears to have little if any postmortem delay in cooling, whilst in Fig. 2.19 it can be speculated that from the rectal cooling curve that a plateau does exist. This has some bearing on the calculated postmortem period.

Most formulae that describe postmortem cooling do not take the plateau into account. Olaisen[34] in 1979, reported similar observations as were recorded by Brinkman et al.[35] that an initial plateau does exist in postmortem brain cooling, but concluded that the brain still had obvious advantages over the more traditional body temperature measurement sites. The

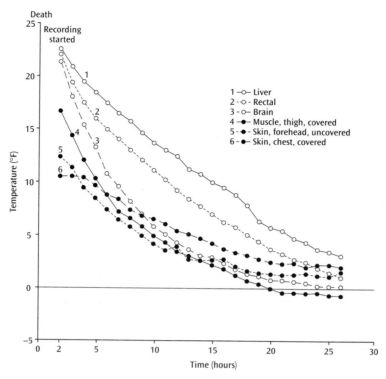

Figure 2.17 *Cooling curves from six body sites.*

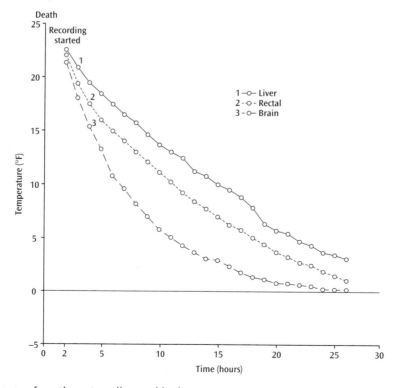

Figure 2.18 *Cooling curves from the rectum, liver and brain.*

major disadvantage of using the brain as a site for temperature measurement is its relative inaccessibility.

The disadvantages of using the rectum as a measurement site include those reported by Mead and Bonmarito[16] and, perhaps more significantly in modern scene-of-crime procedures, is the desire not to disturb the anus because of possible sexual abuse that may have occurred to the victim before death.

In 1986, Nokes *et al.*[26] reported five cases where the tracheal temperature was recorded during a finite postmortem period. They pointed out the following disadvantages:

- The uncertainty of the original trachea temperature at the time of death.

- The possibility of a cooling plateau, which is not taken into account in the technique.
- The precise position of the thermocouple must be known.

It is difficult – if not impossible – to state with any degree of confidence that one body site is preferable to another when recording and analysing postmortem cooling. In an ideal situation, the temperatures should be recorded external to the corpse, but be sufficient to measure the cooling of a particular point deep within the body that is not influenced by the environment. The recorded cooling curve should be in the form of a pure exponential in order that a simple mathematical formula can be developed to estimate the time since death.

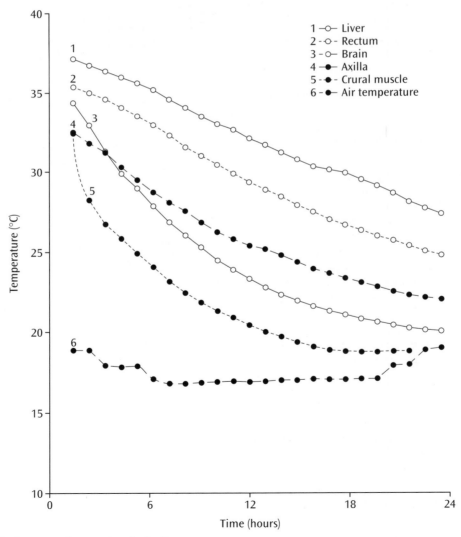

Figure 2.19 *Cooling curves from various body sites.*

Outer-ear (tympanic) temperature in estimation of time since death

BERNARD KNIGHT

In France, Baccino has carried out extensive experiments using the temperature in the deep auditory canal, against the tympanic membrane, for estimating time since death.[36,37] This approach is claimed to be more accurate than the Henssge nomogram used alone.

The claimed advantages include avoidance of using the rectum for thermometry at the scene of death, with its attendant problems of contamination before sampling for sexual interference. The head is also known to cool independently of the clothing on the body and other modifying factors; only the thickness of the head hair affects the cooling rate. The problem of the temperature plateau is also avoided as the relatively small, globe-shaped head cools uniformly, with no significant delay in the establishment of a temperature gradient.

The temperature at the tympanic membrane has been shown to be the same as the hypothalamus, and thus can be accepted as being equivalent to the core temperature of the head. The shape of the probe used by Baccino is such that aberrations from external air temperature passing down the meatus are avoided. The probe often actually penetrates the tympanic membrane. Many hundreds of test estimations were made on deceased hospital patients where the time of death was accurately known. One sample of 138 cases was divided into four groups representing different ambient temperatures during postmortem storage, and regression formulae were derived from ear temperature and known time since death. Both ears were used, and mean temperature was used as a single parameter. Serial temperatures were not employed.

Results were better than were obtained with five other methods also used singly (rectal temperature, vitreous and cerebrospinal fluid potassium, and blood sodium, potassium and chlorides), but were less accurate than a multivariate equation using a combination of several of these other methods. An equation expressing the postmortem interval (PMI) as a function of ear temperature and ambient temperature was derived.

On a second cohort of 141 cases, the PMI was calculated using this equation, and compared with three other temperature methods: the Henssge nomogram; the 'Rule of Thumb 1' (PMI = fall in rectal temperature in °F/1.5); and 'Rule of Thumb 2' (PMI = fall in rectal temperature in °C + 3). This regime was applied to both the four ambient groups and to three varying ranges of PMI. In all cases, the ear temperature method gave better results than all three methods, and contrasted especially with the Henssge method and Rule of Thumb 1. No postmortem temperature plateau was observed in bodies kept at ambient temperatures above 15°C.

Where ambient temperatures are between 16 and 23°C, the formula is:

$$\text{PMI (minutes)} = 56.44 \, (37 - \text{tympanic temperature, °C}) - 150.$$

The 66% confidence interval is ± 25%, and the 95% interval is ± 40%.

Baccino has emphasized that the method's simplicity makes it especially suited to use at the scene of death, as no interference occurs with either the perineal or liver area. Moreover, a PMI result is immediate, without recourse to delay for weighing the body or sending samples for biochemical analysis, although combined methods may eventually provide a more accurate result. No penetration of the cranium is required, as in other published methods using brain temperature.

Errors in estimating time since death

BERNARD KNIGHT

Apart from the inherent fallacies and inaccuracy of the actual models and algorithms used to calculate the postmortem interval, a number of external factors also contribute to errors in the final estimation. It is not possible to introduce compensatory corrections for some of these when making the calculation, usually because the magnitude of the effect of the factor is incalculable, especially when that effect varies in an unknown fashion during the postmortem period. For example, a body may lie before discovery in an ambient temperature which varies considerably due to weather changes, the opening of doors, changes in central heating, etc. Even if the effect of a factor upon the chosen algorithm is accurately known (which is rare), the variation in magnitude and the times during which these variations have operated cannot be known retrospectively in operational conditions, so marked errors can be introduced into the calculations.

Factors that can introduce errors into the calculations include:

- The ambient temperature, which can vary widely and rapidly in certain conditions and can swing both higher and lower than the final temperature as measured on discovery of the body. The temperature of the environment is, of course, partly determined by some of the other factors listed below.
- Wind and draughts affect body temperature by increasing convection and conduction from the surface and by evaporating moisture.
- Rain, humidity and snow, apart from the direct temperature effect, alter the evaporative properties of the skin and clothing.
- The body posture alters the rate of heat loss, by varying the effective exposed surface area per unit mass available for convection and conduction.
- The body size also alters the mass/surface area ratio. Infants and children cool more quickly for this reason, as the heat gradient from the core is steeper.
- Naturally, clothing (or its lack) makes a very great difference to cooling rates. Other coverings, such as bedclothes, other fabrics, even debris or another adjacent body, can dramatically alter the cooling characteristics.
- In the same way as clothing, body fat acts as an insulator, and its deficiency or absence accelerates cooling, and vice versa.
- However debatable the applicability of Newton's law of cooling might be to human cooling, there is no doubt that original body temperature at the time of death affects the progress of heat loss. This is partly by the Newtonian principle of a higher cooling rate where the excess of body temperature above ambient is large, but also from the smaller fall of temperature remaining above ambient.

The errors introduced by these variables in most methods of estimation of the postmortem interval can be gross and, even more disturbing, usually incalculable. This means that not only do the investigating officers receive an inaccurate time of death but, where they realize it is inaccurate, they cannot know the possible range of inaccuracy within wide limits. Most recent workers in this area have estimated their 'confidence limits', a prime example being Henssge et al.,[14] whose meticulous research is contained in later chapters of this book.

However, even accepting the veracity of the underlying theory and calculations, the result of providing a 95% confidence limit (i.e. indicating that the calculation will produce results that will lie with the time range offered 95 times out of each 100) is that a wide safety margin has to be incorporated into the method. This is to be applauded, as false accuracy is worse than no estimation at all, but naturally reduces the evidential value of the estimation. All research is directed at increasing the usefulness of the technique by decreasing the width of the confidence limits.

One of the few published accounts of an estimation of actual errors was made by James and Knight.[13] In this investigation, 110 bodies with a known time of death were examined by one of two experienced forensic pathologists, each pathologist making the estimation alternately with no knowledge of the real time of death. The estimates were then compared with the true interval to evaluate the errors. Although the rectal temperature was used to obtain the first estimate of the time since death, this was modified by other factors in the light of the pathologist's experience, to arrive at a final estimation. The factors used were clothing, height, weight, intraocular pressure, skin discoloration, rigor mortis and hypostasis. The examiner was also told where the body had been since death, in order to try to duplicate the information that would be available at a real scene of suspicious death. The investigation took place over 1 year, and the climatic conditions were known to the pathologists.

The first 100 cases were estimated on the basis of a single rectal temperature, whilst a further 10 were subjected to the Fiddes and Patten[3] calculation using two or more temperature readings over a minimum of 3 hours.

The single temperature method was a 'rule of thumb' test in which the fall of the rectal temperature from 37°C was multiplied by a factor which varied with the 'average' ambient temperature in which the body had spent most of the time since death. These factors were 1.0, 1.25, 1.5, 1.75 and 2.0 for average temperatures of 0, 5, 10, 15 and 20°C, respectively. The results of this scheme showed that under-estimations of the postmortem interval were considerably more frequent than over-estimations – in other words, the body had more often been dead considerably longer than the pathologist estimated. This error increased as the true interval exceeded 36 hours. Of the 100 bodies, the true time since death was correctly estimated in only 11 cases, whilst under-estimations occurred in 57 and over-estimations in 32. In 35 of the 100, the error was less than 10%, in 54 less than 20%, in 70 less than 30%, in 90 less than 40% and in 95 was less than 50%. In two cases, there was an error of 100%.

The absolute error increased as the interval grew longer but, in percentage terms, appreciable errors can also exist even near the time of death. For instance, a 1.5-hour estimate of a true 45-minute interval would imply 100% error.

As mentioned earlier, 10 extra cases were tested using both a single and a Fiddes and Patten[3] double-temperature estimation. Times of death were calculated for each method for all 10 cases and the results compared. In five cases the single temperature method gave the best result, in four cases the double method was more accurate, and in one case they were equally inaccurate.

The general experience gained from this investigation was that in deaths which occurred less than 4 hours before estimation, the major problem was the variable 'plateau', with seven bodies having rectal temperatures at or even above 37°C up to 4 hours postmortem – a phenomenon constantly encountered since the early days of research in the mid-nineteenth century.

Analysis of algorithms in actual cases

LEONARD NOKES

The use of eight different temperature methods to determine the time since death for eight corpses was examined. The various calculations may give the reader a useful insight into which method might best suit their particular circumstances.

Again, it is important to point out that it is not the intention to establish which is the most accurate method. The objective is to show the various calculations for each algorithm applied to practical case examples. The choice of the algorithms was based on the desire to illustrate the wide variation in application. Some require little mathematical ability by the user, whilst others require numerous calculations. For detailed explanations of how each algorithm was derived, the reader is referred to the appropriate references listed at the end of the chapter.

SUBJECTS AND METHODS

After admission to the mortuary, the bodies (of which the time of death was accurately known) were stripped, weighed and measured. They were then taken to a room where they were placed in a supine position on a plastic tray. Rectal temperatures were recorded using a calibrated thermocouple, connected to a recorder which printed temperature readings every 30 minutes. The thermocouple was inserted approximately 6 cm into the rectum.

Table 2.3 shows the data from eight corpses, required to apply the eight algorithms. For ease of comparison, the first temperature reading (i.e. Temp 1) corresponds to the actual postmortem interval of 10 hours for each corpse.

APPLICATION OF ALGORITHMS

The following calculations correspond to corpse 1 in Table 2.3. The remaining corpses were similarly analysed and the results are presented in Table 2.4. All estimates were rounded to the nearest hour (h).

Rule of thumb[38]

The general method used by many to calculate the postmortem period involved the following two formulae. Note that the first rule of thumb method is in degrees Fahrenheit. If required, conversion from degrees Centigrade to degrees Fahrenheit is achieved by $(C \times [9/5]) + 32$.

METHOD A

$$\text{Time since death (TSD)} = \frac{\text{Rectal temperature at time of death (°F)} - \text{Rectal temperature at time } t1 \text{ (°F)}}{1.5}$$

$$\text{TSD} = \frac{98.6 - 80.6}{1.5} = 12 \text{ hours}$$

Table 2.3 *Data from eight corpses used to apply the eight algorithms*

Corpse	Age (years)	Height (m)	Weight (kg)	Temp 1 (T_1) (°C)	Temp 2 (T_2) (°C)	Interval between T_1 and T_2 (h)	Average environmental temp (°C)
1	95	1.65	48	27.0	26.2	1	15.0
2	93	1.72	80	27.6	26.8	1	15.5
3	69	1.60	70	29.4	29.0	1	19.0
4	90	1.60	60	32.2	31.3	1	17.5
5	80	1.50	50	30.7	29.8	1	15.4
6	77	1.67	82	31.9	31.2	1	16.0
7	70	1.67	50	30.8	29.9	1	18.0
8	79	1.57	64	31.4	30.7	1	16.0

Temp 1 is the rectal temperature after an actual postmortem interval of 10 hours.

Table 2.4 *Results of applying eight algorithms to data from eight corpses presented in Table 2.3*

Corpse	Rule of thumb (a)	Rule of thumb (b)	De Saram et al.[10]	Fiddes and Patten[3]	Marshall and Hoare[4]	Green and Wright[30]	Al-Alousi and Anderson[31]	Henssge et al.[14]
1	12	13	12	11	9	13	10	10
2	11	12	12	11	11	12	10	15
3	9	11	19	9	10	20	8	13
4	6	8	7	6	7	8	4	7
5	8	9	7	10	7	9	7	7
6	8	8	7	5	8	11	4	9
7	7	9	7	11	7	8	7	8
8	7	9	8	14	7	11	4	8

All estimates rounded to nearest hour. Actual postmortem interval is 10 hours.

METHOD B

$$TSD = \left(\begin{array}{c} \text{Rectal temperature at} \\ \text{time of death (°C)} \end{array} \right) - \left(\begin{array}{c} \text{Rectal temperature at} \\ \text{time } t1, \text{ (°C)} \end{array} \right) + 3$$

where '+ 3' is often included as compensation for possible delay in cooling, i.e. plateau.

$$TSD = (37 - 27) + 3 = 13 \text{ hours}$$

Method of De Saram et al.[10]

$$\frac{TSD}{t2 - t1} = \frac{\log \theta 0 - \log \theta 1}{\log \theta 1 - \log \theta 2} \text{ (all temperatures in °F)}$$

$\theta 0$ = rectal temperature at time of death; $\theta 1$ = rectal temperature at $t1$ after death; $\theta 2$ = rectal temperature at $t2$ after death; $t2 - t1$ = time interval between $t2$ and $t1$, i.e. 1 hour.

$$TSD = \frac{\log 98.6 - \log 80.6}{\log 80.6 - \log 79.2} = 11 \text{ hours previous to } t1.$$

De Saram suggests that, in order to take into account any delay in cooling, 45 minutes should be added to the calculation, so TSD ≈ 12 hours.

Method of Fiddes and Patten[3]

This method involves the use of the graph shown in Fig. 2.20.

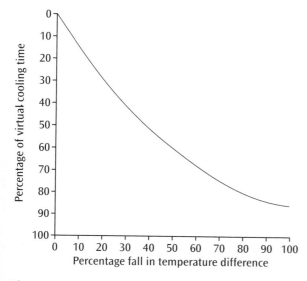

Figure 2.20 *Graph of percentage fall in temperature difference against percentage of virtual cooling time.*

Rectal temperature at time of death = 37°C.
Environmental temperature at time of death = 15°C.
The temperature difference between rectum and environment at time of death = 22°C.
The rectal temperature at $t1$ = 27°C.

There is therefore a drop of 10°C between the rectal temperatures at the time of death and $t1$.

The drop in rectal temperature compared with the difference between the rectal and environmental temperatures at time of death is calculated as a percentage:

$$\% \text{ drop in rectal temperature (at } t1) = \frac{10}{37 - 15} = 45\%$$

Similarly, an hour later, at $t2$, the rectal temperature is 26.2°C.

$$\% \text{ drop in rectal temperature (at } t1) = \frac{10.8}{37 - 15} = 49\%$$

With reference to Fig. 2.20, a fall through the first 45% of the temperature difference occupies approximately 33% of the virtual cooling time; a fall through 49% of the temperature difference occupies approximately 36% of the virtual cooling time. If 3% (36% − 33%) of the virtual cooling represents 1 hour, i.e. $t1$ to $t2$, then the virtual cooling time is approximately 33 hours. At $t1$, 33% of the virtual cooling time had elapsed:

$$TSD = 33 \times 0.33 = 11 \text{ hours}.$$

Method of Marshall and Hoare[4]

$$= B \times \exp (-Zt) + \frac{C}{Z - P} \times \exp (-Pt)$$

$$= \text{Temperature difference between rectum and environment at } t1$$

$$= 27°C - 15°C = 12°C.$$

B, C, Z and P are constants for the corpse under investigation.

Determination of constants

CONSTANT Z

$$\text{Size factor} = \frac{0.8 \times \text{area of corpse}}{\text{mass of corpse}}$$

From the graph shown in Fig. 2.21, the area of corpse is 1.5 m².

$$\text{Size factor} = \frac{0.8 \times 1.5}{48} = 0.025 \text{ m}^2/\text{kg}.$$

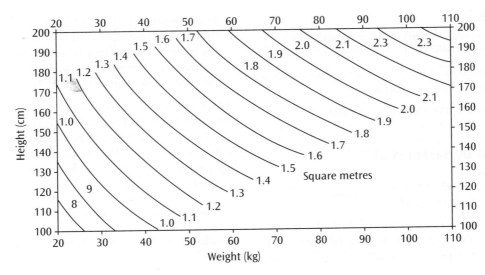

Figure 2.21 *Relationship between height, weight and body surface area.*

From the graph shown in Fig. 2.22, the cooling factor *Z* from the rectal temperature is approximately 0.1.

CONSTANT C

Rectal temperature at time of death is assumed to be 37°C:

θd = Temperature difference between rectum and environment at the time of death

= 37 − 15°C = 22°C.

$$C = \theta d \times Z$$
$$= 22 \times 0.1$$
$$= 22°C.$$

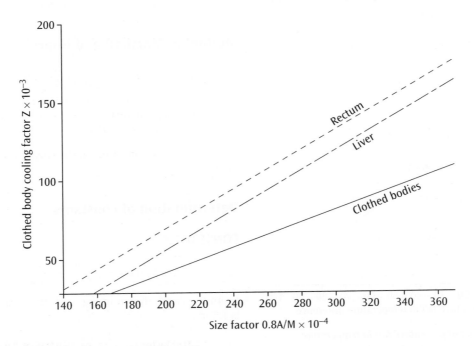

Figure 2.22 *Graph of size factor against body cooling.*

CONSTANT P

If death was thought to have occurred many hours before the first temperature recording, then the value of P should be approximately 0.6. This reduces the effect of the second exponential term on the calculations. The second exponential term represents the early postmortem period on the cooling curve. Conversely, if death was thought to have occurred close to the time of temperature measurement, an appropriate value of P would be 0.275.

In practice, it is difficult to know which value of P is appropriate; therefore it is recommended that a value of 0.4 be used unless reliable information is available on the possible time of death. Therefore:

$$\frac{C}{Z - P} = \frac{2.2}{0.1 - 0.4} = -7.33°C \text{ (to two decimal places)}.$$

CONSTANT B

$$B = \theta_0 - \frac{C}{Z - P}$$
$$= 22°C + 7.33°C$$
$$= 29.33°C$$

Returning to Marshall and Hoare's original formula (see earlier):

$$12 = 29.33 \exp(-0.1t) - 7.33 \exp(-0.4t)$$

A value for t is required which, when substituted into the above equation makes the right-hand side of the equation approximately equal the left-hand side, i.e. 12. By trial and error, if $t = 9$ hours, a satisfactory solution is obtained:

$$TSD = 9 \text{ hours}$$

Method of Green and Wright[30]

θ_1 = rectal temperature at $t1$.
θ_2 = rectal temperature at $t2$.
θ_0 = rectal temperature at death.

$$\text{Gradient } G = \frac{\theta_1 - \theta_2}{\text{time interval between readings}}$$
$$= \frac{27 - 26.2}{1} = 0.8 \text{ °C/hour}$$

$$\text{Abscissa } A = \frac{\theta_1 + \theta_2}{2} - F$$
$$= \frac{27 + 26.2}{2} - 15 = 11.6°C$$

$$\text{Reduced } \theta = \frac{\theta_1 - (\theta_0 + \theta_2)/2}{\theta_0 - F} = \frac{37 - 26.6}{37 - 15}$$
$$= 0.47$$

From the graph shown in Fig. 2.23, the numerical function F is approximately 0.9:

$$TSD = F + \frac{A}{G} + 0.9 + \frac{11.6}{0.8} = 13 \text{ hours}$$

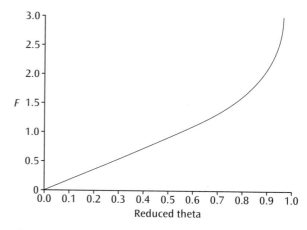

Figure 2.23 *The theoretical reference curve relating reduced theta with the numerical function F.*

Method of Al-Alousi et al.[31,32]

θ_1 = rectal temperature at $t1$.
θ_0 = rectal temperature at death.
$\theta F1$ = environmental temperature at tl.

$$\text{Temperature difference ratio} = \frac{\theta_1 - \theta F1}{\theta_0 - \theta F1} = \frac{27 - 15}{37 - 15} = 0.54$$

From the graph of the average cooling curve for the rectum (naked) shown in Fig. 2.10:

$$TSD \text{ (mean)} = 10 \pm 3 \text{ hours}$$

Although the rectal temperatures were used in this example, the above technique can be applied using liver and brain temperatures. The corresponding cooling curves associated with the brain and liver are shown in Fig. 2.10.

Method of Henssge[39]

This technique relies upon the use of a nomogram shown in Fig. 2.24a. Note that Fig. 2.24a is constructed for environmental temperatures below 23°C. Figure

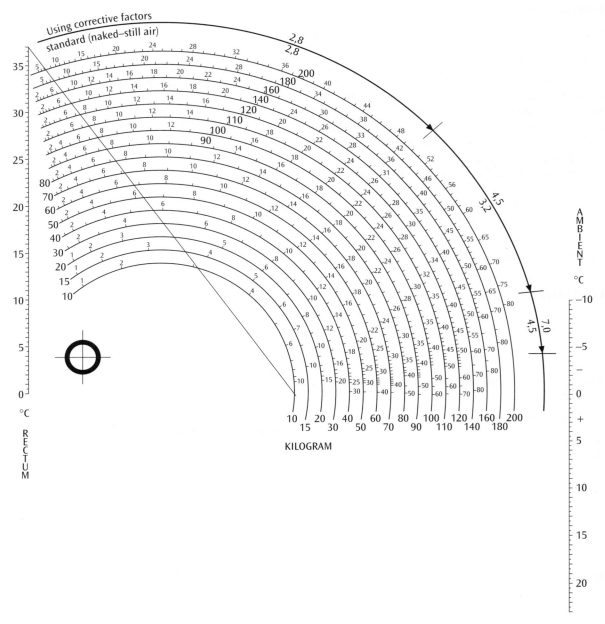

Figure 2.24a *Temperature–time of death relating nomogram (for ambient temperatures up to 23°C. Permissible variation of 95% (± h).*

2.24b is for use at environmental temperatures above 23°C:

Rectal temperature at $t1 = 27°C$.
Average environmental temperature
    during cooling = 15°C.
Naked body weight = 48 kg.

To use the nomogram in Fig. 2.24a, a line is drawn between the rectal temperature and the ambient temperature (dotted in Fig. 2.25). Another line is drawn between the centre of the circle and the bisection point of the two lines on the nomogram (closed in Fig. 2.25). The time since death is then read at the point corresponding to the weight of the body. Following the

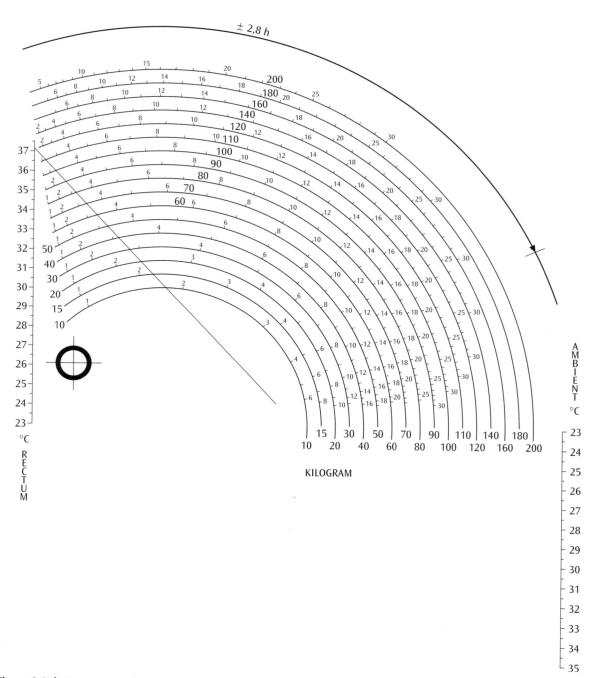

Figure 2.24b *Temperature–time of death-relating nomogram (for ambient temperature above 23°C. Permissible variation of 95%.*

above procedure illustrated in Fig. 2.25, the following interval was derived:

$$TSD = 10 \pm 3 \text{ hours}$$

Henssge suggests that, if the values for ambient and/or body weight are uncertain, corrective values may be useful in widening the limits of the postmortem period. Table 2.5 provides a list of corrective factors which should be multiplied by the body weight for various boundary conditions. The corrected body weight value is then used in place of the original body weight when constructing the lines on the nomogram.

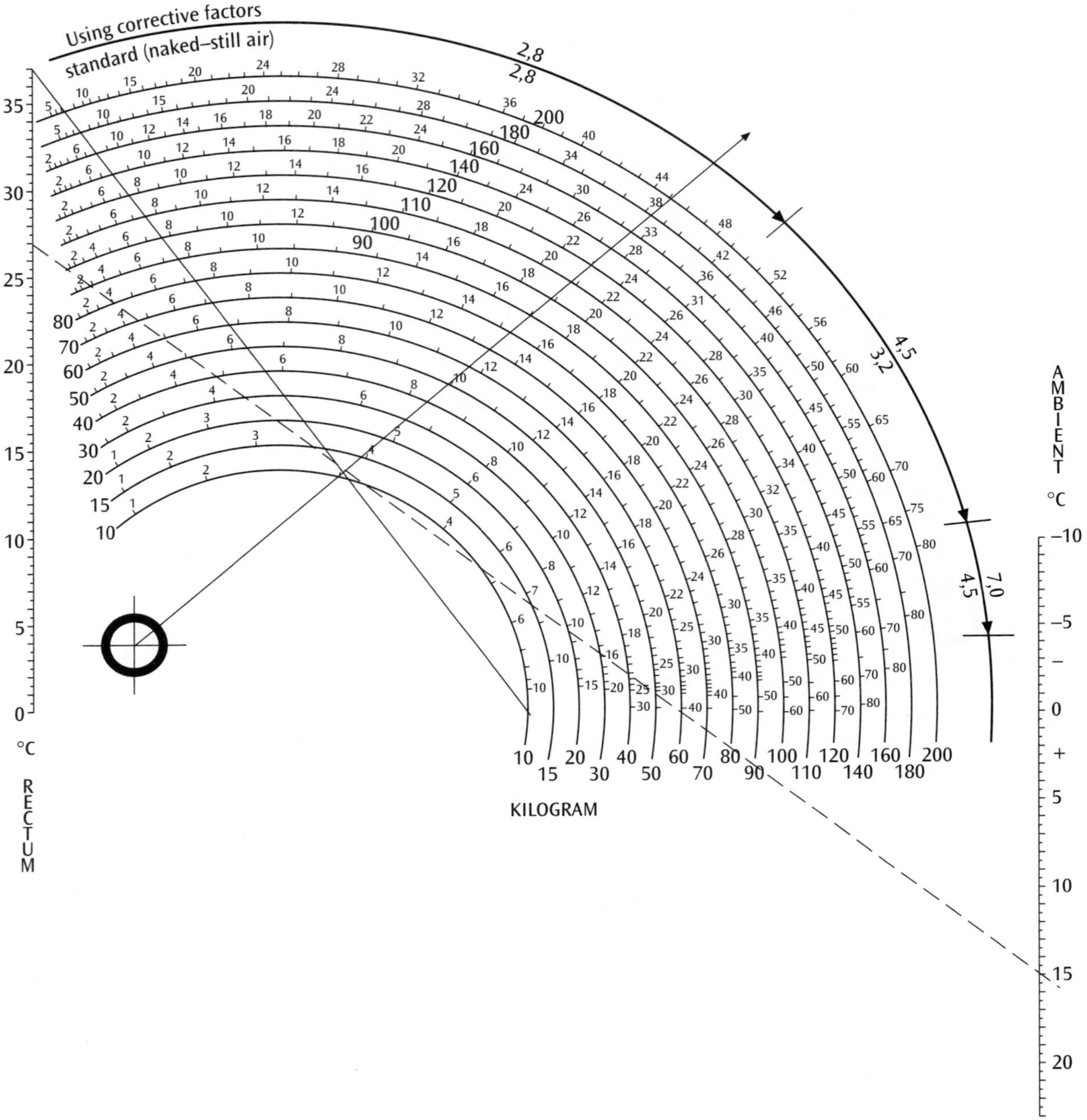

Figure 2.25 *Example of completed 'Henssge' nomogram for case under examination.*

For simplicity, no corrective factors have been included in the calculations for this case study.

Henssge advised that the techniques should not be used under the following conditions:

- strong radiation (sun, heater, cooling systems);

- suspicion of general hypothermia;
- the place where the body was found is not the place of death;
- uncertain severe changes of cooling conditions during the period between the time of death and examination.

Table 2.5 *Empiric corrective factors of the body weight*

Dry clothing/ covering	In air	Corrective factor	Wet through clothing/covering wet body surface	In air	In water
		0.35	Naked		Flowing
		0.5	Naked		Still
		0.7	Naked	Moving	
		0.7	1–2 thin layers	Moving	
Naked	Moving	0.75			
1–2 thin layers	Moving	0.9	2 or more thicker	Moving	
Naked	Still	1.0			
1–2 thin layers	Still	1.1	2 thicker layers	Still	
2–3 thin layers		1.2	More than 2 thicker layers	Still	
1–2 thicker layers	Moving or still	1.2			
3–4 thin layers		1.3			
More thin/thicker layers	Without influence	1.4			
Thick bedspread plus clothing		1.8			
combined		2.4			

Note: For the selection of the corrective factor of any case, only the clothing or covering of the lower trunk is relevant.

RESULTS

Table 2.4 lists the calculated postmortem intervals for eight corpses using eight temperature-based time-since-death algorithms.

Figures 2.26 and 2.27 are graphs of error for all corpses by algorithm and errors for all algorithms by corpse, respectively.

DISCUSSION AND CONCLUSION

It is important to stress that the aim of this part of the chapter is to show how eight different time-of-death algorithms can be applied. With such a small sample size, it would be incorrect to advocate which is the most accurate. However, with reference to Figs 2.26 and 2.27, the following observations were made:

- With corpses 4 and 5, the time since death was under-estimated by all methods (Fig. 2.27).
- Algorithms 3 and 6 produced, for one corpse, very large errors between actual and calculated postmortem intervals (93% and 98%, respectively; Fig. 2.27).
- On average, the rule of thumb method B produced the most consistent results over all

corpses, with a maximum error of approximately 30% (Fig. 2.26).
- Rule of thumb method A was better than rule of thumb method B when the time since death was over-estimated. However, rule of thumb method B was better than rule of thumb method A when the time since death was under-estimated.

No definite conclusions can be made, but it appears that even with the increased complexity of the algorithms, this does not guarantee any greater accuracy of the calculated times compared with the actual time of death. The simple rule-of-thumb methods were devised over 100 years ago. Based on the results presented, they compared favourably with the temperature-based methods since introduced. This leads to the question of whether research using temperature-based algorithms to determine the time since death is valid. There are many who would question the continued efforts to devise new temperature-based algorithms. The introduction of user-friendly computers considerably lightens the arithmetic manipulation previously carried out by hand. Recent studies by Madea and Henssge[40] have suggested that a multiprocedure approach involving temperature-based algorithms combined with electrical excitability of muscle after death may be the most useful way forward in accurately determining the postmortem period.

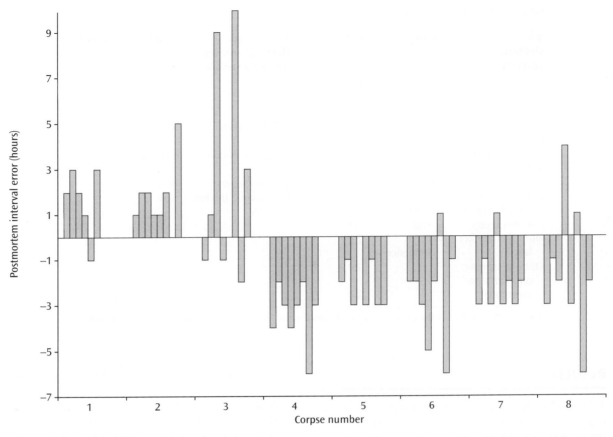

Figure 2.26 *Errors between actual and calculated postmortem interval for all corpses by algorithm. The error in postmortem period is shown for each corpse. The algorithms 1 to 8 are displayed left to right.*

The authors hope that this exercise will be useful with respect to the application of temperature-based algorithms to calculate the postmortem period. The choice of algorithm depends upon the individual using it. For the non-numerate, the best technique may involve graphical solutions, whilst the mathematically inclined may wish to use the more complex procedures, which can easily be pre-programmed into a pocket calculator. It may be advantageous to apply more than one algorithm to obtain an 'average' time since death. Whatever method is applied, the calculated times should not be accepted blindly as the 'true' time of death. The derived times should be combined with a degree of common sense, to indicate the centre point of a range of probability, the width of which will vary according to the particular circumstances of the case, and the confidence limits of the particular algorithm.

REFERENCES

1 Taylor A, Wilkes D. On the cooling of the human body after death. *Guy's Hosp. Rep.* 1863; **9**: 180–211.
2 Rainy H. On the cooling of dead bodies as indicating the length of time since death. *Glasg. Med. J.* 1868; **1**: 323–30.
3 Fiddes F, Patten TA. Percentage method for representing the fall in body temperature after death. *J. Forensic Med.* 1958; **5**: 2–15.
4 Marshall T, Hoare F. Estimating the time of death – the rectal cooling after death and its mathematical representation. *J. Forensic Sci.* 1962; **7**: 56–81.
5 Knight B. The evolution of methods for estimating the time of death from body temperature. *Forensic Sci. Int.* 1988; **36**: 47–55.
6 Knight B. *Forensic Pathology.* London: Edward Arnold, 1991.

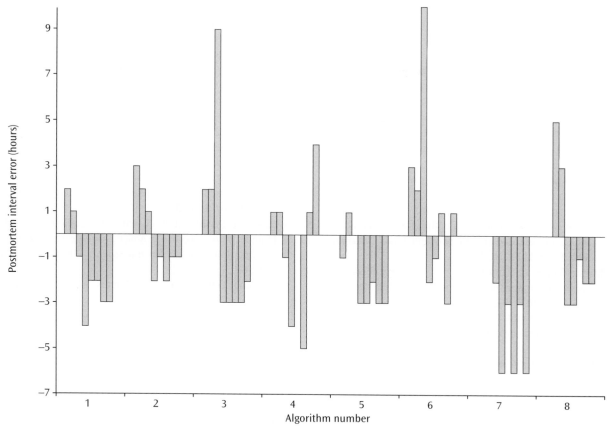

Figure 2.27 *Errors between actual and calculated postmortem interval for all algorithms by corpses. The error in the postmortem period is shown for each algorithm. The corpses 1 to 8 are shown left to right.*

7 Goodhard JF. Thermoelectric observations in clinical medicine. *Guy's Hosp. Rep.* 1870; **15**: 365–419.

8 Burman J. On the rate of cooling of the human body after death. *Edin. Med. J.* 1880; **25**: 993–1003.

9 Womack F. The rate of cooling of the body after death. *St. Bart's Hosp. Rep.* 1887; **23**: 193–200.

10 De Saram G, Webster G, Kathirgamatamby N. Post-mortem temperature and the time of death. *J. Crim. Law, Criminol. Police Sci.* 1955; **1**: 562–77.

11 Lyle H, Cleveland F. Determination of the time since death by heat loss. *J. Forensic Sci.* 1956; **1**: 11–24.

12 Sellier K. Determination of the time of death by extrapolation of the temperature decrease curve. *Acta Med. Leg. Soc.* 1948; **2**: 279–301.

13 James W, Knight B. Errors in estimating time since death. *Med. Sci. Law* 1965; **5**: 111–16.

14 Henssge C, Madea B, Gallenkemper E. Death time estimation in casework; integration of different methods. *Forensic Sci. Int.* 1988; **38**: 77–87.

15 Marshall TK. Estimating the time of death. *J. Forensic Sci.* 1962; **7**: 189–210.

16 Mead J, Bonmarito L. Reliability of rectal temperature as an index of internal body temperature. *J. Appl. Physiol.* 1949; **2**: 97–109.

17 Selkurt E. *Physiology.* Boston: Little Brown & Co., 1971.

18 Joseph A, Schiekele A. A general method for assessing factors controlling post-mortem cooling. *J. Forensic Sci.* 1970; **15**: 364–91.

19 Shapiro H. The post-mortem temperature plateau. *J. Forensic Med.* 1965; **12**: 137–41.

20 Hutchins G. Body temperature is elevated in the early post-mortem period. *Hum. Pathol.* 1985; **16**: 560–1.

21 Brown A, Marshall T. Body temperature as a means of estimating the time of death. *Forensic Sci. Int.* 1974; **4**: 125–33.

22 Nokes L, Hicks B, Knight B. The post-mortem temperature plateau – fact or friction. *Med. Sci. Law* 1985; **25**: 263–4.

23 Lundquist F. Physical and chemical methods for the estimation of the time of death. *Acta Med. Leg. Soc.* 1956; **9**: 205–13.

24 Simonsen A, Voigt J, Jeppesen N. Determination of the time of death by continuous post-mortem temperature measurement. *Med. Sci. Law* 1977; **17**: 112–21.

25 Kuehn L, Tikuisis P *et al.* Body cooling after death. *Aviat. Space Environ. Med.* 1980; September: 65–9.

26 Nokes L, Hicks B, Knight B. The use of trachea temperature as a means of determining the post-mortem period. *Med. Sci. Law* 1986; **26**: 199–202.

27 Corlslaw HS, Jaeger JS. *Conduction of Heat in Solids.* Oxford: Clarendon Press, 1959.

28 Botezatu GA. On examination of the time of death based on the rectal temperature data, the biomechanical indices of the blood and the pericardial fluid. *Sudebno. Med. Expert* 1977; **20**: 1–8.

29 Hiraiwa K *et al.* Estimation of post-mortem interval from rectal temperature with the use of computer. *Med. Sci. Law* 1980; **20**: 115–25.

30 Green M, Wright J. Post-mortem interval estimation from body temperature data only. *Forensic Sci. Int.* 1985; **28**: 35–6.

31 Al-Alousi LM, Anderson RA, Worster DM, Land DV. Multiple-probe thermography for estimating the post-mortem interval: I. Continuous monitoring and data analysis of brain, liver, rectal and environmental temperatures in 117 forensic cases. *J. Forensic Sci.* 2001; **46**: 317–22.

32 Al-Alousi LM, Anderson RA, Worster DM, Land DV. Multiple-probe thermography for estimating the post-mortem interval: II. Practical versions of the triple-exponential formulae (TEF) for estimating the time of death in the field. *J. Forensic Sci.* 2001; **46**: 323–7.

33 Kuroda F, Hiraiwa K, Oshida S, Akaishi S. Estimation of post-mortem interval from rectal temperature by use of computer – thermal conductivity of the skin. *Med. Sci. Law* 1982; **22**: 285–9.

34 Olaisen B. Post-mortem decrease in brain temperature. *Z. Rechtsmed.* 1979; **83**: 253–7.

35 Brinkman B. Merizel S, Reimann G. Post-mortale organ-temperatures unter verschiedenen umweltbedingungen. *Z. Rechtsmed.* 1978; **81**: 207–17.

36 Baccino E, De Saint Martin L, Schuliar Y, Guilloteau P, Le Rhun M, Morin J, Leglise D, Amice J. Outer ear temperature and time of death. *Forensic Sci. Int.* 1996; **83**: 133–46.

37 Baccino E. Letter to the Editor. *Forensic Sci. Int.* 1997; **87**: 173.

38 Moritz A. *Pathology of Trauma*, 2nd edn. Philadelphia: Lea & Febiger, 1954.

39 Henssge C. Death time estimation in case work. I. The rectal temperature time of death nomogram. *Forensic Sci. Int.* 1988; **38**: 209–36.

40 Madea B, Henssge C. Electrical excitability of skeletal muscle postmortem in casework. *Forensic Sci. Int.* 1990; **47**: 207–27.

3

Temperature-based methods II

CLAUS HENSSGE

INTRODUCTION

The main topic of this chapter is the rectal temperature 'nomogram method' for determining the time of death, which was developed for practical use at the scene of death. It provides a time range immediately at the scene, and may considerably assist criminal investigations at their earliest stage. Beyond that, evidence may be provided as to the guilt or innocence of a suspect, due to the denial or corroboration of an alibi.

The main object is to be able to use the method in a wide spectrum of casework. For that, the circumstances at the scene of death must be analysed thoroughly and the findings taken into account. This requires personal experience. Additional rapid methods used at the scene are helpful for reducing the range of the interval limited by the nomogram, and will be described in Chapter 7.

This chapter is divided into two main parts: first, basic physical considerations, mathematically modelling body-cooling by two exponential equations and verifying them on experimental body and dummy cooling under various controlled conditions. The second part describes the practical means of applying the 'nomogram method' in casework, with references to the first part where essential.

SCIENTIFIC INVESTIGATION OF EXPERIMENTAL BODY COOLING UNDER CONTROLLED CONDITIONS

Basic conditions

Body cooling occurs due to non-stationary heat conduction inside a body of low thermal diffusivity.

1. With failure of circulation, convectional transport of heat inside the body ceases. (In hanged bodies, hypostasis could theoretically distort rectal temperature by warm blood descending from above, but this has no practical significance.)

2. Exchange of heat between the core and the surface of the body takes place only by conduction. (Heat transfer inside the body by radiation and convection is negligible.)

3. The postmortem rate of heat production is very low. (Heat is produced mainly by anaerobic glycolysis, which is on-going for about the first 10 hours postmortem, in a non-linear fashion. Lundquist[51] calculated roughly that heat release per gram glycogen was 0.4 kcal, so the glycogen store of the body (350 g) corresponds to 140 kcal heat release. A body of about 70 kg and a specific heat of 0.8 kcal/kg would be heated by 2.5°C over the first 10 hours after death. With that, one-sixth of the postmortem temperature plateau could be explained as a rough estimation. The rate of heat release from autolysis and putrefaction is even lower during the early postmortem phase of cooling the body to ambient temperature, so that its influence on cooling is negligible. A fulminant putrefaction in the early postmortem period may markedly decelerate the cooling.)

4. The thermal diffusivity of body tissues is much lower than that of metals. (Thermal diffusivity of water = 0.00143, of fat = 0.001, of aluminium = 1.0 $[10^{-4}\ m^2\ s^{-1}]$. Note the small difference between water and fat. Because of its lower thermal conductivity, fat conducts heat more slowly than muscle. Because of its lower specific heat and specific weight, the fall in temperature is greater when leaving a hotter object. Since the thermal diffusivity is the quotient from thermal conductivity and specific heat times specific weight, only a small difference results between water and fat (e.g. Sellier[31])).

5. The cooling of a body is nearly 'non-stationary' and unsteady. As a consequence, the 'thermal diffusivity' is the measure of any heat transfer inside the body, but not the 'thermal conductivity'.

6. The body is not 'thermally thin'.

7. Newton's law of cooling is not adequate to describe the cooling curve of any central probe site.

8. With the start of cooling, a temperature gradient develops from the surface to the core of any part of the body.

9. First, heat is lost from the most superficial layers of the body, whereas the deeper layers are initially unaltered. Because of the low velocity of heat transport inside the body, it takes some time for heat to be conducted from the deeper layers to the more superficial (colder) layers, until, eventually, the temperature gradient reaches the core.

10. The temperature gradient has an almost radial direction. The cooling curve of any central temperature probe site has a sigmoidal shape with the physically determined 'postmortal temperature plateau' occurring during the first cooling phase.

COOLING DUMMY

Any solid body consisting of a substance of low thermal diffusivity and without significant heat release cools in the same manner. Thus, a body figured like a human trunk, consisting of a layer of coated material or caoutchouc and filled with a gel mixture of glycerine (47.5%), water (47.5%) and agar (5%) (Fig. 3.1)

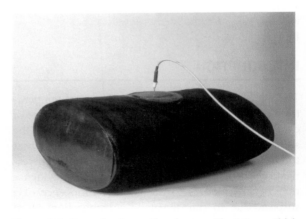

Figure 3.1 *Example of a cooling dummy. The 1.5 mm-thick wrap is made of caoutchouc. It is filled with a gel mixture ('Wirodouble' from BEGO, Emil-Sommer-Strasse 7–9, D-2800 Bremen 41; 47.5% glycerine and water, 5% agar) at 90°C, at which it is molten. At lower temperatures the consistency becomes solid-elastic. The dimensions are 19 cm (sagittal), 38 cm (transverse) and 50 cm (longitudinal). The real weight is 31 kg. The temperature probe is inserted in the middle, 9.5 cm deep, corresponding to half of the sagittal diameter.*

provides cooling curves which resemble those of cadavers, including the plateau (Fig. 3.2). Similarly, the two exponential equations (see eqns 3.4 and 3.14), though investigated empirically on dead human bodies, also apply to the dummy (Fig. 3.3). This is due to the similar thermal diffusivity and the similar relationship between surface area and volume of both dead human bodies and dummies. Therefore, a dummy cools under controlled conditions like a cadaver of a specified body weight, dependent on its cross-sectional dimensions (Table 3.1; Fig. 3.4.) The conformity of cooling curves of bodies and dummies has been confirmed in numerous experiments conducted under different conditions (see Fig. 3.18). Therefore, test coolings of dummies can replace bodies.[1–7]

HEAT EXCHANGE TO SURROUNDINGS

The actual mechanisms of heat exchange between body and surroundings (conduction, convection, radiation, evaporation) depend on the individual circumstances at the scene and, therefore, cannot be stated in generally valid terms for any cooling conditions.

Conductive heat exchange results from the temperature difference between the body and the surroundings, the intermediate material between the body surface and the surroundings (e.g. clothing, covering), as well as the surrounding medium (e.g. water, air). At the contact zones of the body with the supportive

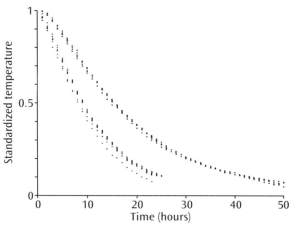

Figure 3.2 *Cooling curves of two different-sized dummies. Abscissa: time (hours) after taking the 37°C heated dummy out of the incubator. Ordinate: standardized temperature (central temperature of the dummy – ambient temperature) divided by (37°C – ambient temperature). Each of six test coolings under chosen standard conditions at each of three different places in nearly constant ambient temperatures between 0.1 and 14.1°C. The upper cooling curves are as good as the curve of a 73 kg body, the lower curves of a 42 kg body when cooling under comparable 'standard' conditions. Even the 'postmortal temperature plateau' is equally developed. The model curves of a 73 kg and a 42 kg body computed according to eqn 3.14 would fit into the middle of each of the six curves (see Fig. 3.3).*

Table 3.1 *Mean radius of cross-section of some different-sized dummies and the resulting body weight ('virtual weight') calculated from the Newtonian coefficient B of the cooling curves according to eqn 3.3 (see Fig. 3.4)*

Real weight (kg)	Mean radius (mm)	Virtual weight (kg)	Wrap
0.70	42.8	6.9	0.5 mm-thick
1.02	49.6	14.3	PVC-coated
2.82	67.8	17.3	material
3.35	78.1	32.8	or
8.20	110.9	36.8	0.5 mm-thick
10.00	115.6	38.0	transparent
21.80	152.9	64.8	PVC foil
22.00	152.9	66.5	
27.50	161.2	72.5	
24.00	162.3	72.4	
25.00	162.3	76.5	
31.00	177.0	67.0	1.5 mm-thick caoutchouc

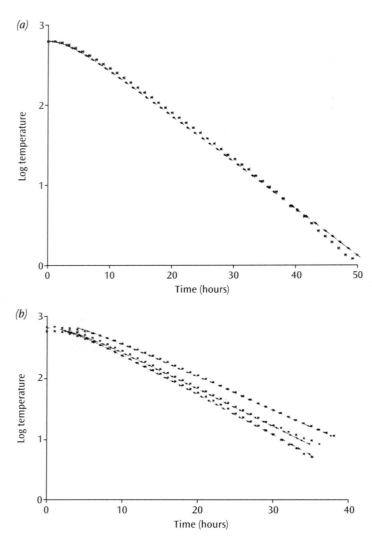

Figure 3.3 *Experimental cooling curves of dummies and their modelling by the two exponential equations using the figures of constants investigated on bodies (eqns 3.5 and 3.14) 10 years before the dummies were 'born'. Abscissa: time (hours); ordinate: logarithm of (central temperature of the dummy – ambient temperature). (a) Cooling curve of the dummy in Fig. 3.1. The 36.5°C heated dummy cooled in nearly constant mean ambient temperature of 20.1°C. The stars without connecting lines are the original values of measurements. The crosses coupled by connecting lines represent the model curve of a 67 kg dead human body. The differences between the real and the model-computed cooling times do not exceed – 0.8 to 1.1 hours up to the 40th hour. After this, the differences increase to 1.8 hours. (b) Experimental cooling and model curves of a dummy and two bodies under identical circumstances. Naked bodies lying on a wood board in a closed room:*

	Uppermost body	**Intermediate body**	**Lowest dummy**
Ambient temperature (°C)	19.5	20.5	20.6
First measurement			
hpm	3	1	0
°C	35.7	37.6	36.5
Real body weight (kg)	80.8	67.0	–
Calculated body weight (eqn 3.3)	78.0	69.8	64.6
Cooling coefficient	−0.0558	−0.0618	−0.0663

hpm = hours postmortem.

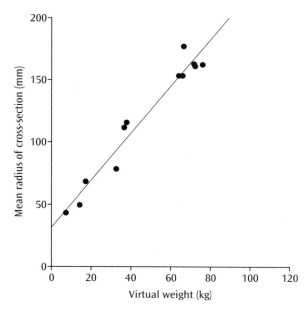

Figure 3.4 *Close relationship between mean radius of cross-section and 'virtual weight' of some different-sized dummies (see Table 3.1). The virtual weight results from the Newtonian coefficient B of the cooling curves set in eqn. 3.3.*

surface, conductive heat exchange plays the decisive role. The heat capacity and the thermal conductivity of the supporting surface must be noted (see Figs 3.19–3.21).

At non-contact areas of naked bodies the convectional mechanism of heat exchange dominates, even without forced convection such as wind. In the case of a naked body, the heat exchange at the non-contact surface usually exceeds that of the contact surface (see Figs 3.7, 3.8, 3.22), unless the supporting base conducts heat exceptionally well (see Fig. 3.19).

Under standard conditions, heat exchange by radiation is extensive for the first hour postmortem, but it decreases during the later process of cooling, depending on the rapid decrease in skin temperature[8,9]. However, under special conditions, such as sun radiating on the body, the net exchange of heat between body and surroundings will be influenced to a large degree. There are no reports about this in the literature.

The loss of heat from the dry surface of the body by evaporation does not have any significant influence on the cooling. The loss of heat would correspond to 580 kcal/L of evaporated water. The weight of the body does not diminish during the early postmortem interval to such an extent that a considerable acceleration of cooling would result from such fluid loss.

Noting the almost radial direction of heat conduction inside the body, it is essential to take into account which parts of the body contribute to total heat transfer.

HEAT FLOW MEASUREMENTS ON BODY SURFACES

By utilizing new, highly sensitive heat flow sensors (HY-CAL Engineering Sensable®; 1205 Los Nietos Rd., Santa Fe Springs, CA 90670. Types used: BI-6 and LO-6) (Fig. 3.5), the heat exchange on both the con-

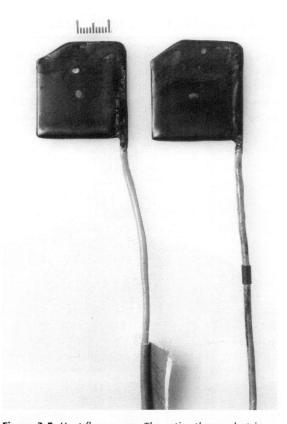

Figure 3.5 *Heat flow sensor. The active thermoelectric sensor transduces the whole absorbed or emitted heat flow of a surface area into a voltage. The sensitivity of the two sensors was 149 and 46 mV per 500 Btu ft^{-2} h^{-1}. The range of measurements was limited from minus to plus 11.38 Btu ft^{-2} h^{-1} and the discrimination was set to 0.01 Btu ft^{-2} h^{-1}. Into each heat flow sensor a thermocouple (10 mV/°C) is integrated to measure the surface temperature beside the heat flow. The gauge can be attached easily using double-sided tape.*

tact and the non-contact surfaces can be investigated in combination with superficial and central temperatures (Figs 3.6–3.8). Using the analogy of Ohm's law, the heat flow corresponds with the power of an electric current. With the temperature measurements corresponding to the voltage, the resistance can be calculated as the third, but unknown, quantity of Ohm's law. Thus, a complete circuit of the heat exchange between body and environment can be established (Fig. 3.9). Heat flow measurements on body surfaces support the incorporation of influencing factors of body cooling such as clothing, wetness or supporting surfaces.[4,5,7]

RECTAL TEMPERATURE PROBE SITES

Keeping the non-stationary heat conduction inside a body of low 'thermal conductivity' in mind, the time course of any body temperature depends first of all on the temperature probe site. Since surface temperatures may be susceptible even to transient, minute alter-

ations of the actual cooling circumstances, they seem to be unsuitable for measuring 'the' body temperature. [The measurement of surface temperatures is problematic (e.g. Newitt C, Green MA., *J. Forensic Sci. Soc.* 1979; **19**: 179–81). In addition, surface temperatures approach the ambient temperature more quickly and complicate the procedure once more.] At present, the deep rectal temperature and central brain temperature are the most investigated probe sites. Because of the greater radius of the trunk compared with the radius of the head, the cooling curve of the rectal temperature probe site has a shallower slope and therefore gives information about the time since death over a longer postmortem interval than the steeper cooling curve of the brain. On the other hand, in general, the steeper the cooling curve, the more exact the calculated time since death. Therefore, temperature probe sites on different parts of the body having a different radius are not alternative methods but can complement each other, e.g. brain and rectal probe site[10] as well as multiple probe sites (see Chapter 2).

Besides the location of the temperature probe,

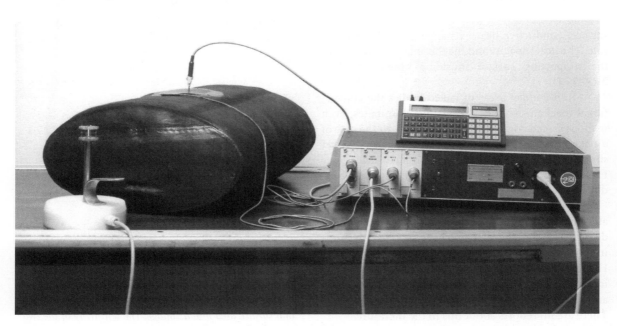

Figure 3.6 *Experimental arrangement for measurements of ambient temperature (air and base), the central temperature of the dummy, surface temperatures and heat flow on both the contact and non-contact surfaces. To control and store the seven automatic measurements, the hand-held computer HP 71B is used. This picks up the measurements in optional intervals from the data logger at the right. After the programmed end of measurements the HP 71B is connected to a plotter, a printer and a digital cassette drive. To analyse the data, special algorithms corresponding to the given equations are utilized. Development of the device including construction of the probes, integration of thermocouples into the heat flow sensors (Fig. 3.5) and calibration: BMT Messtechnik GmbH – Dr. Ing. F. Wallner, Arghentinische Allee 32a, D-14163 Berlin).*

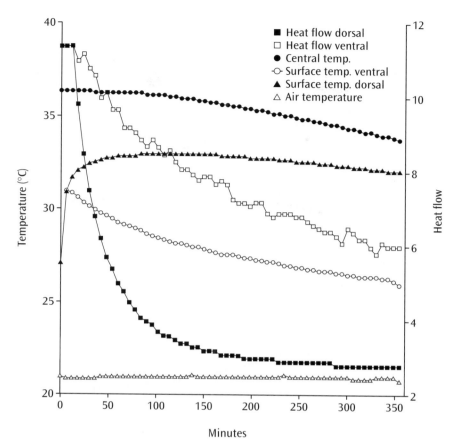

Figure 3.7 *Heat flow measurements on the surfaces of the dummy of* Fig. 3.6. *Central temperature, ventral (non-contact) and dorsal (contact), both surface temperatures and heat flow curves of a 36.5°C heated dummy during the first 6 hours of cooling in still air of 21°C. The supporting base was a wood board 2 cm thick. Left ordinate: temperature (°C); right ordinate: heat flow Btu ft^{-2} h^{-1}. Abscissa: cooling time (min). Interval of measurements: 6 minutes. The initially great heat flow at the contact surface (dorsal) heats the base quickly (see the curve of dorsal surface temperature). The subsequent very low dorsal heat flow is combined with a very slow decrease of the dorsal surface temperature, indicating that the wood board has a low thermal conductivity. The curves of ventral heat flow and surface temperature initially show the heating of the bound layer and afterwards, with the start of thermic air movement (convectional heat exchange), the greater heat loss combined with a steeper fall of the ventral surface temperature compared with the dorsal surface. Note the more irregular curve of the ventral ('naked') heat flow in comparison with the dorsal one.*

another question should be discussed: the infliction of injuries by measuring brain temperature and the disturbance of traces such as semen during measurement of rectal temperature. The injuries caused by central brain temperature measurements are minute and discernible.[11–14]

The disturbance of traces by rectal temperature measurement can be avoided by taking a swab before inserting the temperature probe into the sphincter. The securing of micro-traces by the criminal investi-

gators must be finished before any removal of the clothing or cutting through the crotch area of trousers can be done. Co-operation is required with other investigators to avoid conflict of interests.

In my opinion, the rectal probe site provides the most reliable determination of the time since death, compared with other probe site measurements.

Nevertheless, there is some discussion concerning the exact probe site in the rectum. Joseph and Schickele[15] suggest that variation of the exact location

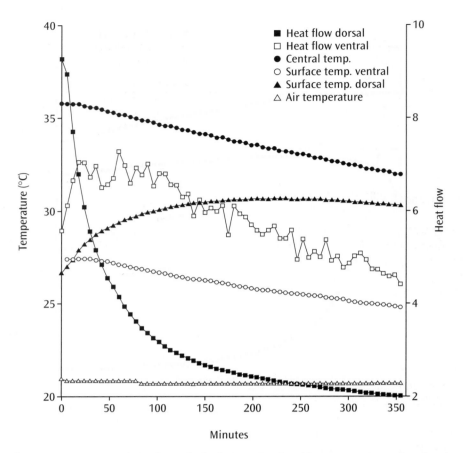

Figure 3.8 *Heat flow measurements on the surfaces of a body. Rectal and ambient temperatures, dorsal and ventral surface temperatures and heat flows of a naked 69.5 kg body lying on a wood board 2 cm-thick in still air of 20.7°C. Left ordinate: temperature (°C); right ordinate: heat flow (Btu ft⁻² h⁻¹). Abscissa: cooling time after the start of measurements 3.1 hours postmortal with a rectal temperature of 35.8°C. Interval of measurements 6 minutes. Considering the death time of 3.1 hours at the beginning of measurements with advanced postmortal plateau, the curves agree well with those of the dummy in* Fig. 3.7. *The more irregular curve of the ventral heat flow curve is apparent, indicating that it is unsuitable for short interval analysis, at least on naked surfaces.*

of thermometers in the rectum from body to body (and from one experiment to another) could explain the wide variation of Marshall's cooling curves.[16] They criticize the rectal probe site for not being at the centre of the body, and they propose as a convenient standardized location – a more defined point 2.5 cm (1 inch) above the symphysis – at which the thermometer would be inserted through an incision to a depth half the distance of the anteroposterior diameter. However, this impracticable procedure could cause injury, for example of the bladder, possibly followed by an outflow of urine into the peritoneal cavity.

The site of a straight, non-flexible probe inserted at least 8 cm inside the anal sphincter[16] is in fact not at the centre of the lower trunk but at a level corresponding to the junction between the posterior third and anterior two-thirds of the anteroposterior diameter of the trunk, at a longitudinal level that is not defined exactly.[17] If a straight, non-flexible probe is inserted deep into the rectum via the anal sphincter without undue force, a convenient standardized point is given; a great variation of the 'location factor' (so-called by Joseph and Schickele) from body to body is not of practical significance, in our opinion.

Hiraiwa *et al.*[18] analysed the location of the rectal probe by computed tomography in 10 patients after

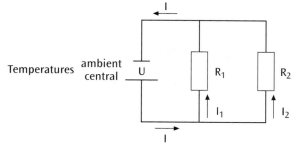

$$R = \frac{U}{I} = \text{Resistance} = \frac{\text{difference temperature}}{\text{heat flow}}$$

Figure 3.9 *Circuit of heat exchange between body and environment analogously to Ohm's law. Calculating both the total and the parts of resistance (R_1, R_2) and flow (I_1, I_2) at lying and non-lying surfaces the parts of their surface areas must be taken into account.*

inserting the thermometer about 10–15 cm beyond the anus close to the anterior wall of the sacrum. The ratio of the length between the centre of the rectum and the middle of the back to the distance between the surface of the lower abdomen and the middle of the back was found to have a mean of 0.27. Our own simple measurements of the sagittal and transverse diameter of the lower trunk at the level of the greater trochanter and the anterior inferior iliac spine (corresponding to the actual level of a straight rigid temperature probe when inserted via the anus into the rectum as deep as possible without resort to force) resulted in ratios between 0.42 and 0.47, depending on whether the insertion was more ventral or more dorsal.

Standardization of the temperature probe site is absolutely necessary and much more important than its exactly central location. All experience of death-time estimation from body cooling is limited to a distinct probe site. Experience can be extended more by systematic measurements based on a few standardized probe sites than by a surfeit of 'new' temperature probe sites. I therefore decided to adhere to Marshall's procedure,[16] including the rectal probe site as described above, when I started my studies of body cooling in 1975.

The rectal temperature and the ambient temperature were measured on-line by an electronic device within an accuracy of 0.1°C.

MODELLING MATHEMATICALLY THE RECTAL COOLING CURVE BY THE TWO EXPONENTIAL FORMULAE OF MARSHALL AND HOARE

In 1962, Marshall and Hoare[16] published a formula for modelling rectal body cooling mathematically using different notation:

$$Q = \frac{Tr - Ta}{To - Ta}$$

$$= A \times \exp(B \times t) + (1 - A) \times \exp\left(\frac{A \times B}{A - 1} \times t\right) \quad (3.1)$$

where Q = standardized temperature; Tr = rectal temperature at any time t; To = rectal temperature at death ($t = 0$); Ta = ambient temperature; A = constant; B = constant; and t = time of death.

There are two exponential terms: the first (with the constant B as exponent) expresses the exponential drop of the temperature after the plateau according to Newton's law of cooling (Fig. 3.10). The second (with the constant A as a part of the exponent) describes the 'postmortal temperature plateau'.

The formula by Marshall and Hoare is the ultimate success in modelling body cooling for the purpose of

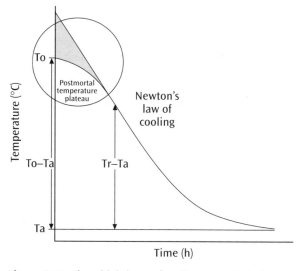

Figure 3.10 *Sigmoidal shape of cooling curve. A single exponential term like Newton's law of cooling is insufficient to describe this mathematically. The two-exponential term (eqn 3.1) of Marshall and Hoare provides a close mathematical description. The quotient Tr–Ta/To–Ta (standardized temperature) is a good measure of the progress of cooling.*

estimation of the time since death. The formula requires only two constants besides the body temperature at death but, nevertheless, it provides a sufficient mathematical description of real cooling curves of different parts of the body (e.g. rectum, brain) as well as of the cooling dummy. As demonstrated by Brown and Marshall,[19] more than two exponential terms complicate the model without improving results.

Though there are some difficulties in identifying the individual values of the only two constants in any specific case, the solution is not to look for a better model, but for the best way to identify the individual values of the constants A and B. They are dependent on the body build and the ambient cooling conditions, including the thermal factors on the surface of the body. Besides great variation of body build, the cooling conditions at the scene may vary over a wide range. In addition, some of the actual influencing factors at the scene may be unknown to the forensic pathologist. Furthermore, the ambient conditions can change between the time of death and the time of investigation. The question of identifying the representative values of the required constants seems to be insoluble.

First, we must accept that the problem cannot be solved in all cases. Second, we must accept that the problem cannot be solved *exactly* in many cases. However, we can at least *approximate* the value of the required constants.

There are two different ways to identify the individual values of the constants. The first is to estimate the values by analysing the whole experimental cooling curve. Then we can decide if a short part of the cooling curve is able to give representative values of the constants for the whole curve. The second way uses the effect of the constants on whole cooling curves, as a means to find rules approximating the representative individual values of the constants indirectly by taking the most important features of body build and ambient cooling conditions into account.

Theoretically, both ways have some inherent advantages and disadvantages. The decision whether the first or the second way is better can only be made under the conditions of practice at the scene in many cases.

Though the formulae of Marshall and Hoare validate the earlier observation of Rainy in 1868[20] that bodies would cool more slowly in the first phase after death than expected by Newton's law of cooling, and though the excellent papers of Marshall and Hoare gave an adequate and easily applied mathematical expression of postmortem cooling, including the postmortal plateau, progress concerning their application

to the important field of forensic practice was incomprehensibly insignificant. Instead, for example, pathologists continued to use simplistic methods such as the rule of thumb that bodies would cool 1°C per hour: this persisted as if Rainy,[20] as well as Marshall and Hoare,[16] had not existed. Only James and Knight [21] reported errors in estimating the time since death in coroner's cases, and Prokop[22] stated that Marshall and Hoare's data would be much more useful than the earlier data of Schwarz and Heidenwolf,[23] who produced a sigmoidal curve of rectal body cooling in 1953.

As has been said, the main question is to identify the individual values of the constants A and B in individual cases at the scene where the circumstances do not allow extensive measurements. The constant B has greater significance to the reproduction of the cooling curve from the measurement at the scene to the moment of death, since it describes the cooling rate for as long as there is a difference of temperature between the body and the ambient. In comparison, the constant A is of less significance; it expresses the relative duration of the plateau phase and ceases its function after that. Both these are discussed below.

THE INDIVIDUAL VALUE OF THE CONSTANT B (THE NEWTONIAN COOLING COEFFICIENT)

Estimation of B by multiple temperature measurements

The individual value of B can be exactly computed by a linear regression line with time t (h) as the independent variable (X) and logarithm of temperature difference between rectum and ambient $\ln (Tr - Ta)$ as the dependent variable (Y) of the cooling curve after the plateau (Fig. 3.11c). The exact estimation of B as the slope of the regression line (regression coefficient b_{yx}) requires a long period of temperature measurements after the plateau, without any change of the cooling conditions (including constant ambient temperature). The more slowly the body cools (e.g. high body weight, covering with thick clothing or bedclothes), the more the requirement has to be met. Shorter periods of temperature measurement of the order of 1 to 4 hours and/or actual changes of the cooling conditions shortly before or during the measurements may result in erroneous values of B. The inability to estimate reliably the representative cooling

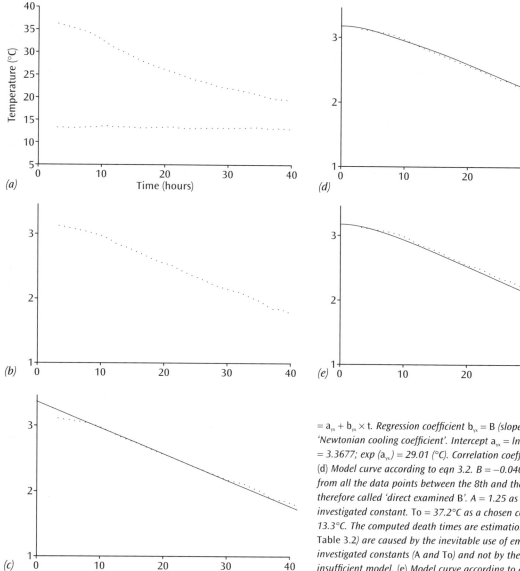

Figure 3.11 *The cooling of a body and its modelling. Hourly measurements of rectal (Tr) and ambient (Ta) temperatures from the beginning of the third hour postmortem of a naked body of 99.5 kg lying extended on the back on a thermally indifferent base in a closed room. Abscissa: time since death (t) in hours; ordinate: temperature (°C). Compare with Table 3.2. (a) Data points of rectal and ambient temperatures in linear measures. The mean of the ambient temperature is 13.3°C (Ta). (b) Logarithm of temperature differences 'rectal–ambient'. There is apparently a linear relationship between 'time' and 'ln temperature difference' from the 8th to the 28th hour postmortem. (c) Regression line 'time' (X) against 'ln temperature difference' (Y) computed from the data points between the 8th and the 28th hour postmortem: ln (Tr − Ta)*
$= a_{yx} + b_{yx} \times t$. *Regression coefficient* $b_{yx} = B$ *(slope) = −0.0408 'Newtonian cooling coefficient'. Intercept* $a_{yx} = ln$ (Tr − Ta) *at* $t_o = 0$ *= 3.3677; exp* (a_{yx}) *= 29.01 (°C). Correlation coefficient r = 0.9996. (d) Model curve according to eqn 3.2. B = −0.0408 as computed from all the data points between the 8th and the 28th hour; therefore called 'direct examined B'. A = 1.25 as an empirically investigated constant. To = 37.2°C as a chosen constant; Ta = 13.3°C. The computed death times are estimations. The errors (see Table 3.2) are caused by the inevitable use of empirically investigated constants (A and To) and not by the use of an insufficient model. (e) Model curve according to eqns 3.1 and 3.2. Instead of the use of the real existing figure of B (−0.0408), which can only be known exactly by many hourly data points after the postmortal plateau and without any tendency-change of cooling conditions, B = −0.0439 is used as calculated from the real body weight (99.5 kg) according to the empirically investigated eqn 3.2; therefore called 'indirect estimated B'. The real figure of B (−0.0408) would be calculated (eqn 3.2) from a body of 106.6 kg according to eqn 3.3. The difference between the real, direct examined figure of B (−0.0408) and the body weight-related, indirect estimated figure of B (−0.0439) causes additional errors in computation of the time of death (see Table 3.2). The error increases with the progress of cooling, as in this case. This disadvantage yields a great gain for practical application in casework. Now, the time of death can be computed from a single measurement of rectal temperature at any time in the process of cooling.*

rate B to the whole period between death and time of investigation by multiple temperature measurements within a few hours at the scene is the main reason why these methods give unsatisfactory results in estimating the time since death (Table 3.2).

Without any question, it would be an important breakthrough, similar to that of Marshall and Hoare,[16] to obtain a measurement of the individual slope of the temperature drop of any case, instead of evaluating it indirectly from the 'size factor'[16] or the body weight with 'corrective factors' for particular circumstances (nomogram method, see page 84).

Table 3.2 *The cooling of a body and its modelling. Data from* Fig. 3.11. *Mean ambient temperature* = 13.3°C

Time (h)	Real temperatures (°C)		Model error (h)	
	Rectal	1*n* difference	$B = -0.0408$ (*Fig. 3.11(d)*)	$B = -0.0439$ (*Fig. 3.11(e)*)
0	–	–	–	–
1	–	–	–	–
2	–	–	–	–
3	36.1	3.1274	0.9	0.6
4	35.7	3.1097	0.7	0.4
5	35.4	3.0962	0.2	−0.1
6	35.0	3.0780	−0.1	−0.5
7	34.6	3.0594	−0.4	−0.9
8	34.2	3.0405	−0.8	−1.3
9	33.4	3.0015	−0.5	−1.1
10	32.8	2.9712	−0.6	−1.2
11	32.0	2.9293	−0.4	−1.1
12	30.9	2.8687	0.3	−0.5
13	30.3	2.8341	0.3	−0.6
14	29.7	2.7982	0.2	−0.7
15	28.9	2.7482	0.6	−0.5
16	28.3	2.7090	0.6	−0.6
17	27.7	2.6682	0.6	−0.6
18	27.1	2.6257	0.7	−0.6
19	26.5	2.5813	0.8	−0.5
20	26.1	2.5506	0.6	−0.8
21	25.7	2.5189	0.4	−1.1
22	25.1	2.4693	0.7	−0.9
23	24.7	2.4349	0.5	−1.1
24	24.1	2.3809	0.9	−0.9
25	23.7	2.3432	0.8	−1.0
26	23.5	2.3238	0.3	−1.5
27	22.9	2.2633	0.8	−1.2
28	22.5	2.2208	0.8	−1.2
29	22.3	2.1989	0.4	−1.7
30	21.9	2.1535	0.5	−1.6
31	21.7	2.1300	0.1	−2.1
32	21.5	2.1059	−0.4	−2.5
33	21.1	2.0560	−0.1	−2.4
34	20.9	2.0301	−0.5	−2.8
35	20.5	1.9761	−0.2	−2.6
36	20.1	1.9191	0.2	−2.3
37	19.7	1.8586	0.7	−1.9
38	19.7	1.8586	−0.3	−2.9
39	19.5	1.8269	−0.5	−3.2
40	19.3	1.7942	−0.7	−3.4

The methods of De Saram *et al.*,[24] Fiddes and Patten,[25] Marshall and Hoare[16] and, more recently, Green and Wright,[26,27] are based on the principle of measurement of the individual slope, by measuring the temperature at least twice. The most sophisticated method of this type is that published by Green and Wright.[26,27]

We, therefore, examined these methods, especially that of Green and Wright,[26,27] on all our experimental material, as well as on the more problematic part of our casework.[28]

Experiments on a series of 30 cooling curves of dummies under different, but controlled, constant conditions[29] gave the same results as in body cooling[30] – we obtained worse results than with the nomogram method (see page 84).

In my opinion, there are three main reasons for these inferior results from multiple temperature measurements:

1. There is only a small decrease in the rectal temperature over an interval of 1 to 3 or 4 hours, especially in cases of obesity, thick clothing or high ambient temperature: thus even a small mismeasurement of either one or both rectal temperatures, of the order of 0.1°C, may lead to a relatively large error in the cooling rate. In computing the time of death, this small error in the rate is multiplied and may result in a large error in the calculated time of death. To reduce this source of error, Marshall and Hoare[16] recommended taking the second measurement 3 or 4 hours apart. To avoid any inaccuracy of the rate by small mismeasurements, Green and Wright[26,27] used, in addition to a double measurement, an 11-fold measurement of the rectal temperature, with measurements taken at intervals of 6 minutes over a period of 1 hour for computing a regression line, but without success, as demonstrated by the experiments of Koppes-Koenen.[29]

2. The actual measured rate of the decrease in rectal temperature is valid only for the cooling conditions during the period of measurement. When the cooling conditions* – including the ambient temperature – have been changed, even shortly before, the body cooling rate also changes. Nevertheless, it is used multiplicatively for the whole period between time of death and time of investigation. There is no way to take into account even well-recognized changes of the cooling conditions* – including the ambient temperature. Figures 3.12 and 3.13 illustrate the great change in the cooling rate *B* after the cooling conditions had been altered. The cooling conditions inevitably change at the scene of death, since the forensic pathologist is never the first to arrive. The question is, whether we can recognize and reconstruct the changes in cooling conditions more or less approximately. If not, no temperature-based method can be applied. If this is possible, the method used should be able to take the changes into account, even approximately (compare the recommended strategy of the nomogram method; see Fig. 3.38). So the main advantage of the enlightened method of Green and Wright[26,27] – measuring instead of *evaluating* the individual factors – is reduced by the impossibility of taking into account even known changes of the cooling conditions.

3. The plateau must have ended before estimating constant *B*. In casework at the scene, the doctor cannot decide whether the plateau is over or not. Only the method of Green and Wright[26,27] avoids this particular problem, which could introduce great errors during the very early phase after death.

The real inability to estimate reliably the representative cooling rate *B* by multiple temperature measurements within a few hours at the scene led to the concept of indirect estimation of the individual values of the constants *A* and *B* by ascertaining rules from a mass of experimental body cooling under various controlled conditions. This took the main influencing factors of body cooling into account in calculating the time since death at the scene of death.

Indirect estimation of *B* under chosen standard conditions of cooling

As said earlier, the values of the constants *A* and *B* are dependent on the body build and the ambient cooling conditions, including the thermal factors on the sur-

---

* Common situations at the scene: a thick bedspread was taken off the body; the ambient temperature is changed by the investigators opening windows and doors or using special lamps, which generate heat; or by the sun rising and shining on the body. Such changes can occur before the temperature measurements of the body can be made.

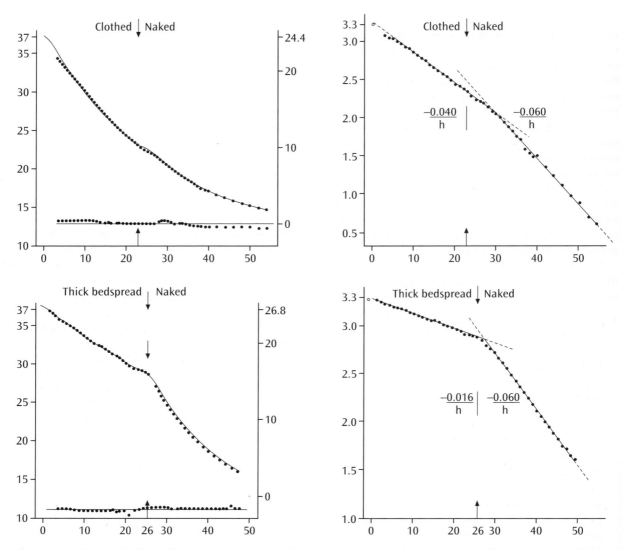

Figure 3.12 *'Broken' cooling experiments. Change from clothes to naked (upper graphs) and from being covered by a thick bedspread to naked (lower graphs). On the left: rectal and ambient temperature (scale in the left margin) and temperature difference 'rectum–ambient' (scale in the right margin) in linear measures. On the right: logarithm of the temperature difference 'rectal–ambient'.*[34,46]

face of the body. To investigate empirically the dependency of the constants on the body build, I at first kept the other influencing factors uniform, except for the ambient temperature, which was relatively constant during a single experiment but was at different levels (between 5.8 and 22°C) in different experiments.

The chosen standard conditions (Fig. 3.14) of the cooling used in this sequence of experiments are the same as described by Marshall and Hoare:[16]

- Naked body – lying extended – on the back – on a thermally indifferent base – in still air – in a closed room – without any sources of strong heat radiation.

In the first sequence of experimental body cooling under almost identical conditions of the chosen standard (same investigator, room and random circumstances), I estimated the true value of *B* by the procedure shown in Fig. 3.11c, and investigated it in

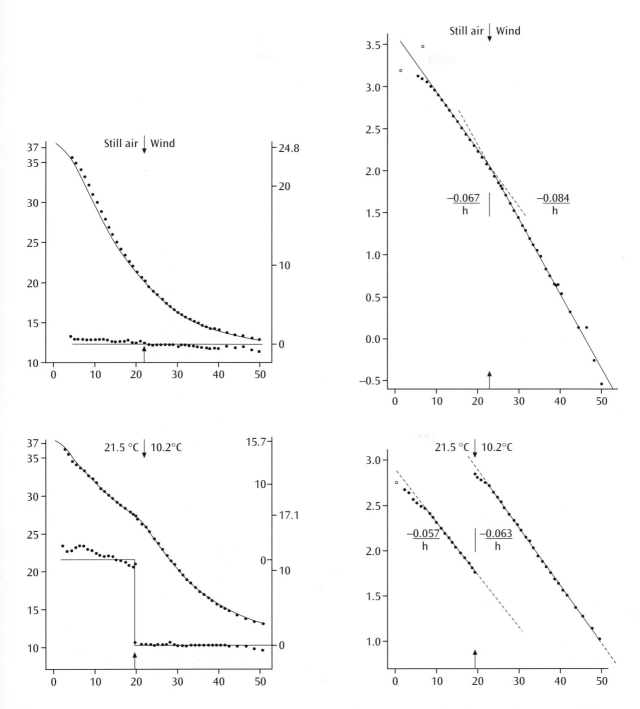

Figure 3.13 *'Broken' cooling experiments. Change from cooling in still air to permanently moving air ('wind'; upper graphs). As a control experiment (lower graphs): change of the ambient temperature only, from 21.5 to 10.2°C.*[34,46] *For further details see* Fig. 3.12.

relation to some measures of body build. The strongest correlation was found between the 'body weight to the power of −0.625' and the 'directly estimated' value of B (Fig. 3.14; eqn 3.1).

The correlation between the 0.8-fold of the quotient 'body surface/body weight' ('size factor' according to Marshall and Hoare[16]) and the value of B was less strong but not significantly so in this sample of 29 bodies, which ranged between 30 and 112 kg body weight.[28,31] I concluded that the body build described as the relation of height and weight (by the size factor) does not give a more precise estimation of the cooling coefficient B than the more simple measure of the body weight (bw) in kg only. Therefore, I preferred the simpler procedure of calculating the value of B from the body weight. In addition, the quantity of fatty tissue of a body had no apparent influence on the value of B, in accordance with theoretical aspects.[32] (see footnote d, p. 63)

A combined series of 53 body-cooling experiments by different investigators conducted at different places (though under the chosen standard conditions of cooling) confirmed this correlation. The variance was greater than in the first series because of similar, but not identical, cooling conditions.[33] In consequence, the individual value of B can be computed under 'chosen standard conditions' of cooling by:

$$B = -1.2815 \, (bw^{-0.625}) + 0.0284 \qquad (3.2)$$

The power of −0.625 seems to be an analogy to the 'rule of surface': the surface is proportional to the body weight to the power of 0.67 according to the cubic root of the squared body weight. If the individual value of B is investigated experimentally from the whole cooling curve of the body (Fig. 3.11c), the body weight can be computed[28] by solving for the variable body weight (bw) in eqn 3.2:

$$bw \, (\text{kg}) = \left[\frac{-1.2815}{B - 0.0284} \right]^{1.6} \qquad (3.3)$$

In 46 cases this agreed with the real body weight within a standard deviation of ±6.1 kg. That means that body weight-related estimation of the value of B results in a rather moderate inaccuracy, compared with the direct estimation by multiple temperature measurements over a period of a few hours, possibly after a change in the cooling conditions. Nevertheless, this moderate inaccuracy can lead to a moderate systematic error in computing the time since death, which increases with progress of cooling related to the standardized temperature, Q.

A typical but pronounced example is the case of Fig. 3.11. The body of 99.5 kg cooled somewhat slower than expected compared with the body weight-related value of B according to eqn 3.2, which would be −0.0439, so providing a progressive over-estimation of the calculated time since death, as can be seen by comparing Fig. 3.11d/Table 3.2 with Fig. 3.11e/Table 3.2. The actual observed value of B (−0.0408) would correspond to a body weight of 106.6 kg according to eqn 3.3.

Indirect estimation of B under cooling conditions differing from the chosen standard

See Figs 3.12 and 3.13.

INVESTIGATIONS ON BODIES

For a clear decision as to whether there is a significant influence of clothing, covering and wind on the body cooling[16,34] or not,[32,35] I performed some special

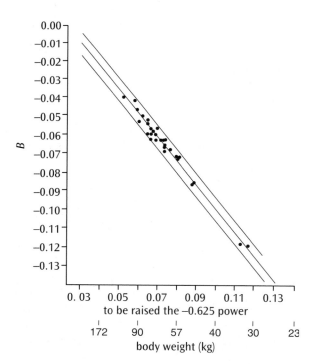

Figure 3.14 *Relation between the exponent B (eqn 3.2) and the body weight to the power of −0.625 under chosen standard conditions of cooling. Regression line and permissible variation of 95%.*[34,46]

'broken' experiments (see Figs 3.12 and 3.13). A body was allowed to cool for the first few hours clothed or covered, the covering was removed and the body then cooled naked in still air (chosen standard) (see Fig. 3.12). The graphs on the left show the original points of measurement with the computed cooling curves (lines) according to eqns 3.1 and 3.2 using the individual calculated values of the constant *B*, which can be seen in the graphs on the right. These graphs demonstrate the cooling curves as the logarithm of the temperature difference between the rectum and the surroundings. Here, the given lines are the regression lines and the given figures are the slopes, which are identical to the constant *B* of each of the two parts of the cooling curves (Fig. 3.11c).

Figure 3.12 clearly illustrates the results. The clothed body (upper graphs) cools with a slope of *B* = −0.04, which corresponds to the slope of a naked body of 109 kg according to eqn 3.3. After taking the clothing off the body, the same body now cools with a slope of *B* = −0.06, corresponding to 72 kg. The actual body weight was 76 kg. The influence of the clothing (underwear, shirt, suit and thicker coat) is significant. The influence of a covering such as a thick bedspread (lower graphs of Fig. 3.12) is much more pronounced: the body cools with *B* = −0.016, corresponding to 217 kg. After taking the covering off the body, it cools with *B* = −0.06, corresponding to 72 kg. The actual body weight was 73 kg. In analogy (see Fig. 3.13, upper graphs), if a body first cools naked in still air (chosen standard), then later in permanently moving air (by switching on a small fan; 25 watts, mounted on the ceiling at a distance of about 2 metres from the body surface giving only a very slight air movement), the slope *B* equals −0.067 (64 kg) under the chosen standard conditions (still air), and is closely related to the real body weight of 65 kg. This changes to *B* = −0.084 under the conditions of moving air corresponding to 49 kg. The conclusion of this experiment indicates that even a slight but permanent air movement results in a significant acceleration of the cooling of a naked body.

Conversely (see lower part of Fig. 3.13) there is no significant change in the slope of the cooling curve when the ambient temperature changes only rectangularly. As a control experiment, this naked body of 71 kg body weight cooled in still air, first in an ambient temperature of about 21.5°C and later, after a quick transfer to another room, in about 10°C ambient temperature. The slope *B* changed from −0.057 (76 kg) to −0.063 (68 kg), which is insignificant.

The principle of corrective factors of the body weight

Taking as an example the upper part of Fig. 3.12, a clothed body cools like a naked body 1.4 times heavier: 109 kg/76 kg = 1.4. This corrective factor of the body weight (*C*) equals the body weight calculated according to eqn 3.3 from *B* of the cooling curve (*bw calc*) divided by the real body weight (*bw*):

$$C = \frac{bw\ calc}{bw} \tag{3.4}$$

So, eqn 3.2 is now:

$$B = -1.2815\ (C \times bw)^{-0.0625} + 0.0284 \tag{3.5}$$

where *C* = corrective factor of the body weight taking into account any difference of the cooling conditions from the chosen standard.

In the case of the lower part of Fig. 3.12 (thick bedspread):

$$C = \frac{217\ kg}{73\ kg} = 3.0$$

In the case of the upper part of Fig. 3.13 (wind):

$$C = \frac{49\ kg}{65\ kg} = 0.75$$

In the case of the lower part of Fig. 3.13 (chosen standard; rectangular change of the ambient temperature only):

$$C = \frac{76\ kg}{71\ kg} = 1.07,\ \text{and}\ \frac{68\ kg}{71\ kg} = 0.96$$

In comparison with the chosen standard (*C* = 1), thermic insulation conditions will result in a corrective factor greater than 1. Conditions that cause an acceleration of the cooling will result in a corrective factor less than 1.

After the pilot experiments, we made several series of cooling experiments under various cooling conditions, all differing from the chosen standard, using naked bodies in constantly moving air, different types of dry clothing and covering,[33,36] wet clothing, wet, naked body surface with or without wind[37] and body cooling in still water.[38] From each experimental body cooling curve, the real value of *B* (analogous to the graphs on the right in Figs 3.12 and 3.13), the corresponding body weight according to eqn 3.3 and the resulting corrective factor according to eqn 3.4 were calculated.

Body cooling in constantly, even slightly moving, air

The cooling curves of ten naked bodies of actual body weight between 52 and 89 kg, lying extended on the back beneath a 25-watt fan mounted at a distance of 2 metres on the ceiling of the room and producing a slight movement of air, provided values of B equal to 0.75 times the real body weight on average (Table 3.3). The corrective factor varied only a little, from 0.66 to 0.81, corresponding to lower errors of computed death times (standard deviation ± 0.9 h) in comparison with body cooling in still air (standard deviation ± 1.3 h) in the same series of body coolings.[34]

The cooling of clothed bodies

The data of experimental cooling of clothed bodies in still air (Table 3.4) show the relationship between the verbal description of clothing and the corrective factor. However, they also show that this relationship is not without exception and, therefore, it is not possible to estimate a corrective factor true to within ± one-tenth from a verbal description. A further conclusion is that only the clothing of the lower trunk is relevant for the retardation of rectal body cooling. The almost radial direction of heat transfer inside the body and the rectal temperature probe site theoretically support this conclusion.

Clothed bodies in moving air

A study of Table 3.3 (naked bodies in moving air) and Table 3.4 (clothed bodies in still air) shows that the influence of moving air on clothed bodies becomes less as the clothing or covering becomes thicker. Moving air accelerates cooling in very thinly clothed bodies (Table 3.5; H12, H15), compensates the slightly decelerating influence of thin clothing (H14, H11) and

seems to be without any accelerating influence on thicker-clothed bodies (B66, B67). Moving air accelerates the cooling by forced convection of heated air from the body surface. Clothing decelerates the cooling, mainly by fixation of a layer of heated air at the surface of the body. This principle should be borne in mind when estimating a corrective factor in cases of clothed bodies lying in moving air.

Covered bodies in still air

The corrective factors for taking usual coverings into account are rather uniform, though it is pointed out that the cooling experiments listed in Table 3.6 were made by laying the bodies on 'thermally indifferent' bases, e.g. on a simple covered stretcher. When bodies are lying on more thermally insulating bases (couch, divan, bed), somewhat higher corrective factors may be required, even in covered bodies. The corrective factors of bed-like covered bodies are rather non-uniform. In Table 3.6, the different corrective factors for cases H09 and H06, and H08 and H10 may be explained by the great difference in body weight, as the cooling conditions were nearly identical in these cases. This is one clue that lower corrective factors are necessary for higher thermic insulation conditions (e.g. a bedspread) on heavier bodies, and vice versa (see page 56).

Body cooling in still water

Nineteen bodies (body weights between 48.5 and 108.5 kg) were suspended undressed in a tub holding 1000 L of almost still water at temperatures of approximately 20 and 10°C, from the third hour postmortem (Table 3.7). The rectal temperature was measured, usually until the 33rd hour postmortem. The bodies cooled as quickly as naked bodies of half the real body mass in still air of the same temperature, correspond-

Table 3.3 *Body cooling in permanently moving air*[34]

Case	Body weight	B_{wind}	bw_{calc}	Corrective factor
01	52.0	−0.095	42.3	0.81
02	57.0	−0.098	40.7	0.71
27	65.0	−0.094	42.8	0.66
28	65.0	−0.084	49.1	0.76
29	66.5	−0.082	50.5	0.76
30	89.0	−0.063	68.4	0.77
38	56.0	−0.091	44.3	0.79

Body weight calculated according to eqn 3.3.

Table 3.4 *Corrective factors for clothed bodies lying on a 'thermally indifferent' base in still air*[28,33]

Case number	Whole clothing	Clothing of lower trunk	Real bw	Calculated bw	Corrective factor
B61	Work jacket, trousers displaced up-, downward, vest, short pants	Short pants	92.0	92.0	1.0
B63	Vest, panties	Panties	110.0	121.0	1.1
H66	Sweater, vest, drawers, short pants	Drawers, short pants	92.5	94.4	1.02
B64	Shirt, displaced upward, vest, short pants, trousers	Short pants, trousers	82.0	90.2	1.1
B58	Trousers, thin sweater, two vests, short pants	Trousers, short pants	68.0	74.8	1.1
B37	Open anorak, sweater, trousers, drawers	Trousers, drawers	79.0	85.3	1.08
B57	Anorak, jacket, sweater, vest, trousers, drawers	Trousers, drawers	76.5	86.4	1.26
H2	Jacket, sweatshirt, shirt, vest, short pants, trousers	Trousers, drawers	84.5	110.7	1.31
H6	Sweater, shirt, vest, trousers, two drawers	Trousers, two drawers	68.0	72.8	1.07
B53	Parker, jacket, waistcoat, shirt, vest, trousers, drawers	Parker, trousers, drawers	79.0	104.3	1.32
H4	Jacket, vest, roll-on panty, two short pants, trousers	Trousers, roll-on panty, two short pants	86.5	102.9	1.19
B60	Waistcoat, shirt, two vests, short pants, trousers, corselet, tights	Trousers, corselet, tights; short pants	55.5	79.4	1.43
B54	Jacket, shirt, long cardigan, vest, trousers, thick drawers	Long cardigan, trousers, thick drawers	63.5	91.4	1.44
B36	Woollen coat, jacket, waistcoat, vest, shirt, short pants, trousers	Woollen coat, trousers, short pants	85.0	126.7	1.49
B59	Jacket, sweater, vest, drawers, trousers, truss with pad	Trousers, drawers, truss with pad	78.5	125.6	1.6
B60	Lining trench coat, thick woollen dress, slip, short panty, tights	Lining trench coat, thick woollen dress, slip, short panty, tights	52.0	93.6	1.8

Table 3.5 *Corrective factors for clothed bodies in permanently moving air*[28]

Case number	Clothing of lower trunk	Real bw	Calculated bw	Corrective factor
H12	Nightwear, short panty	73.3	55.7	0.76
H15	Short panty	67.5	60.8	0.9
H14	Trousers, drawers	78.0	75.6	0.97
H11	Trousers, drawers	73.0	80.3	1.10
B66	Thin trench coat, short panty, trousers	78.5	110.7	1.41
H13	Dress, slip, short panty, roll-on panty, truss	63.7	77.7	1.21
B67	Thick coat, skirt, slip, corselet, tights, short panty	83.5	138.7	1.66

ing to a corrective factor of 0.5 as a mean (ranging from 0.36 to 0.63). However, 10 further bodies (body weights between 44 and 95 kg), suspended in nearly still water at approximately 0°C, yielded a distinctly smaller temperature decrease, which was especially marked at rectal temperatures below about 11°C in all bodies, without regard to body mass. In bodies of great body weight and small body surface in proportion to body mass, the lower cooling rate was pronounced, the cooling curve corresponding to corrective factors tending to 1.0. This can be explained by a decrease in the thermal conductivity of the subcutaneous adipose tissue with a decrease in tissue temperature.[38]

Table 3.6 *Corrective factors for covering of naked and partly clothed bodies respectively* [28]

Case number	Clothing	Covering	Real bw	Calculated bw	Corrective factor
Thinner covering – thermically indifferent supporting base					
B62	Naked	Simple cover	66.0	79.2	1.2
B51	Naked	Double cover	91.0	106.2	1.17
B56	Drawers, short panty	Simple cover	92.5	119.3	1.29
B52	Drawers, short panty	Simple blanket	74.0	100.2	1.34
Bed-like covering – mattress on supporting base					
B33	Short panty	Thick bedspread	73.0	157.7	2.16
H08	Naked		77.0	110.4	1.44
H07	Nightwear		93.0	124.0	1.33
H10	Trousers, drawers	Two thick blankets	113.0	152.2	1.35
H06	Skirt, drawers		64.5	127.0	1.97
H09	Two napkins, short panty		6.3	16.4	2.6
			6.25	25.0	4.0

Body cooling in flowing water

Brown and Marshall[19] characterize the cooling curve of a very small body (size factor: 320 cm²/kg) suspended in flowing water (velocity 5 m/h) by a four-exponential model. Transcribed to the two-exponential eqn 3.1 and the body weight relation of *B* according to eqn 3.2, this would result in a corrective factor of the body weight in order of 0.35 which relates well to all the other corrective factors.

Body cooling in cases of wet clothing or covering, or unclothed wet body surface

Some cooling experiments of 'wet-through' clothed or covered bodies, and of naked bodies with a wet body surface were made in a closed room, and by night in the open air under a cloudless sky when reconstructing a special case.[37]

According to the accused husband, his wife had fallen from a boat into the water and drowned. The real time of death could not have been earlier than 22:10 h and not later than 22:20 h, averaging 22:15 h according to his declaration. Some 15 minutes later, the body was detected by the husband and salvaged by witnesses. The body was lain on a lawn. At 00:23 h the deep rectal temperature was measured as 28°C, and at 00:40 h as 27.5°C. The law court decided on 28.3°C rectal temperature at 00:23 h after examining the thermometer. The body weight of the woman was 53 kg and her height 159 cm. Until the temperature measurement, the body was clothed with a slip, a corselette, silastic trousers, a shirt, a brassiere and a long waterproof anorak. The day

in August was sunny. During the windless night there was a cloudless sky. The weather station stated the following temperatures: 20.7°C (16:00 h), 20.1°C (19:00 h), 15.6°C (21:00 h), 14.3°C (22:00 h), 13.8°C (23:00 h), 12.6°C (00:00 h) and 11.9°C (01:00 h). From these data there resulted a mean temperature of 12.8°C between 23:00 h and 01:00 h. The water temperature within the harbour measured approximately 20°C. The decisive question was whether the rectal body cooling to 28.3°C at 00:23 h could be compatible with a death-time at 22:15 h.

To solve this question, some cooling experiments were made (Table 3.8), which led to the following conclusions:

1. Naked bodies suspended in water for a short time (~10 minutes) cool in still air as a result of their wet body surface at the same rate as bodies 0.75 times the real body weight.
2. Bodies with thin but 'wet-through' clothing/covering seem to cool in moving air like bodies of 0.7 times the real body weight.
3. Bodies with more layers of wet-through clothing/covering seem to cool in moving air like bodies of the real body weight without any corrective adjustment.
4. One layer of thin, wet-through clothing/covering does not seem to have a marked influence on the velocity of body cooling in still air, compared with cooling under chosen standard conditions. Therefore, no corrective adjustment of the real body weight is necessary. On the other hand,

Table 3.7 *Body cooling in still water*[38]

Case number	Body weight (kg)	B_{stand}* calc.	Temp. water (°C)	B_{water} real	bw_{calc} (kg)	Corrective factor
01	65.0	−0.066	19.3	−0.128	28.9	0.445
20	68.0	−0.063	20.0	−0.107	36.5	0.536
21	59.5	−0.071	20.3	−0.137	26.6	0.447
22	84.5	−0.052	20.2	−0.091	44.6	0.528
24	108.5	−0.040	20.2	−0.074	57.4	0.529
25	100.5	−0.043	19.8	−0.082	50.5	0.502
27	97.5	−0.045	19.7	−0.084	49.0	0.503
28	77.5	−0.056	19.9	−0.113	34.1	0.439
30	71.5	−0.061	20.5	−0.111	35.0	0.489
						0.491 ±0.036
02	92.0	−0.048	9.8	−0.074	57.4	0.623
03	48.5	−0.085	9.8	−0.156	22.2	0.457
04	75.0	−0.058	10.0	−0.098	40.7	0.543
05	58.5	−0.063	9.9	−0.104	36.4	0.631
08	88.0	−0.050	10.2	−0.103	38.2	0.435
10	70.0	−0.062	10.2	−0.127	29.2	0.417
11	83.5	−0.052	10.0	−0.099	40.2	0.482
12	77.5	−0.056	8.3	−0.133	27.5	0.355
13	56.5	−0.075	10.0	−0.150	23.5	0.415
14	85.5	−0.051	9.1	−0.092	44.3	0.518
						0.488 ±0.086
06	44.2	−0.092	0.6	−0.140	25.8	0.583
07	75.5	−0.058	0.0	−0.071	60.3	0.798
09	83.5	−0.052	0.0	−0.079	52.9	0.633
15	95.5	−0.046	0.0	−0.044	99.7	1.040
16	79.0	−0.055	0.0	−0.092	44.0	0.557
17	80.0	−0.054	−0.1	−0.055	79.0	0.988
18	49.0	−0.084	−0.1	−0.121	31.1	0.638
19	69.5	−0.062	0.0	−0.073	57.6	0.828
23	58.0	−0.073	0.0	−0.090	44.9	0.775
29	66.5	−0.065	1.2	−0.082	50.6	0.761
						0.760 ±0.155

*$B_{standard}$ according to eqn 3.2; body weight$_{calculated}$ according to eqn 3.3; corrective factor according to eqn 3.4.

thick, wet-through clothing/covering, especially of several layers, provides a reduced velocity of body cooling in still air that is similar to dry clothing/covering and corresponding to corrective factors between 1.1 and 1.4.

On the basis of these results, corrective factors from 1.1 to 1.4 were used to test the husband's account of events. However, another technical expert maintained

that the body would have cooled more because of the influence of radiation against the cloudless sky at night, which would be equal to a corpse at −30°C. To examine this argument, the cooling experiments of cases 80, 81 and 82 in Table 3.8 were made by night in the open air under a cloudless sky by laying the bodies on a wet lawn. The results were the same as for a closed room, showing that radiation from the surface of the body to the cloudless sky by night had no marked

Table 3.8 *Body cooling under wet-through clothing/covering and respective wet body surface*[37]

Case number	Cooling conditions	Real body weight	Corrective factor
Closed room, still air, wet body surface			
50		45.0	0.77
52		65.0	0.75
Wet-through covering or clothing			
41	1 smock	84.5	1.00
42	2 smocks	57.2	1.10
51	Roll-on panty, trousers, 3 smocks	69.5	1.10
44	Roll-on panty, trousers, 3 smocks	65.0	1.30
Permanently moving air			
68	Drawers, trousers, skirt, pullover, jacket	64.5	0.7
55	Drawers, trousers, pullover, coat	91.0	0.9
47	3 smocks	91.5	0.7
Under cloudless sky, wet lawn, still air			
80	Drawers, dress, 1 smock	59.5	1.2
81	Drawers, skirt, 1 smock	67.5	1.4
82	Drawers, dress, 1 smock	58.0	1.4

influence on body cooling. The computation was made using the following:

- mean ambient temperature 12.8°C;
- body weight 53 kg;
- averaged corrective factor 1.2;
- rectal temperature 28.3°C;
- rectal temperature at death 36.5°C (as agreed by the law court).

This equals (according to eqns 3.1 and 3.5) 9.4 hours before 00:23 h as a mean value. Using the range of corrective factors from 1.0 to 1.4, which might be possible according to the special cooling experiments (Table 3.8), the time of death ranges between 5.6 hours (corrective factor = 1.0) and 13.5 hours (corrective factor = 1.4), corresponding to 3.8 hours around the mean of 9.4 hours, which is in close agreement with three times the experienced standard deviation of cooling experiments under various conditions (see Figs 3.29, 3.30 and Table 3.14). Therefore, a time of death at 22:15 h (22:10 to 22:30 h) could be excluded.

INVESTIGATIONS ON DUMMIES

Using dummies to replace bodies of average weight, we obtained results which correspond well with the corrective factor for various cooling conditions. An exception was experiments with wet-surfaced dummies and dummies suspended in water, where somewhat lower corrective factors were found compared with bodies (Fig. 3.15).

Dependence of corrective factors on the body weight[1,6]

Though the corrective factors established on bodies include a wide spectrum of frequently occurring cooling conditions, nearly all these experiences resulted from bodies of average body weight. Only a few cases support the assumption that bodies of a very high body weight and, at the same time, strong thermic insulation conditions (see Table 3.6) would require lower corrective factors and, conversely, bodies of a low body weight would require higher corrective factors. To correct these deficiencies, 98 cooling experiments on five different-sized dummies under five different cooling conditions, besides standard ones, were made. The dummies were cooled under standard conditions equivalent to human bodies of 14, 33, 41, 83 and 104 kg, respectively.

Characteristics of the cooling conditions

The dummies were lain on a thick, foam-upholstered supported base and exposed permanently to a slightly moving air, produced by a small fan (25 watts)

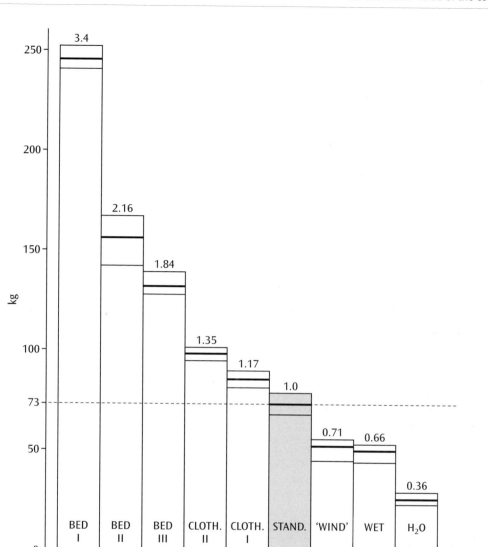

Figure 3.15 *Comparison of corrective factors investigated on bodies and on a dummy cooling under various, but very similar, conditions. The dummy replaces a body of 73 kg. The corrective factors resulting from dummy experiments are given at the top of the columns. Beneath the baseline the corrective factors of bodies are shown as they resulted from the above reported experimental body investigations.*[3]

mounted on the ceiling at a distance of approximately 2 metres.

- Clothing I: two layers. One layer was thin (cotton textile, like pants) and the second layer was rather thick (blue jeans).
- Clothing II: three layers. Additional to 'clothing I', a second thin layer was applied.
- Covering I: A wool blanket, loose-fitting.

- Covering II: A thick feather eiderdown. The dummies were laid down on an additional mattress, which was placed on the upholstered support base used for the other dummies.

After repeated test cooling measurements under chosen standard conditions, the coefficient B was calculated. From these 'experimental' values of B, 'virtual' weights were calculated according to eqn 3.3. The virtual weight represents the weight of a body whose cooling curve is identical to cooling under standard conditions.

Just as under standard conditions of cooling, a close linear relationship results between 'experimental' B and 'virtual weight' to the power of −0.625 for each condition differing from the standard (Fig. 3.16).

Due to the common point of intersection, the dependence of B for each cooling condition is differentiated only by the slope S. Therefore, the coefficient B can be calculated for each cooling condition, depending on the body weight (standard) according to its own slope S:

$$B_{condition} = [(bw^{-0.625} - 0.028)\, S_{condition}] - 0.007 \quad (3.6)$$

$B_{condition}$ can be used to calculate the body weight (kg) by:

$$bw_{condition} = [-1.2815/B_{condition} - 0.0284]^{1.6} \quad (3.7)$$

The bw condition represents the weight that is apparently changed due to the special cooling conditions. Dividing the virtual weight (standard) by the apparently changed weight, the corrective factor can be determined. Conversely, the virtual weight of the dummy (standard) multiplied by the corrective factor provides for a special cooling condition.

The corrective factors of the investigated cooling conditions can be calculated universally for any virtual weight (Fig. 3.17):

$$\left[\frac{-1.2815}{(S_{condition} \times bw_{standard} + I_{condition}) - 0.0289} \right]^{1.6} \Big/ bw_{standard} = F \quad (3.8)$$

where $S_{condition}$ = slope; $I_{condition}$ = intercept from Table 3.9; $bw_{standard}$ = virtual weight under standard conditions.

The dependence of the corrective factors on the virtual dummy weight (acting for body weight) is evident. If the dependence on body weight did not exist, the lines for all the cooling conditions in Fig. 3.17 must be horizontal, just as they are for the standard condition and, approximately, for the cooling condition 'wind'. The dynamics of the dependence on body weight become pronounced with the power of the thermic insulation. The curves of Fig. 3.17 demonstrate a non-linear regularity of the cooling conditions. The dependence between virtual weight and the corrective factor of the investigated cooling conditions can also be used to interpolate the relation to non-examined cooling conditions of any distinct weight, as shown in Fig. 3.18 for an average body weight of 70 kg. The 'best fit' curve of

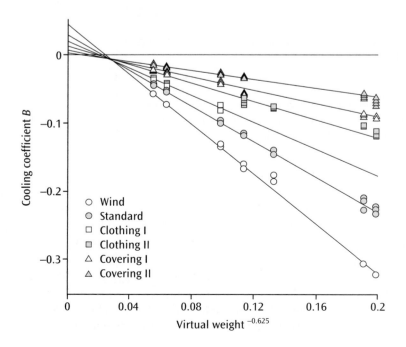

Figure 3.16 *Regression lines (Table 3.9) of the dependence of cooling coefficient B (ordinate) on virtual weight to the power of −0.625 (abscissa) for the various cooling conditions. The common point of intersection has the coordinates Y = −0.007 and X = 0.028.*[1.6]

Table 3.9 *Regression lines of cooling coefficient* B *(ordinate) against virtual weight to the power of −0.625 (abscissa) for the various cooling conditions (see Fig. 3.16)*[1,6]

Condition	Number of experiment	Regression line slope 'S'	Intercept
Wind	20	−1.8083	0.0436
Standard	24	−1.2815	0.0289
Clothing I	07	−0.9591	0.0199
Clothing II	12	−0.6431	0.0110
Covering I	17	−0.4828	0.0065
Covering II	18	−0.3218	0.0020

the measurement points drawn is expressed mathematically:

$$S = 3.24596 \times \exp(-0.89959 \times C_{70}) \qquad (3.9)$$

where S = slope to calculate the cooling coefficient B from body weight to the power of −0.625 (Fig. 3.16); and C_{70} = corrective factor valid for a special cooling condition to a body of 70 kg.

The interpolation can only be made, in the first instance, on the range of the actually investigated cooling conditions (from wind to thick bedspread) and for those corrective factors (from 0.75 to 3.0) valid for 'average' body weights.

Using the same principle, the corrective factor (C) can be calculated for any actual body weight (kg) according to eqn 3.8, provided that the corrective

factor for an 'average body weight' of 70 kg (C_{70}), for any actual cooling condition, is known:

$$\left[\frac{-1.2815}{(bw^{-0.625} - 0.028)(-3.24596 \times \exp(-0.89959 \times C_{70})) - 0.0354} \right]^{1.6} = C \qquad (3.10)$$

Using eqn 3.10, the corrective factors were calculated for body weights ranging from 4 to 150 kg, related to the corrective factors of 70 kg (see Table 3.17).

Equation 3.10 can be used to demonstrate that spe-

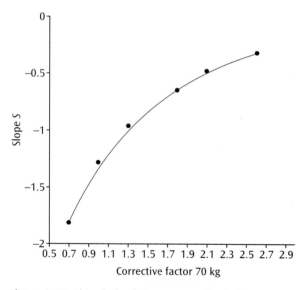

Figure 3.18 *The relation between corrective factors (abscissa) and slope S of the correlation between cooling coefficient and weight according to* Fig. 3.16 *and* Table 3.9 *(ordinate) for a dummy of approximately 70 kg. The points represent, from below: wind, standard, clothing I, clothing II, covering I, covering II.*[1]

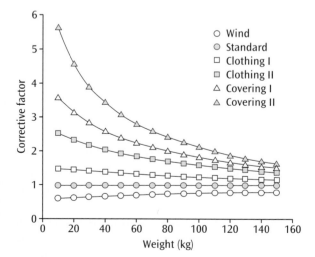

Figure 3.17 *Generalization of the dependence of the corrective factors on the virtual weight of dummies (acting for body weight) for the investigated cooling conditions.*[1,6]

cial thermic insulating conditions, which require a corrective factor of 2.0 on a dummy of 70 kg virtual weight, would require a higher corrective factor of approximately 3.2 on a dummy of virtual 10 kg; and, in the case of a 110-kg dummy, a lower corrective factor of 1.7. In these experiments, the corrective factor for one of the different-sized dummies of one of the applied cooling conditions can be calculated by eqn 3.10 if the corrective factor of a different-sized dummy is known.

Because of the close conformity of the previous investigations in comparing the cooling of dummies and bodies under various conditions (see Fig. 3.15) it is concluded that the result of the dependence of corrective factors on the body weight is applicable to bodies.

Intuitively, it appears obvious that, in the case of a 150-kg body, a special bedspread does not cause a deceleration of cooling proportional to the body weight corresponding to 525 kg (3.5×150 kg), such as in a case of a 4-kg body corresponding to 14 kg (3.5×4). The physical explanation for this effect is, however, more difficult. The model of a cylinder of infinite length[39] applied to body cooling[17,18,32] may be helpful. A special bedspread has a distinct layer thickness. The enlargement of the radius is, in the case of a 4-kg body, relatively much greater than in the case of a 150-kg body; it is not proportional to the radius of the body, but enlarges the radius cumulatively. In addition, the bedspread causes a deceleration of heat loss by its comparatively smaller heat conductivity against body tissues. The effect of this component on the velocity of body cooling is proportional to the surface area of the body. The surface area itself is proportional to the body weight to the power of 0.67 (see Fig. 3.4; 'geometric likeness'). Therefore, it may be concluded that the deceleration of body cooling by a bedspread is provided by the enlargement of the radius of a body as an additive component, as well as by the low heat conductivity as a proportional component.[1,6]

However, although these considerations may be helpful in understanding, they do not lead to practicable solutions useful for casework.

Influence of the type of supporting base on body cooling[4,5,7]

In a series of cooling experiments utilizing heat flow sensors (see Figs 3.5–3.9), 'naked' dummies were lain on supporting bases with very different thermic features (Table 3.10; Figs 3.19–3.21).

Related to a 'thermally indifferent base', insulating bases slow down the cooling rate by corrective factors of up to 1.3. As may be seen in Table 3.10, it was not possible to slow down the cooling beyond this level by adding more insulating material (see experiment numbers 200 to 310) but not covering the dummies' flanks. On the other hand, some bases accelerate the cooling, requiring corrective factors in the order of 0.75 to 0.5.

Figure 3.19(a–c) demonstrates not only the dependence of the heat flow at the contact surface but also the slope of central temperature on that type of base. Even the heat flow at the non-contact surface is slightly influenced by the type of base, which is comprehensible in view of the parallel circuit of the surfaces in Fig. 3.9. This also explains why the cooling cannot be further decelerated by adding more insulating features to the supporting base. Lastly, the heating of the ground by the heat flow from the contact surface of the dummy to the base itself, immediately after contact, causes a more reduced temperature difference between base and contact surface, as can be clearly seen in the first parts of the curves in Figs 3.7 and 3.8. In accordance with this, there is a linear relationship between central temperature (X) and heat flow at the contact surface (Y) during cooling after the plateau. The slope of this regression line best characterizes the influence of the type of base on the cooling velocity, since there is a strong correlation with the cooling coefficient B (Fig. 3.21), which means the slope of logarithm of temperature difference against cooling time (see Fig. 3.11c).

In a second series of experiments by Unland[7] with different-sized dummies, it was shown that this relation depends on the size of dummy (Fig. 3.21). According to Fig. 3.21 the cooling coefficient B can be computed for any body weight and any kind of base by:

$$B = (bw \times 0.4774 + 13.3462)^{-0.725} \times$$
$$sFT - (bw \times 0.3210 + 1.5299)^{-0.98} \quad (3.11)$$

where bw = body weight in kg; and sFT = slope of central temperature against the heat flow at the lying surface.

The importance of eqn 3.11 is the replacement of the estimation of a corrective factor for any cooling condition, by the measurement of the heat flow at surfaces, in addition to the measurement of ambient and central (rectal) temperatures and body weight.

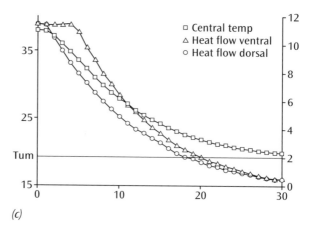

(a)

(c)

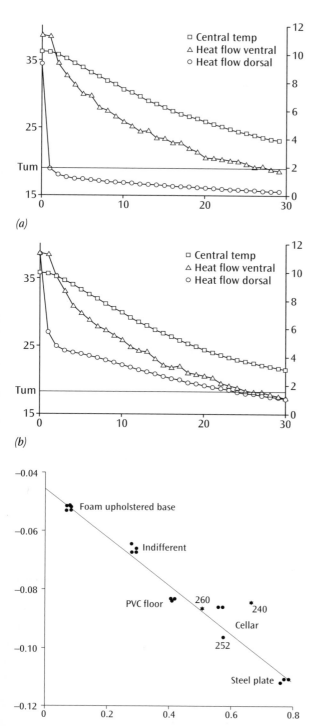

(b)

Figure 3.19 *Heat flow on the contact and the non-contact surfaces of a 'naked' dummy in still air lying on different supporting bases. Abscissa: cooling time (hours); ordinate: heat flow (Btu ft^{-2} h^{-1}).[4] (a) Isolating base. Experiment number 201 from Table 3.10. (b) Indifferent base. Experiment number 211 from Table 3.10. (c) Well-conducting base. Experiment number 292 from Table 3.10.*

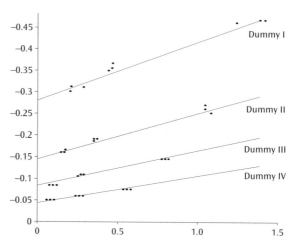

Figure 3.20 *Relationship between the slope of central temperature against heat flow on the contact surface (abscissa) and cooling coefficient B (ordinate) of the experiments with different thermal features of the base listed in Table 3.10.[4]*

Figure 3.21 *Relationship between the slope of heat flow against central temperature (abscissa) and cooling coefficient B (ordinate) investigated in four different-sized dummies (I = 6.9 kg; II = 17.3 kg; III = 36.8 kg; IV = 72.5 kg) and three thermally different bases (double-covered table; thick, foam-upholstered base; concrete cellar floor).[7]*

Table 3.10 *Type of supporting base and its influence of cooling of a 'naked' dummy related to a 'thermally indifferent base' as used at 'standard conditions'*

Experiment number	Supporting base	Real B	bw calculated	Corrective factor
	Thick foam-upholstered base			
200		−0.0514	84.9	1.31
201		−0.0524	83.3	1.29
202		−0.0528	82.6	1.28
270	Thick foam-upholstered base + styropor plate	−0.0529	82.4	1.27
300	Thick foam-upholstered base + styropor plate + cushion	−0.0514	85.0	1.31
310	Armchair	−0.0526	82.9	1.28
	Table + cover 'indifferent'			
210		−0.0646	66.4	1.03
211		−0.0669	63.9	0.99
212		−0.0659	65.1	1.01
225		−0.0672	63.6	0.98
	Floor of a room covering with PVC			
230		−0.0840	49.1	0.76
231		−0.0838	49.2	0.76
232		−0.0829	49.9	0.77
	Loft			
	Ground of cellar			
240		−0.0859	47.8	0.74
250		−0.0863	47.5	0.73
251		−0.0864	47.5	0.73
252		−0.0953	42.1	0.65
260	Stone slab outside	−0.0867	47.3	0.73
	Steel plate on concrete-ground wash round			
290		−0.1095	35.4	0.55
291		−0.1106	34.9	0.54
292		−0.1116	34.5	0.53

Calculation of the body weight (bw) according to eqn 3.3. Calculation of the corrective factor according to eqn 3.4 with an average 'standard' weight of 64.7 kg. The nearly constant ambient temperatures ranged between 14 and 19°C, except in experiment number 260 where it was 6.1°C.[4]

THE INDIVIDUAL VALUE OF THE PLATEAU-RELATED CONSTANT A

Estimation of A on bodies

The empirical investigation of the dependency of the constant A in experimental body cooling was much more difficult than that of the constant B, because A describes the 'postmortal temperature plateau'[40] and the temperature at death was really unknown in our cases, since the bodies which were investigated came in between 0.8 and 6 hours postmortem. In the first series of experiments, the duration of the plateau varied from 5 to 14 hours, which is equivalent to a period

without any drop of the rectal temperature between 1 and 6 hours.[31] Nevertheless, there was a significant relationship between the duration of the plateau and the rate of the temperature drop after the plateau. Bodies with a low rate (high body weight) also had a longer plateau phase than bodies with a high rate (low body weight). There is a relationship between the values of the exponent of the first and second terms of the model (see eqn 3.2). Within the investigated range of the ambient temperature, between 5 and 22°C, the value of the second exponent was found to be five times the value of the first exponent (B), resulting in an approach of $A = 1.25$ as a mean.[31] In the example of the body in Fig. 3.11, the temperature measurement began 3 hours after death. The intercept of the regression line (Fig. 3.11b) was 3.3677, corresponding to 29.01°C above ambient temperature (13.3°C) in a linear measure. The best fit of the curve was made using a value of *A* equal to 1.25, assuming a starting temperature at death of 37.2°C (see Fig. 3.11d).

If the value of *A* really equals 1.25, then the starting temperature must have been 36.5°C, since (29.01/1.25) + 13.3 gives 36.5°C. On the other hand, if the starting temperature was 37.2°C, then the value of *A* must equal 1.21 (29.01/[37.2 – 13.3]). This example demonstrates the difficulties in investigating the 'true' value of *A* in bodies where the starting temperature at death is unknown.

Marshall and Hoare[16] did not discover any distinct relation between the first exponent (*B*) and the second one (inherent in *A*). In practice, they set the value of the second exponent at a fixed value of –0.4 for all bodies, independent of its general cooling velocity. This procedure leads to additional errors in calculating the time since death, especially in cases of a greater or a lower cooling rate *B*. This error is avoidable by linking the second exponent to the first one, which is provided by a distinct value of *A*.

Using the value 1.25 for *A*, the rectal cooling curves published in 1955 by De Saram *et al.*[24] (which were obtained in ambient temperatures between 26 and 31°C) systematically over-estimated the time of death. The reason for this was solely an over-estimation of the relative length of the plateau related to *A* = 1.25. By means of an approach of *A* = 1.11 (where the value of the second exponent is ten times that of the first), corresponding to a relatively shorter length of the plateau, the over-estimation was removed. Theoretically, the plateau also depends on the magnitude of the difference in temperature between the rectum and surroundings at death,[15] so that the empirical result in modelling De Saram's cooling curves would establish a real dependency of the value of *A* (relative length of the postmortal temperature plateau) on the ambient temperature. The ambient temperatures of our own experimental body coolings (*A* = 1.25) did not usually exceed 23°C. In De Saram's material it ranged between 26 and 31°C (*A* = 1.11). The dependency of *A* on the ambient temperature seems to be non-linear but pronounced in ambient temperatures above 23°C. Certainly, a jump in the value of *A* from 1.25 to 1.11 at 23°C, or at any other level of an ambient temperature, is not to be expected but, lacking more experimental data of rectal cooling curves in higher ambient temperatures, we were unable to pursue the matter any further.

Determination of *A* on dummies

The rule of the close relationship between the first exponent (*B*) and the second exponent of eqn 3.1, corresponding to the value of A according to:

$$\text{Second exponent} = A \times B/A - 1 \qquad (3.12)$$

can be better studied on dummies than on bodies because of the exact measurement of the starting point of cooling (*To*) immediately after removing the dummy from the incubator since:

$$A = \exp (a_{yx})/To - Ta \qquad (3.13)$$

whereas the *To* of bodies is usually unknown.

By extrapolation of the later part of the cooling curves to *t* = 0 according to the procedure shown in Fig. 3.11c, the value of 'exp (*a*$_{yx}$)' is easy to obtain.

Dividing exp (*a*$_{yx}$) by *To* – *Ta* gives the value of *A*.

Cooling curves of a dummy corresponding to a body weight of 70 kg in ambient temperatures of 2 and 28°C (Fig. 3.22) show an identical duration of the plateau if the value of *A* remains the same at 1.25. The plateau is equivalent to a period of 3.7 hours without any drop of the central temperature, independent of the ambient temperature. However, the cooling curves of two dummies of different body weights (10 and 110 kg) show a different duration of their plateaux (Fig. 3.23), equivalent to periods of 6.3 hours (110 kg) and 0.8 hours (10 kg) without any drop of central temperature, assuming the same value of *A* (1.25). These

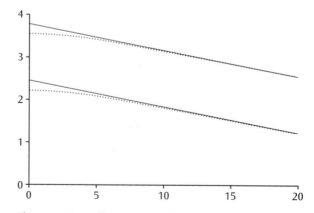

Figure 3.22 *Cooling curves equivalent to a 70 kg body (B = –0.0617) starting at 37.2°C in ambient temperatures of 2°C (upper curve) and 28°C (lower curve) with identical values of A (1.25). The regression lines reach 37.2°C at the same time of 3.7 hours. Abscissa: time (h); ordinate: ln (T$_r$ – Ta).*

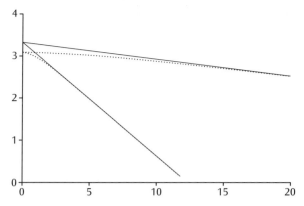

Figure 3.23 *Postmortal temperature plateau dependent on the body weight. Cooling curves are equivalent to a 110 kg body (B = −0.0395; upper curve) and a 10 kg body (B = −0.2755; lower curve) both starting at 37.2°C in 15°C ambient temperature. The value of A is 1.25. The regression line of the 110 kg body reaches 37.2°C as late as 5.7 hours after the start of cooling, but that of the 10 kg body reaches 37.2°C 0.9 hours after start of cooling. Abscissa: time (h); ordinate; ln (Tr − Ta).*

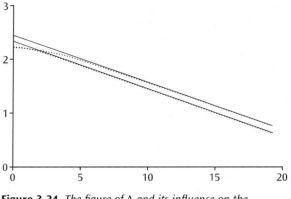

Figure 3.24 *The figure of A and its influence on the duration of postmortal plateau in model curves. Model cooling curves of a 50 kg body (B = −0.0827) starting at 37.2°C in an ambient temperature of 28°C. Modelling with A = 1.25 (upper curve); modelling with A = 1.11 (lower curve). The time till regression lines reaching 37.2°C are different: 2.7 hours (A = 1.25) and 1.3 hours (A = 1.11), respectively. After the end of the plateau the curves proceed in parallel with a time difference of 1.4 hours.*

data are comparable to those of our first sequence of cooling experiments on 29 bodies with real body weights between 30 and 112 kg, which led to the best fit of the actually observed durations of the plateau using 1.25 as value of A. If the plateau is really shorter (Fig. 3.24) as it is in De Saram's cooling curves, a value of A lower than 1.25 must be chosen, e.g. 1.11, for best fitting the plateau.

From 216 cooling experiments conducted on dummies corresponding to body weights of between 7 and 104 kg, and under different ambient temperatures and a wide range of different cooling conditions (including variable conditions such as clothing, covering, wind, wet surface, grounds of very different thermal conductivity and capacity), a mean value of A of 1.16 with a standard variation of ± 0.14 was found. A systematic analysis[41] could not confirm any dependence of the figure of the constant A on the ambient temperature as supposed in body cooling. Nevertheless, the magnitude of A showed a slight dependence on the virtual weight of dummies in cooling experiments under standard conditions. The magnitude of A also varied with the magnitude of B resulting from the virtual weight and the corrective factor for various cooling conditions differing from standard. The cooling curves could not be modelled more accurately mathematically

using these 'new' results than using the 'old' value of 1.25 for the constant A.

The value of A may also depend on the homogeneity of body temperature when death occurs. If the superficial layers of the body are already cool because of the peripheral vasoconstriction, e.g. during haemorrhagic shock without any central hypothermia, a gradient in body temperature, directed from the shell to the core of the body, is present when death occurs; the postmortem temperature plateau, so to speak, has started during life. The real postmortem plateau will be shorter in such cases than in cases with a short duration of agony. This particular event cannot be reproduced by dummies.

THE TEMPERATURE AT DEATH, *To*

The temperature at death, *To*, is the third constant of Marshall and Hoare's formula.[16] Any temperature-based method for calculating the time since death needs a distinct value of this constant. If the rectal temperature at death is unknown, as is usual in casework at the scene, it is necessary to use a fixed value. As the central body temperature has a circadian rhythm, a detailed discussion about the 'true' value of *To*, which should be used as the fixed value in the formula, is meaningless – the more so as physiological mechanisms can change the central temperature, e.g. the menstrual cycle or strong physical activity shortly before death. We used the same fixed value (37.2°C) as used by Marshall and Hoare.[16]

In giving evidence at court, one can extrapolate the rectal temperature to limiting values of the physiological range of rectal temperature (36.5 to 37.5°C), instead of using the fixed value. Actually, this would be an unimportant part of the overall range of uncertain factors (mean ambient temperature, corrective factor of the body weight, approximation of the constants *B* and *A*) in calculating the time since death in any particular case. In addition, the overall limits of error resulting from many investigated body coolings include the partial errors due to the physiological range of rectal temperature. One of the most discussed sources of error in calculating the time since death by extrapolating the body temperature is 'fever at death'. Equation 3.1 is open for electing a greater value than 37.2°C if there is actual information concerning a fever of the decedent (this usually comes from the physician, other witnesses and/or as a result of autopsy) (examples in Fig. 3.25). Nevertheless, this is an exception to the rule.

On the other hand, an unrecognized rise of temperature antemortem during agony may be present in certain cases (especially in intracranial injuries, certain poisonings, febrile illness without any pathomorphological findings, struggle or physical work shortly before death). What errors can be expected in cases of unrecognizable fever? The error due to fever is greatest during the first hours postmortem, and decreases with time. Because of the higher gradient between the rectal

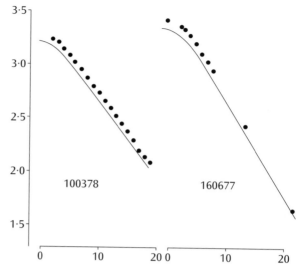

Figure 3.25 *Real cooling curves and model curves according to eqn 3.2 with stated 37.2°C as 'To' of two bodies with fever at death.[28] Abscissa: time of death in hours; ordinate: ln (rectal – ambient temperature). Case 100378: measured temperature 37.8°C 2 hours postmortem and 37.0°C 3 hours postmortem, respectively. Result of autopsy: acute tuberculosis of the lungs with pneumonia and pleuritis. Case 160677: chronic leukaemia with final blast crisis. Last measured temperature 4 hours before death occurred was 39.6°C.*

and the ambient temperature, the drop of the rectal temperature is at first steeper than the stated value of 37.2°C at death (Fig. 3.26; Table 3.11). As long as the measured rectal temperature is 37.2°C or above, the decedent is 'still alive' according to the formula's value

Table 3.11 *Errors caused by fever or slight hypothermia at death. Errors of computed death-times (eqn 3.1) using 37.2°C as the value for To if the temperature at death is really 40.2 and 34.2°C, respectively. Example of a 70 kg body in 15°C ambient temperature (see Fig. 3.28)*

Measured rectal temperature (°C)	Stated 37.2°C at death	Really 40.2°C at death		Really 34.2°C at death	
	Time of death	Calculated	Error	Calculated	Error
37.2	0.0	4.6	−4.6	—	—
37.1	0.8	4.8	−4.0	—	—
34.2	5.0	7.6	−2.6	0.0	5.0
34.0	5.4	7.8	−2.4	1.2	4.2
28.0	12.2	14.4	−2.2	9.8	2.4
22.0	22.4	24.4	−2.0	20.0	2.4

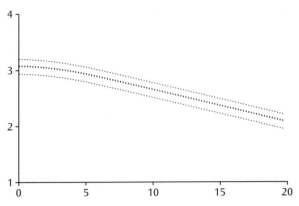

Figure 3.26 *Errors caused by fever or slight hypothermia at death. Model cooling curves of a 70 kg body (B = −0.0617) in 15°C ambient temperature starting at 40.2°C (upper curve), 37.2°C (middle curve) and 34.2°C (lower curve), respectively. The errors of computed death-times according to eqn 3.2 using 37.2°C as the value for To are to be seen in Table 3.11.*

of 37.2°C. When the rectal temperature falls to 37.1°C, the real possibility of an error due to a fever exists. In the example of Table 3.11, the death-time is 0.8 hours in a case of 37.2°C at death. In a case with a real starting point of 40.2°C, the death-time would be 4.8 hours and, in using eqn 3.1 with the stated starting point of 37.2°C, an error of −4 hours would result. This is the maximum error in this case. However, this error should be recognized by rigor mortis, hypostasis and the reduced mechanical and electrical excitability after a real time since death of about 5 hours (see Chapter 7).

Later on, when the rectal temperature decreases further, the error due to a fever diminishes to a level of about 2.5 to 2 hours (Table 3.11).

More serious, in relation to large errors of calculated time since death, is a fall of rectal temperature during the period between fatal injury and death (or general hypothermia). This is because an antemortal decrease of rectal temperature can become greater than any increase due to fever. As long as the antemortal decrease of rectal temperature is of the same order, but with changed sign, the over-estimation of the calculated death-time is also of the same order (see Table 3.11 and Fig. 3.26). Nevertheless, if there is any suspicion of general hypothermia, any temperature method of calculating the time since death must not be used. Hypothermia should be suspected if a long agonal period existed under ambient conditions conducive to hypothermia. In the very early postmortem interval of the first 10 hours, a threatened error can be avoided by applying other tests of death-time estimation (especially the examination of mechanical and electrical excitability of skeletal muscle), which gives results inconsistent with the low rectal temperature in cases of hypothermia (see Chapter 7).

ACCURACY OF CALCULATED TIME SINCE DEATH

When plotting the errors in calculated death-time against the postmortem time-scale, there was first a decrease in error, which reached a minimum about 16 to 22 hours postmortem in a series of 28 bodies between 31 and 112 kg body weight.[31] This phenomenon is mainly due to the use of a fixed (but actually unknown) value of rectal temperature at death To of 37.2°C, which provides larger errors in the early cooling phase than later on, as discussed above (Table 3.11). A second reason was the usually unknown cooling conditions between death and the beginning of examination, before the body had been transported to mortuary. This was called 'preanalytic error'.[13]

After the minimum phase of error there is a continuous increase in error, because the mean value of the constants A (1.25) and B (eqns 3.2 and 3.5, respectively), as well as the low accuracy of temperature measurements, become progressively more disturbing as the temperature difference between body and ambient temperature decreases. In addition, even small changes of ambient temperature, as well as of any other cooling condition, cause larger errors, as the difference between body and ambient becomes lower.

Plotting the errors against the progress of death-time is not a good way of obtaining information about errors because of the great variation in the time taken to reach the ambient temperature, which is dependent on the body weight (Table 3.12). The body of a baby reaches the ambient temperature corresponding to increased errors in a much shorter time than the obese body of an adult, where the larger errors develop much later.

In summarizing cases of different body weights, the errors of computed death-time should not be plotted against the progress of death-time, but against the progress of cooling – which is the real

Table 3.12 *Death-time at defined levels of the standardized temperature 'Q' dependent on the body weight*

Level of Q	Body weight (kg)				
	30	50	70	90	100
0.5	7	11	15	19	23
0.3	12	17	23	29	36
0.2	15	22	30	38	46

cause of the increase in errors. A good measure of the progress of cooling is the standardized temperature Q (see Fig. 3.10 and eqn 3.1). Its value is 1 at death, and 0 when the rectal temperature has reached the ambient temperature. So, a value of 0.5 means that the original difference between the rectal and the ambient temperature at death has been reduced to 50%. Dependent on the body weight, a defined value of Q corresponds to different times of death (Table 3.12). Relating the errors of calculated time since death to the standardized temperature, Q, the values from bodies of very different weights become comparable. In our own experiments under controlled conditions in ambient temperatures between 5 and 22°C, the computed time of death, according to eqns 3.1 and 3.2 (see eqn 3.14), had errors which could be classified into three groups (Figs 3.27 and 3.28; Table 3.13). These corresponded to values of Q between 1 and 0.5 – the permissible variation of 95% is ± 2.8 hours. For more progressive cooling, corresponding to values of Q between 0.5 and 0.3, the permissible variation of 95% is ± 3.2 hours. For values of Q between 0.3 and 0.2, the permissible variation of 95% is ± 4.5 hours.[33] Below a Q-value of 0.2, we obtained very large errors in some cases. Therefore, and in compliance with Fiddes and Patten,[25] the reliability of computing the time since death cannot be assessed.

Computing the time since death of De Saram's[24] cooling curves in ambient temperatures between 26 and 31°C according to eqn 3.15, the standard deviation was ± 1 hour,[25] which corresponded to the permissible variation of 95% of about ± 2 hours. Nevertheless, we recommend the use of the given permissible variation of 95% of our own experimental cooling curves in lower ambient temperatures, because the computation of death-time ended at 8 hours postmortem in De Saram's material.

In computing the time since death of the experimental body cooling under various cooling condi-

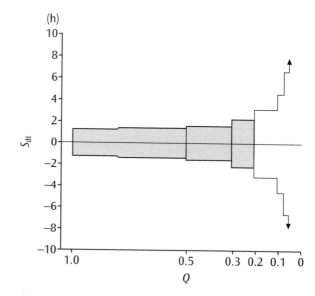

Figure 3.27 *Standard deviation* s_{dt} *of calculated death-time dependent on the progress of cooling Q. Chosen standard conditions of cooling. Fifty-three bodies were used; body weights 9–112 kg; age 1–87 years; ambient temperature 5.8–22°C; start of temperature measurement 0.8–6 hours postmortem to end 10–75 hours postmortem. The majority of bodies were cases of a sudden unexpected death, all of them with time of death known to within some minutes. Calculation of the death-time according to eqns 3.1 and 3.2.*[33,46]

tions, and the resulting error statistics (Table 3.14), we assumed a variation in the corrective factor of ± 0.1 around the real one. If the investigated corrective factor was, for example, 1.4 in a case, we also supplied 1.3 and 1.5. This was done in casework where the selection of a corrective factor is really somewhat uncertain. Dependent on the progress of cooling Q, we obtained the listed permissible variations (Table 3.14; Figs 3.29 and 3.30).[32]

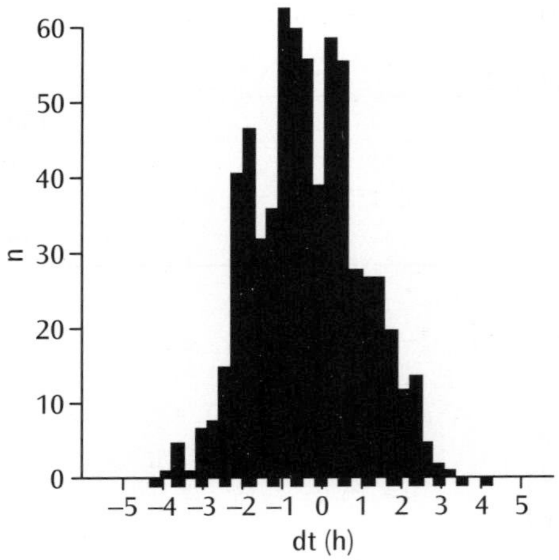

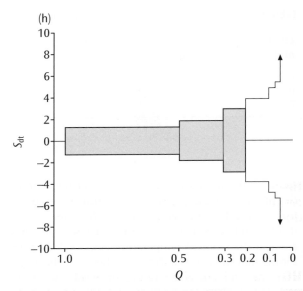

Figure 3.28 *Histogram of the errors of calculated death-time for 1 > Q > 0.5 in addition to Fig. 3.27. Standard conditions of cooling.*[33,46]

Figure 3.29 *Standard deviation S_{dt} of calculated death-time dependent on the progress of cooling Q. Various cooling conditions differing from the chosen standard. Twenty-six bodies were used. Calculation of the death-time was according to eqns 3.2 and 3.6. For further details see Fig. 3.30.*[33,46]

Table 3.13 *Standard deviation of 'calculated – real death-time' dependent on the progress of cooling Q of 53 bodies under chosen standard conditions of cooling. In comparison to the calculation of death-time according to the two exponential formulae, the figures are also given for calculation of the death-time according to the rule of thumb '1°C decrease of rectal temperature per hour plus 3 hours'*[33]

Q range	n	Calculation according to:	
		Eqns 3.1 and 3.2	Rule of thumb
1.0 > Q > 0.90	117	1.3	1.4
0.9 > Q > 0.80	126	1.3	2.0
0.8 > Q > 0.70	142	1.4	2.5
0.7 > Q > 0.60	140	1.4	3.2
0.6 > Q > 0.50	155	1.4	4.0
0.5 > Q > 0.40	181	1.6	5.1
0.4 > Q > 0.30	208	1.6	6.7
0.3 > Q > 0.20	208	2.2	10.8
0.2 > Q > 0.10	224	3.1	16.1
0.1 > Q > 0.07	67	4.5	18.1

Table 3.14 *Standard deviation of 'calculated – real death-time' dependent on the progress of cooling Q of 26 bodies under various cooling conditions (for the 'rule of thumb' see Table 3.13)*

Q range	n	Calculations according to:	
		Eqns 3.2 and 3.5	Rule of thumb
1.0 > Q > 0.5	464	1.3	3.9
0.5 > Q > 0.3	142	2.2	9.2
0.3 > Q > 0.2	42	3.4	18.3

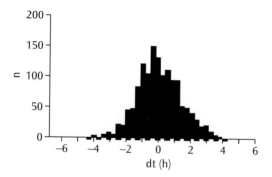

Figure 3.30 *Histogram of the errors of calculated death-time for 1 > Q > 0.5 in addition to Fig. 3.30. Various cooling conditions differing from the chosen standard.*[33,46]

HOW IS THE DEATH-TIME OBTAINED?

To apply all the basic considerations raised by mathematical modelling of the body cooling, and the experience of experimental body and dummy coolings to casework, a simple means is required for the quick calculation of the interval of death at the scene without any mental arithmetic.

The basis for calculating the time of death is eqn 3.1, which has the three constants To, B and A, and the two measures Tr (rectal temperature) and Ta (ambient temperature). As discussed above we defined:

- To as 37.2°C.
- B as $[-1.2815 \times$ (corrective factor $\times$ body weight$)^{-0.625} + 0.0284]$ (eqn 3.5).
- A for ambient temperatures up to 23°C as 1.25. Equation 3.1 can now be written as:

$$Q = \frac{Tr - Ta}{37.2 - Ta} = 1.25 \times \exp(B \times t) - 0.25 \exp(5 \times B \times t) \quad (3.14)$$

The cooling curves published by De Saram *et al.*[24] were obtained in ambient temperatures between 26 and 31°C, and could be better fitted by $A = 1.11$, giving:

$$Q = \frac{Tr - Ta}{37.2 - Ta} = 1.11 \times \exp(B \times t) - 0.11 \exp(10 \times B \times t) \quad (3.15)$$

Equations 3.14 and 3.15 cannot be solved to time t, and therefore an approximation is necessary. There are two ways to calculate the time since death at a scene of death, neither of which requires the use of any mental arithmetic:

1. By means of an available computer program.[42]

This acts as a dialogue and takes all rules treated in this chapter automatically into account.
2. By means of nomogram (Figs 3.31 and 3.32).[34,43]

For the first step (Fig. 3.33), the points of the scales of the measured rectal temperature (e.g. 27°C in the left margin) and ambient temperature (e.g. 15°C in the right margin) have been joined by a straight line, which crosses the diagonal of the nomogram at a specific point. For the second step, a second straight line must be drawn passing through the centre of the circle (below left of the nomogram) and the intersection of the first line and the diagonal (Fig. 3.34). The second line crosses the semicircles, which represent the different body weights, each with a calibration of the death time. The time since death (e.g. 13.5 hours postmortem) can be read off at the intersection of the semicircle of the given body weight (e.g. 70 kg). The body weight used can be the real (chosen standard conditions of cooling) or the corrected body weight (using corrective factors). The second straight line touches the outermost semicircle where the permissible variation of 95% can be seen respectively levelling off the range of reliability. In bodies found under standard conditions of cooling the figures 'standard (naked-still air)' are true (see Table 3.13). The figures 'using corrective factors' should be used when the body is found under cooling conditions differing from the chosen standard (see Table 3.14).

INVESTIGATION OF CENTRAL BRAIN TEMPERATURE

Before continuing with the practice of the rectal temperature probe site, the results of our investigation of central brain temperature are interpolated here for practical purposes only, whereas the theory of modelling the central brain temperature mathematically (see eqn. 3.1) is the same as described in connection with the rectal temperature (see eqn 3.1).

The central brain temperature was recorded in 53 bodies, stored at nearly constant ambient temperatures between 10 and 30°C in still air. The measurements were started on average 1.6 hours postmortem and continued for 8 to 50 hours. The diameters of the temperature probes were 0.5 and 1 mm. The probes were inserted via the upper part of the superior orbital fissure into the brain with a depth of half the sagittal diameter of the head. The computation of the time of death according to eqn 3.1 (Tr replaced by Tb = brain

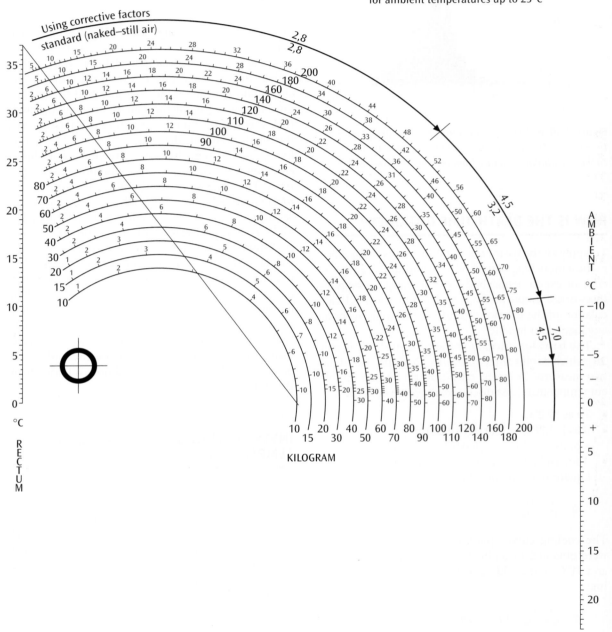

Figure 3.31 *Nomogram for reading off the time of death from a single measurement of rectal and ambient temperature and from the body weight for ambient temperatures up to 23°C according to eqn 3.14. Without any corrective factor the nomogram is related to the chosen standard conditions of cooling.*

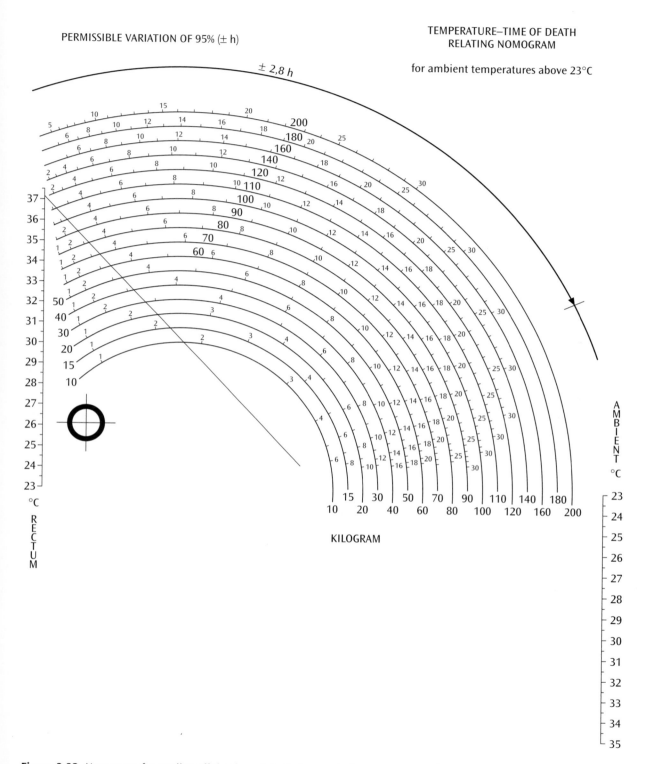

Figure 3.32 *Nomogram for reading off the time of death from a single measurement of rectal and ambient temperature and from the body weight for ambient temperatures above 23°C according to eqn 3.15. Without any corrective factor the nomogram is related to the chosen standard conditions of cooling.*

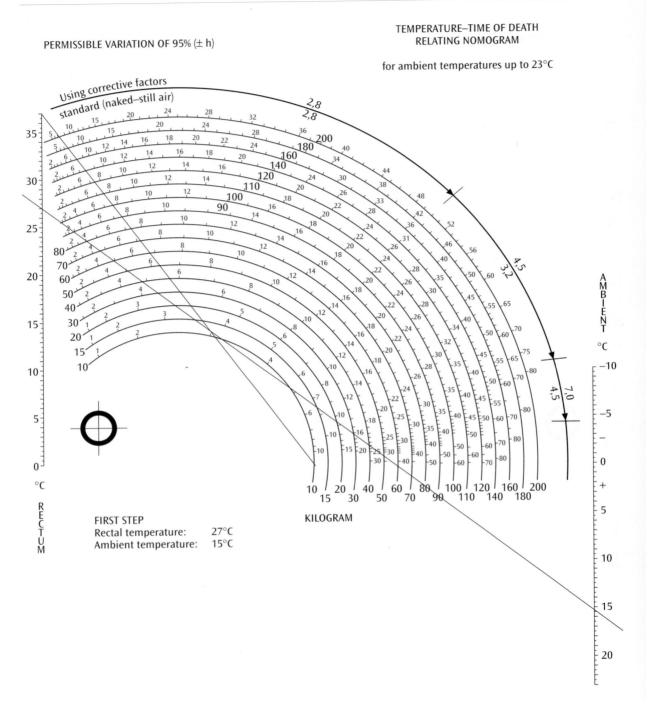

Figure 3.33 *The use of the nomograms. First step.*[46]

temperature) with average values for the starting temperature, T_o (37.2°C), and the constants B (−0.127) and A (1.135) provided margins of error for the 95% tolerance limits of ± 1.5 hours up to 6.5 hours post-

mortem, ± 2.5 hours between 6.5 and 10.5 hours postmortem, and ± 3.5 hours between 10.5 and 13.5 hours postmortem. Compared with the margins of error based on rectal body cooling (see Figs 3.27–3.30;

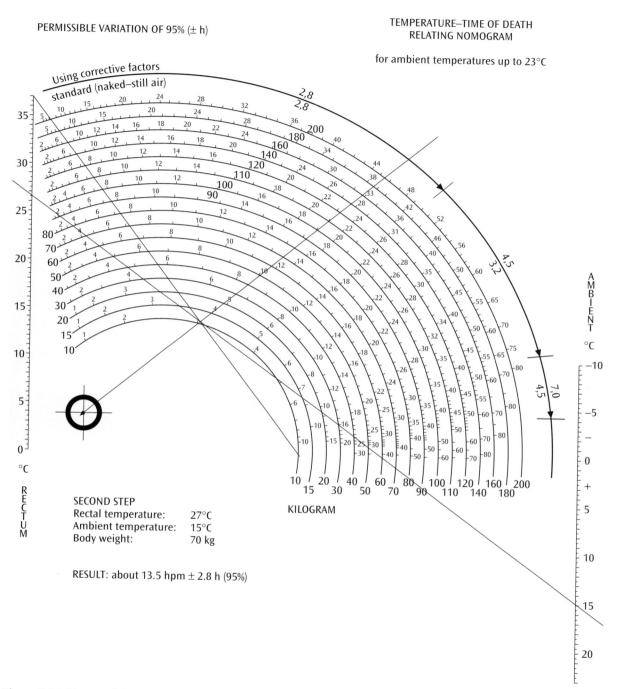

PERMISSIBLE VARIATION OF 95% (± h)

TEMPERATURE–TIME OF DEATH RELATING NOMOGRAM

for ambient temperatures up to 23°C

Using corrective factors standard (naked–still air)

SECOND STEP
Rectal temperature: 27°C
Ambient temperature: 15°C
Body weight: 70 kg

RESULT: about 13.5 hpm ± 2.8 h (95%)

Figure 3.34 *The use of the nomograms. Second step.*[46]

Tables 3.13 and 3.14), a more precise estimation of the time of death can be obtained up to 6.5 hours post-mortem only. For practical applications, a 'brain temperature–time of death nomogram' was constructed (Fig. 3.35). The nomogram is only related to 'standard conditions' of cooling (see page 79). Even uniformly moving air alters the time relations – the constant B changes from –0.127 to –0.158.[28] The cooling coefficient B was also influenced by the amount of hair. Nevertheless, taking this into account, the estimated

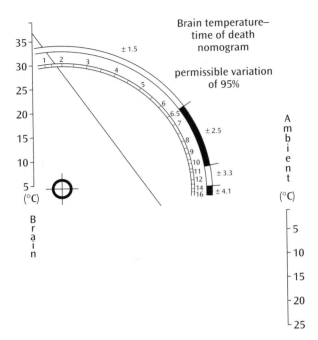

Figure 3.35 *Central brain temperature–time of death nomogram related to 'standard conditions' of cooling. For the first step the points of the scales of the measured brain temperature (in the left margin) and ambient temperature (in the right margin) have been connected by a straight line, which crosses the diagonal of the nomogram at a particular point. The second step is to draw a second straight line through the centre of the circle, below left of the nomogram, and the intersection of the first line and the diagonal. The latter touches the outermost semicircle where the permissible variation of 95% can be seen (see Figs. 3.33 and 3.34).*

the brain. The best method of obtaining a well-standardized probe site was found by Ratermann[14] to be as follows: the probe is placed on the palpebral conjunctive of the lower eyelid within the temporal part of the first medial third of the infraorbital margin at an angle of 50° to 60° to the nasal septum (Fig. 3.36). Using this technique, and using an insertion depth of half the sagittal diameter of the head, the temperature probe will be situated at the centre of the brain. The temperature differences between probes on both sides will be only minutely variable. In a study of 25 bodies using this procedure, the margin of error for the 95% tolerance limits of computed time of death was ± 1.3 hours to 6.5 hours postmortem.

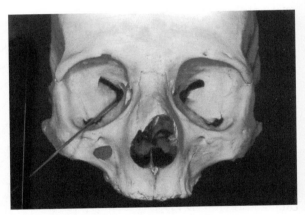

Figure 3.36 *Standardized method of inserting the temperature probe into the 'centre' of brain providing more instant positioning than other procedures of insertion.[14]*

COMBINED BRAIN AND RECTAL TEMPERATURES[10]

Estimating the time of death on the basis of simultaneous measurements of brain and rectal temperatures on 21 bodies cooling under standard conditions, the following margins of error for the 95% tolerance limits were obtained. Up to 6.5 hours postmortem, the most precise computation of time of death was achieved by the exclusive application of brain temperature, which gave a time of death within ± 1.5 hours. Between 6.5 and 10.5 hours postmortem, the brain–rectum combined computation of time of death balanced in the ratio of 6:4 (Fig. 3.37) was the most precise, at ± 2.4 hours. Beyond 10.5 hours postmortem, the most precise computation of time of death was achieved by exclusive application of rectal temperature, and gave a

time of death did not become significantly more accurate. Other influencing factors have not yet been fully investigated. The often-expressed opinion that the cooling curve of the brain would be less affected by factors that could affect the cooling of other temperature probe sites[11,44] cannot be confirmed, either physically or empirically. Nevertheless, they may be correct, as the head is less often clothed or covered than the trunk.

Inserting temperature probes on both sides via the upper part of the superior orbital fissure, the measured brain temperatures differed by up to 1.5°C, corresponding to a difference of computed death times up to 1 hour. This result required further studies into the optimal way to insert the probes into the centre of

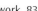

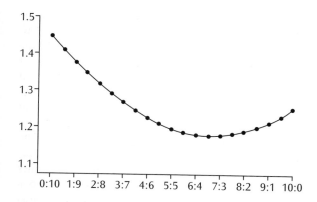

Figure 3.37 *Relationship between standard deviation of errors of the computed time of death (ordinate) and the ratio of the balance of brain to rectal temperatures (abscissa) in combined computation of the time of death during the interval from 6.5 to 10.5 hours postmortem corresponding to the standardized temperature 'Q' (eqn 3.1) of the brain.* [8]

time of death within ± 3.2 hours. These data agree well with those of a series of 53 bodies,[13] which was based on the brain temperature only, as well as of the series which was based on the rectal temperature only.

Integrating eqn 3.1 applied to brain temperature and then again to rectal temperature, to an equation common to both by dividing them into each other, eliminates the starting temperature, To:

$$\frac{Tb - Ta}{Tr - Ta} = \frac{1.135 \exp(-0.127 \times t) - 0.135 \exp(-1.0677 \times t)}{1.25 \exp(B \times t) - 0.25(5 \times B \times t)} \quad (3.16)$$

where Tb = brain temperature; Tr = rectal temperature; Ta = ambient temperature; B = constant; and t = time of death (hours) (see eqns 3.1, 3.2, 3.14 and 3.15).

This procedure may avoid major errors, for example in cases involving fever in the occurrence of death, as in two cases in the above-mentioned series. The rectal temperature, first measured 2 hours postmortem, was in both cases 38°C. The fever-induced errors of computed death times in the later period when the rectal temperature had fallen below 37°C was reduced from about 3 hours (underestimation) to about 1 hour and virtually 0 hours, respectively.

APPLICATION OF THE 'NOMOGRAM METHOD' IN CASEWORK

The estimation of the time since death at the scene of death using the nomogram-form (Figs 3.31–3.34) or computation by means of a computer program[42] requires:

1. Single measurement of the 'deep' rectal temperature (see page 79).
2. Estimation of the body weight.
3. Evaluation of the mean ambient temperature.
4. Evaluation of the corrective factor, if necessary.
5. Consideration of the features where the method must not be used.
6. Calculation of the interval of death.

The nomogram-form itself (or eqns 3.14 and 3.15) are the result of the experimental body coolings under chosen standard conditions of cooling reported above.

The chosen standard conditions of cooling are defined as follows:

- Naked body with dry surfaces.
- Lying extended on the back.
- On a thermally indifferent base.
- In still air.
- In surroundings without any source of strong heat radiation.

If a body is found under conditions similar to or comparable with the chosen standard conditions of cooling, the time of death can be read off according to the measured deep rectal temperature, the mean ambient temperature, and the body weight. Provided it is made as exactly as possible, the time of death read from the nomogram closely approaches the computed time. The given permissible variation of 95% at the outermost semicircle 'standard (naked–still air)' corresponds to the data of Table 3.13 and Figs 3.27 and 3.28.

If the cooling conditions differ from the chosen standard they have to be taken into account by evaluating a corrective factor. The real body weight must be multiplied by the evaluated corrective factor. The time of death has to be read from the nomogram at the semicircle of the corrected body weight. The permissible variation of 95% at the outermost semicircle 'using corrective factors' is then valid corresponding to Table 3.14 and Figs 3.29 and 3.30. By analogy, B must be calculated by eqn 3.5 when computing the time of death.

The successful use of the nomogram method requires experience, as with any medicolegal procedure. It is very easy to read off the time since death from the nomogram, or to compute it. However, especially after computing the time of death without adding the permissible variation of 95%, this gives the impression of high accuracy, which leads to the danger of misuse and misinterpretation.

First, the estimation of the time since death by any method of examination of the body is really the task of a forensic pathologist.

Second, the indicated value read from the nomogram or the computed time of death, is a mean value – a misleading part of the full result. *The interval limited by the permissible variation of 95% is the one and only result: the death occurred, with the probability of 95%, within this interval. A more precise indication of the interval since death cannot be obtained according to all the results of scientific investigations. A central mean value must not be offered.*

Third, when using the nomogram method, the interval of death that is obtained is calculated via factors which are themselves either measures or evaluations. It is possible to use the right rules, but get the wrong results if the factors are wrong. The most important thing is to analyse these factors carefully at the scene of crime.

The estimation of the body weight at the scene of death is rather a question of personal experience. A serious mistake could be remedied quickly by weighing the body after its removal from the scene.

In the following, evaluation of the 'mean ambient temperature' and of the 'corrective factor', as well as consideration of the features where the method must not be used, will be discussed in more detail.

To enable handling of the method, it will be referenced to special cases of a field study which are listed in Tables 3.15 and 3.18. The field study[45] includes 72 consecutive cases of an inspection of the scene of crime by a forensic pathologist before autopsies were carried out. The period of death was estimated by using the nomogram as a primary method (Table 3.15), followed by the use of other non-temperature-based methods to confirm or improve the primary result (see Chapter 7).

Evaluation of the mean ambient temperature

Theoretically, eqns 3.1, 3.14 and 3.15 require a constant ambient temperature. In fact, the mean ambient temperature of the whole period between the time of death and the time of investigation is employed.[28,46] The actual measured ambient temperature at a scene of crime need not necessarily be the mean. At first, the actual ambient temperature should be measured close

to the body, and particularly at the same level above the base. It is recommended that not only the air temperature be measured but also the temperature of the underlying surface itself – if possible probing into the earth, into gaps between stones or beneath a carpet. If there are differences between ambient temperatures around the body, take the mean or use the range (Figs 3.38 and 3.40).

Furthermore, it is advisable to measure the temperature of the wider surroundings of the body, for example in the next room, the corridor and the landing respectively, to obtain a view of temperature distribution (e.g. case 26 in Table 3.15). Some additional observation is necessary: in a closed room, look for the heating system and note its operating state (e.g. case 13 in Table 3.15). Were the windows and doors open or closed when the body was found? What about the outside temperature or sunshine through windows, and its possible influence on the room temperature? (e.g. cases 44, 54 and 56 in Table 3.15). The course of the ambient temperature from night (time of death) to day (finding the body) should be taken into account for evaluation of the mean ambient temperature of the period in question (e.g. cases 27, 42, 49 and 56 in Table 3.15). If the body is found outside, contact the weather station, asking for hourly temperatures and periods of rain, wind and sunshine (e.g. cases 11 and 42 in Table 3.15). Later, for example in court, this can be an advantage if the ambient temperature comes into question. Then consider the mean ambient temperature during the interval between death and the examination of body. The actual measured ambient temperature(s) and the concomitant temperature-related circumstances allow an evaluation of the required mean ambient temperature of the period in question, at least as a range in most cases (Fig. 3.38).

If ambient temperature *decreases* more or less continuously, its mean value for the period in question can be used successfully. A continuous *increase* of the ambient temperature is more problematic if a long death-time comes into question (see below). The difference between rectal and ambient temperature should then be considered. If there is only a small difference, the method should not be used. The progression of cooling can be estimated quickly by calculation of the value of Q (eqns 3.1, 3.14 or 3.15). On the other hand, the calculated mean of the ambient temperature can be used if the progression of cooling is still low ($Q > 0.5$).

When a range of ambient temperature is applied, two death-times are read from the nomogram – a

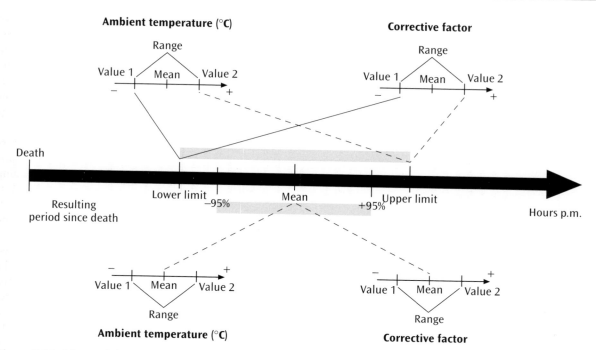

Figure 3.38 *Scheme of the resulting periods since death using: (mode 1) mean values of the elevated ranges of ambient temperature and corrective factor and adding the empirical permissible variation of 95% (Tables 3.13 and 3.14); and (mode 2) the upper and lower brackets of the evaluated ranges of ambient temperature and corrective factor. If the evaluated ranges of both ambient temperature and corrective factor are very wide, the resulting period since death using mode 2 calculation may be greater than that using mode 1 calculation. It is recommended that both modes of calculation be applied and to use the wider period since death for expert opinion.*

shorter time corresponding to the lower ambient temperature, and a longer time corresponding to the higher ambient temperature (Figs 3.38 and 3.40).

A peculiarity is a sudden great change in ambient temperature. Two murder cases in which the bodies had been transported from high ambient temperatures (scene of crime) to low ambient temperature (place of finding the body) were the reason for cooling experiments with a sudden decrease and increase of ambient temperature in the order of 15°C in the course of the cooling process.[47] The experiments were performed with the aforementioned cooling dummies. In the case of a sudden *decrease* in ambient temperature, after cooling in a higher ambient temperature (about 21°C) for several hours to about 4°C, a second 'temperature plateau' occurred which was shorter than the known plateau at the beginning of body cooling. The second plateau at the beginning of the second cooling phase in a sudden decreased ambient temperature required a lower value of the

constant *A* (1.15) compared with the known value (1.25) at the beginning of cooling. The period since death could be computed if the body was transported at a known time from a known high level of ambient temperature to a low ambient temperature by means of the following three-step procedure (Fig. 3.39).

STEP 1

Going from the dummy temperature (T_{r1}) at any time of the second cooling phase (t_1) in low ambient temperature (T_{a2}), the body temperature (T_{r2}) at the known time (t_2) of rapid decrease of the ambient temperature can be calculated by transforming eqn 3.15 using a value of 1.15 for the constant *A*:

$$T_{r2} = \frac{T_{r1} - T_{a2}}{Q} + T_{a2} \qquad (3.17)$$

with

Table 3.15 *Data of instructive cases of a field study*[45]

Case number	Cooling conditions	Correction factor Mean	Range	Real body weight (kg)	Ambient temperature (°C) Measured	Used	Rectal temp. (°C)	Time estimated lower limit (hpm)	upper limit (hpm)	Time ascertained lower limit (hpm)	upper limit (hpm)	Comment
11	Outside, LB on asphalt, trousers, pants, short panty, moving air*	1.1	1.0–1.2	60	16.0/16.3	14.0*/16.3	22.1	16.7	25.7	?	?	*According to local weather station for the period in question; +Stop of destroyed wrist-watch
13	Room, floor, LB, open trousers, short panty	1.1	1.0–1.2	98	19.8/19.8	16.0*/18.0	33.2	07.2	12.8	08.3	+08.3	*Reconstruction of the room temperature by night one day later with automatically turned off central heating system. The body was found in the morning.
15	Street, LL, wet-through track suit-trousers, short panty, rain, moving air	0.7	0.6–0.8	76	12.8/12.8	11.8/13.8	35.0	00.3	05.9	04.3	04.5	
22	Outside, soil, LP, wet-through work trousers, short panty, wind, rain	0.7	0.6–0.8	93	09.9/09.9	08.9/10.9	36.2	00.0	04.9	02.7	2.9	
25	Room, floor, LB, pyjamas, briefs temporarily moving air	1.0	0.9–1.1	56	15.7/17.2	15.7/17.2	25.4	10.7	17.1	12.9	13.0	
26	Concrete staircase ground floor, LB, jeans, short panty	1.0	0.9–1.1	82	07.3/11.1[2]	04.2[1]/11.1	30.2	06.3	11.9	07.4	07.4	[1]Ground floor near the body; [2]Staircase 2nd floor; [3]Outside, open front door
27	Metal road, LL, jeans pulled down to knee-joints, moving air	0.7	0.5–0.9	68	14.2/14.2	07.0*/14.2	30.6	02.8	08.4	01.5	06.3	*Lowest temperature at night before finding in the morning
31	Outside, soil, LL, rests of carbonized # clothing, wet body surface, moving air	0.7	0.6–0.8	57	06.2*/10.3[+]	06.2/10.3	33.3	00.3	05.9	03.8	04.3	*Some minutes after inflammation of the person extinguishing began, first with dry fire-fighting equipment, subsequently with water. #soil; +air. Estimation of the period since death by non-temperature-based methods only; see Table 3.7
	2nd measurement 1 hour later:						31.2	01.4	07.0 method not used	04.8	05.3	
33	LB on bed covered with thick blanket, trousers, boxing shorts, short panty	2.2	2.0–2.4	62	18.5/18.5		41.6	(04.7	10.3) not used inexpertise	00.5	25.5	+On the supposition of malignant hyperthermia with temperature at death of 43.5°C: Subtraction of 6.3°C from the measured rectal and ambient temperatures as the difference between the supposed rectal temperature at death (43.5) and the 37.2°C-norm of the formula (nomogram).
						12.1[+]	35.3[+]					
42	Room of attic flat, floor, open skylight*, jeans, short panty	1.1	1.0–1.2	57	22.5/22.5	12.8*/22.5	24.8	12.6	33.0	15.4	16.2	*Mean temperature at night outside: 12.8°C (weather station). Examination at noon (summer-time).
43	Room, floor, LL, naked, temporarily moving air*	0.9	0.75–1.0	67	19.0/21.0	18.0/22.0	34.5	02.1	07.7	02.7	?	*Open windows
44	Room, floor, carpet, LB, trousers, short panty, moving air*	1.0	0.9–1.1	71.5	15.4/21.3[2]	15.4/21.3	35.5	01.1	06.7	03.6	04.3	*Open windows and doors; [1]At time of examination beside body; [2]Within cupboards, beneath carpets near the body
45	Situation at finding: outside, head-stand-like position within a big bale of straw, jeans, short panty / 4 hours before examination: Outside soil, LB, jeans, short panty, temporarily moving air	1.8? / 1.0	1.5–2.0? / 0.9–1.1	83	18.6[1] / 11.5[2] / 12.2[3] / 16.0–18.0[4]		32.8	Method not used: no experience as to particular cooling condition		04.5	07.5	[1]Within straw; [2]Air at examination; [3]Soil at examination; [4]Air for the period in question (weather station). Estimation of the time since death by non-temperature-based methods only; see Table 3.7

No.	Description											Notes
48	Room, LL on sofa with his back in contact with the back-rest of sofa, blanket between tights, short panty	1.2	1.1–1.3	78	27.3/27.3	25.0*/27.3	33.3	08.8	14.4	11.0	14.0	*According to crime police at coming to the scene 2 hours before examination
49	Outside, soil, LB, jeans, trousers, leggings, panty, moving air	1.35	1.3–1.4	45.5	16.6[1]/20.3[2]	13.0/20.3	25.4	11.2	21.6	16.3	16.8	[1]Soil [2]Air [3]Mean temperature at night before finding the body at the early afternoon
54	Room, LL on couch, tracksuit, short panty, moving air*	1.05	0.9–1.2	77	21.5/21.5	17.0[+]/20.0[+]	29.8	10.5	16.4	04.8	13.8	*Open window. [+]The open window of the very small room was closed by investigators 1 hour before examination. At this time the room temperature was 18.5°C measured by crime police
55	Street, LL on asphalt, jeans, short panty, moving air	0.9	0.8–1.0	80	05.5/07.2[+]	05.5/07.2	33.2	02.2	07.8	03.8	05.2	*Asphalt [+]Air
56	Room, LL on bed, trousers, short panty, moving air*	1.05	0.9–1.2	78	15.7/16.2	10.0[+]/16.2	26.9	11.2	19.1	04.7	20.7	*The window was open at finding the body 4.5 hours before examination. Then it was closed. It was opened again for 30 minutes a short time before examination and was closed again [+]The temperature outside at night before examination at noon was around 0°C
64	Outside LP* on lawn, jeans, short panty, temporarily moving air	1.0	0.9–1.1	98	10.3/11.0	10.3/11.0	33.8	03.9	09.5	06.3	06.6	*Finding LP, changing in LB by first-aid doctor
62	LB on bed, naked	1.15	1.0–1.2	60	18.0/20.5	18.0/20.5	27.5	10.9	17.3	13.2	19.7	
66	Room, LB on bed, covered with eiderdown until 2.5 hours before examination, boxer shorts	1.8	1.6–2.0#	116	26.9*/26.9*	26.4/27.4	33.0	24.1	34.2	24.8	?	*Temperature at any place in the near and wider surrounding of bodies #Because of strong insulation condition and high body weight adaptation to 1.4 to 1.7 according to [1]
72	Behind open entrance-door of shop, floor, LL, trousers, short panty, temporarily moving air	1.0	0.9–1.1	82	17.1/17.5	17.1/17.5	33.9	03.9	09.5	05.1	05.4	

LB = lying back; LP = lying prone; LL = lying lateral.

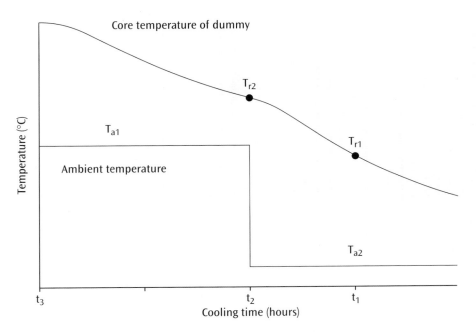

Figure 3.39 *The scheme for the three-step procedure.*

$$Q = 1.15 \times \exp[B \times (t_1 - t_2)] - 0.15 \times \exp[\frac{1.15 \times B}{0.15} \times (t_1 - t_2)] \quad (3.18)$$

STEP 2

Using the calculated body temperature (T_{r2}) at the known moment of moving the body according to eqns 3.17 and 3.18, the unknown period ($t_2 - t_3$) of the first cooling phase in the known higher ambient temperature (T_{a1}) can be calculated by the standard method, either nomographically or by computing as usual according to eqn 3.15.

STEP 3

The whole cooling period (tw) analogous to the period since death results from the addition of times of both cooling phases:

$$t_1 - t_3 = (t_1 - t_2) + (t_2 - t_3) \quad (3.19)$$

The errors of the calculated cooling times were within the known confidence limits of the method. The estimated period of death calculated by the three-step procedure was in agreement with the investigated period in the murder cases. One experimental on-line cooling curve of a body cooling for the first 10 hours at an ambient temperature of 22.5°C, and for the next 9 hours at 7.8°C, could also be sufficiently modelled by the three-step procedure.

On the other hand, the cooling curves of experiments with a sudden *increase* of the ambient temperature from 4°C to 21°C could not be modelled mathematically by the two-exponential model. Heat flows in opposite directions are likely to account for this result. The cooled superficial layers will be re-heated from outside and, at the same time, will be further cooled by the lower temperature of the deeper layers. This means that the nomogram method cannot be used in casework if a body is cooled first for a longer period in low ambient temperature and, thereafter, for a longer period in a significantly higher ambient temperature.

Evaluating the corrective factor

The experience of all the experimental body and dummy cooling reported above is shown in Table 3.16. The listed corrective factors are valid for typical situations whenever a body is found in a roughly extended position, or sitting.

The corrective factor for cooling conditions which differ from the standard conditions should be evaluated under three aspects:

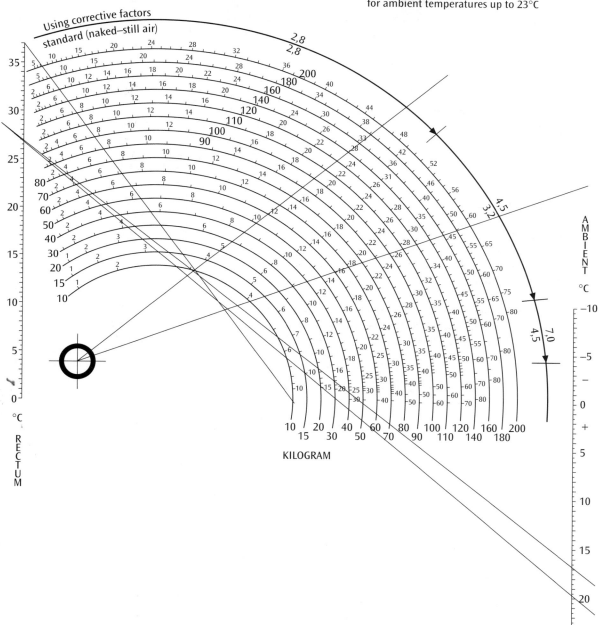

Using corrective factors
standard (naked–still air)

AMBIENT °C

°C
RECTUM

KILOGRAM

Figure 3.40 *The use of the nomogram in a case with ranges of the ambient temperature (17 to 20°C) and the corrective factor (1.2 to 1.5) of a real body weight of 75 kg corresponding to corrected body weights between 90 and 110 kg.*[46]

Table 3.16 *Empirical corrective factors of the body weight for cooling conditions differing from the chosen standard.*[46] *The listed values apply to bodies of average weight (reference: 70 kg), in an extended position on a 'thermally indifferent' base*

Dry clothing/covering	Air	Corrective factor	Wet-through clothing/covering wet body surface	In air	In water
		0.35	Naked		Flowing
		0.5	Naked		Still
		0.7	Naked	Moving	
		0.7	1–2 thin layers	Moving	
Naked	Moving	0.75			
1–2 thin layers	Moving	0.9	2 or more thicker	Moving	
Naked	Still	1.0			
1–2 thin layers	Still	1.1	2 thicker layers	Still	
2–3 thin layers		1.2	More than 2 thicker layers	Still	
1–2 thicker layers	Moving	1.2			
3–4 thin layers	or	1.3			
More thin/thicker layers	Still	1.4			
	Without influence	...			
Thick blanket		1.8			
+		...			
Clothing combined		2.4			
		2.8			

Thermically indifferent bases are e.g.: usual floor of rooms, dry soil, lawn, asphalt.

In comparison, bases which look more thermally insulating or heat-conducting should be taken into account additionally: Excessively thickly upholstered bases require a corrective factor *of 1.3* for naked bodies. In cases of clothed bodies the corrective factor should be increased *by 0.1 units* (thickly clothed) *to 0.3 units* (very thinly clothed). Insulating but not excessively thickly upholstered substrates like e.g. mattress (bed) or thick carpet require a corrective factor of *1.1 to 1.2* for naked bodies. In cases of clothed bodies the corrective factor should be increased *by 0.1 unit*. Bases which accelerate the cooling, e.g. concrete, stony or tiled bases on ground require a corrective factor *up to 0.75* for naked bodies. In cases of clothed bodies the corrective factor should be reduced by 0.1 unit (thicker clothes) respectively by *0.2 units* (very thin clothes).

1. Clothing/covering of the lower trunk, dry (left-hand side) or 'wet-through' (right-hand side).
2. Resting or moving air.
3. Type of supporting base (accelerating or decelerating) compared with 'indifferent'.

Should the occasion arise, it is useful to re-examine the experimental background which provided the corrective factors listed in Table 3.16:

1. With the exclusively radial transfer of heat from the body to surroundings (as well as the probe site within the rectum) in mind, only the clothing or covering and other special cooling conditions (the ground, wetness, wind) of the lower trunk are relevant for evaluating the corrective factor.
2. The corrective factors listed in Table 3.16 were investigated experimentally on bodies lying on a simple covered stretcher, which was declared to be a 'thermally indifferent' base. Different grounds such as floor, asphalt and dry lawn (e.g. cases 11, 55 and 64 in Table 3.15); dummy experiments have shown that insulating bases may require corrective factors up to 1.3, and excessively heat-conducting bases to 0.5 in naked bodies (see Table 3.10). Therefore, the base on which the body lies should be checked for both its thermal conductivity and its heat capacity. For example, a thin sheet-metal has a high conductivity but a low heat capacity, and so will not markedly accelerate body cooling. In contrast, the concrete floor of a cellar has both a higher conductivity and capacity. The cooling of a naked body will be accelerated according to a corrective factor of 0.75. The effect of the type of base on clothed bodies seems to be diminished more (thicker clothes) or less (thin clothes). Instructive examples in Table 3.15 are cases 15, 26, 28 and 46 for accelerating bases; and cases 47, 48, 62 and 70 for insulating bases.

3. The position of the body, i.e. whether it is extended or crouched, will influence the cooling. Exact data are not yet known.

4. The influence of even slow but permanently moving air on body cooling is significant as long as the body is naked, is only thinly clothed (covered) or if the surface of the naked or clothed (covered) body is wet-through. Therefore, attention should be paid to even slightly moving air (e.g. cases 25, 43 and 72 in Table 3.15).

5. The corrective factors listed in Table 3.16 were investigated on bodies of average body weight. Systematic investigations of the cooling of different-sized dummies under various conditions resulted in a clear dependency of the corrective factors on the body weight in cases of a low or high body weight and, at the same time, higher thermic insulation conditions.[1] Higher body weights need lower factors and, vice versa, lower body weights need higher factors, as listed in Table 3.16. Insulation conditions which require a corrective factor up to 1.3 according to the experience on bodies of medium body weights (Table 3.16) – reference 70 kg – can be used independently of the real body weight. Table 3.17 should be used whenever a special case requires a corrective factor of 1.4 or above, according to Table 3.16, and the body weight exceeds 80 kg or falls under 60 kg at the same time. In such a case, evaluation of the corrective factor should be made, in the first instance, relative to the actual cooling conditions by experience from average body weights (e.g. Table 3.16). The corrective factor chosen in the first instance must be applied to the real high or low body weight either by Table 3.17 or by eqn 3.10. Using eqn 3.10 removes the need for interpolation. The above-mentioned computer program[42] automatically takes into account this adaptation whenever the body weight and the corrective factor according to Table 3.16 requires that. Examples can be seen in Table 3.15 (cases 6 and 66) and Table 3.18 (case 37).

6. As in many cases involving cooling conditions significantly different from standard conditions, the initial commitment to an exact corrective factor is impossible, and it is advisable to choose a range for the corrective factor (Figs 3.38 and 3.40). If it is necessary to use Table 3.17 or eqn 3.10, the threshold values of that chosen range of corrective factors must be modified. Once the time of death has been taken from the nomogram at two corrected body weights, the result is a range for the time of death (Figs 3.38 and 3.40).

Example: A scene may lead to the choice of a range of corrective factors, perhaps between 1.8 and 2.2; the choice is based on experience of particular conditions (e.g. a bedspread) for an average body weight (Table 3.16). The actual body weight may be evaluated to approximately 20 kg. Using Table 3.17, a corrective factor range of 2.4 (from 1.8) to 3.6 (from 2.2) would be the result. Using

Table 3.17 *Chart of the dependence of corrective factors on the body weight*[1]

Cooling conditions	Real body weight (kg)																	
	4	6	8	10	20	30	40	50	60	70	80	90	100	110	120	130	140	150
										Average range								
										1.3								
Clothing, more	1.6	1.6	1.6	1.6	1.5					1.4					1.3	1.2	1.2	1.2
layers	2.1	2.1	2.0	2.0	1.9	1.8				1.6				1.4	1.4	1.4	1.3	1.3
Bedspread	2.7	2.7	2.6	2.5	2.3	2.2	2.1	2.0		1.8			1.6	1.6	1.6	1.5	1.4	1.4
	3.5	3.4	3.3	3.2	2.8	2.6	2.4	2.3		2.0		1.8	1.8	1.7	1.6	1.6	1.5	1.5
	4.5	4.3	4.1	3.9	3.4	3.0	2.8	2.6	2.4	2.2	2.1	2.0	1.9	1.8	1.7	1.7	1.6	1.6
Clothing +	5.7	5.3	5.0	4.8	4.0	3.5	3.2	2.9	2.7	2.4	2.3	2.2	2.1	1.9	1.9	1.8	1.7	1.6
bedspread	7.1	6.6	6.2	5.8	4.7	4.0	3.6	3.2	2.9	2.6	2.5	2.3	2.2	2.1	2.0	1.9	1.8	1.7
Feather bed	8.8	8.1	7.5	7.0	5.5	4.6	3.9	3.5	3.2	2.8	2.7	2.5	2.3	2.2	2.0	1.9	1.8	1.7
	10.9	9.8	8.9	8.3	6.2	5.1	4.3	3.8	3.4	3.0	2.8	2.6	2.4	2.3	2.1	2.0	1.9	1.8
										(see Table 3.1)								

The average range of body weight which is the base of the corrective factors 'known by experience' (Table 3.16) has been chosen at 70 kg (bold figures). Below a corrective factor of 1.4 (up to 0.75), the dependence on the body weight can be neglected.

Table 3.18 *Data of paired cases*[45]

Case	Cooling conditions	Correction factor		Real body weight (kg)	Ambient temperature (°C)		Rectal temp. (°C)	Time estimated (hpm)		Time ascertained (hpm)		Comment
		Mean	Range		Measured	Used		lower limit	upper limit	lower limit	upper limit	
6	LB on bed, covered with two thick blankets together about 30 cm thick, night dress, short panty	2.4	2.0–2.8*	89	20.6/20.6	19.6/21.6	36.9	02.0	07.6	01.8	15.0	*Because of strong insulation condition and high body weight: adaption according to Table 3.3: 1.8–2.5
7	Room, hanging at door, short panty	1.05	1.0–1.1	78	20.6/20.6	19.6/21.6	35.0	03.0	08.6	01.8	15.0	The wife was strangled by the husband who committed suicide by hanging thereafter
36	Apartment house, stony staircase, LP, thicker pyjamas	1.0	0.9–1.1	62	15.6/16.1	15.5/16.5	33.1	03.0	08.6	07.1	08.1	The mother and her 3-year-old son were killed by the culprit
37	Room, floor, carpet, thicker pyjamas, disposable nappies	1.5	1.3–1.7*	14	15.8/16.3	15.5/16.5	28.3	02.5	08.1	06.8	07.8	*There is no experience with one-way nappies concerning the correction factor. The used range was speculated. Because of strong insulation condition and low body weight the correction factor of 1.7 was adapted to 2.2 according to [3]
46	Windowless basement room, LP on tiled floor, jeans, bodice	1.0	0.9–1.1	57	22.5/23.0	22.5–23.0	32.8	04.9	10.5	05.8	06.1	The woman was killed by the man who committed suicide immediately thereafter
47	Windowless basement room, leaned back sitting on a pail with a dust-filled bag on it, jeans, short panty	1.3*	1.2–1.4*	77	as 46	as 46	35.5	03.5	09.1	07.3	07.6	*The pail with a dust-filled bag on it looks like a stronger thermic insulation
70	Room, sitting position on thick upholstered couch, back and left region of the lower trunk leaning against thick cushions, pyjamas, pants, in front open bathing-gown	1.3	1.2–1.4	96	18.0/19.0	18.0/19.0	33.5	08.5	14.1	04.0	17.5	The man committed suicide at an unclear time after having killed his wife at a time which could be exactly investigated
71	Room, LL, floor, carpet, pyjamas, briefs	1.2	1.1–1.3	64	18.0/19.0	18.0/19.0	26.5	14.4	23.4	17.2	17.7	

LB = lying back; LP = lying prone; LL = lying in a lateral position.

eqn 3.10, the exact range would be 2.3 to 3.4. The corrected weight, taking the bedspread in the case of a 20-kg body into account, would range between 50 and 70 kg. If the ambient temperature is 18°C and the rectal temperature 29°C, the range of the time of death would be 9.4 hours (50 kg) to 12.6 hours (70 kg) according to the nomogram, corresponding to 11 ± 1.6 hours. However, this range of the time of death resulting from the range of corrective factor is smaller than the ± 2.8 hours permissible variation of 95% given by the nomogram (Figs 3.38 and 3.40). We recommend, in all cases, using the wider range (11 ± 2.8 hours) in official statements to avoid misleading the investigation. In fact, it is impossible to limit that range without loss of reliability. The above-mentioned computer program[42] operates according to this recommendation. On the contrary, the use of additional methods for estimating the time of death is recommended (see Chapter 7).

A few cases of the bodies of babies and infants covered with a bedspread may confirm the data of Table 3.17. The victims of a triple murder were a baby (3.2 kg), a child (8.1 kg) and their mother (44 kg). The bodies of the children were found in bed, fully clothed and covered by a thick bedspread. The body of the mother was found lying on a bed, clothed in ski trousers and covered partly by a bedspread. The time of death would be met exactly in the case of the 3.2-kg body by nomographical read-off of the time of death using a corrective factor of 9.0, which corresponds to 2.8 in the case of a 70-kg body (see Table 3.17). The real time of death would be recorded by the upper limit of the permissible variation of 95% (2.8 hours) to the examined time applying a corrective factor of 4.0, which corresponds to 2.0 in the case of a 70-kg body. Corrective factors of between 7.0 (2.7 at 70 kg) and 3.0 (1.9 at 70 kg) would be correct for the 8.1-kg body. In the case of the 44-kg body, the real time of death would be recorded by the application of 3.2 (1.9 at 70 kg) and 1.4 (1.4 at 70 kg) as corrective factors. The three cases can be solved sufficiently by the combined application of Tables 3.16 and 3.17. Further actual cases (numbers 36 and 37 in Table 3.18) may also confirm adoption of the corrective factor in dependence of the body weight in cases of strong thermic insulation conditions according to eqn 3.10 (Table 3.17).

7. Evaluating the corrective factor of body weight for special cooling conditions differing from the chosen standard conditions is often the most difficult problem, particularly when clothing or covering, special bases, moving air and wetness overlap. The difficulty can be avoided when complying the above-mentioned order of the three aspects in evaluating the corrective factor, namely: (i) clothing or covering; (ii) resting or moving air; and (iii) accelerating or decelerating base. The difficulty can be further avoided if, instead of a point value, a range of corrective factors is chosen which are appropriate to the actual cooling conditions (see Table 3.16 and Figs 3.38 and 3.40). Instructive examples are those of cases 15, 22, 27 and 54 in Table 3.15.

The above-mentioned computer program supports this recommendation; a demonstration version of this can be down-loaded from the internet[42] for self-instruction.

Known changes of cooling conditions

If the changes in cooling conditions are known, they can often be taken into account without loss of reliability and without a significant reduction in accuracy. The one common situation is a change of the cooling conditions by the investigators before the temperature measurements can be made.

Example: A thick bedspread was taken off a body 1 hour before the temperature measurement. Nevertheless, a corrective factor of about 1.8 (Table 3.16) was used for calculating the death-time. Though the drop of the rectal temperature starts to become steeper during the 1 hour after the bedspread was removed from the body, the resulting error will be negligible because it is additive (compare the lower graphs in Fig. 3.13; 26–28 hours postmortem). Certainly, if such a significant change of the cooling conditions has lasted several hours, it can no longer be neglected. The probable cooling curve should then be reconstructed from the time of temperature measurements, using a computer.

Sometimes, the ambient temperature is significantly changed by the person who found the body, or by the investigators (e.g. closing or opening windows, using special lamps which heat a small room quickly), a short time before temperature measurement. If the ambient temperature was changed 1 or 2 hours before body temperature measurement, the body cooling becomes accelerated or decelerated after the change of ambient temperature, then the resulting error will again be negligible so far as the ambient temperature before its change is used.

A second temperature plateau provides a lag of the 'reaction' of the rectal temperature curve (see example of Fig. 3.39). If such a significant change of the ambient temperature has lasted for several hours, the range or the mean ambient temperature should be used as discussed above.

Uncertainty in the value of corrective factors

There is often uncertainty about point values of mean ambient temperature, body weight and, especially, corrective factors for special cooling conditions. It is a good strategy to evaluate possible upper and lower limits (Fig. 3.38). The nomogram (Fig. 3.40) or a computer program helps in this calculation by taking a range of each factor. The available computer program[42] requires range on principle.

Example (Fig. 3.40): For a body of 75 kg actual body weight and a rectal temperature of 27°C, evaluate a mean ambient temperature between 17 and 20°C and a corrective factor between 1.2 and 1.5 for special clothing. Using the nomogram, draw 2 × 2 straight lines: connect a 27°C rectal temperature with both 17 and 20°C. Now draw two more lines crossing the semicircles. Read off the time since death on both lines at the two intersections of the following semicircles: $75 \times 1.2 = 90$ kg and $75 \times 1.5 = 112.5$ (110) kg. The result will be four values for a death-time: about 19, 23.5, 23 and 28.5 hours postmortem. Thus it could be stated that death occurred between 19 and 28.5 hours before the time of investigation, which means 23.5 ± 4.5 hours. This example also demonstrates clearly that the given permissible variation at the outermost semicircle (± 4.5 hours, Fig. 3.40) includes some uncertainties.

This method is recommended if the points of contact (mean ambient temperature, corrective factor, body weight at scene) are not closely defined, so that a range must be taken into account.

The above-mentioned computer program[42] generally computes the period of death in two ways (see Figs 3.38 and 3.40):

1. The time of death is computed using the mean values of the chosen ranges of corrective factor, and mean ambient temperature, respectively. The period of death results by adding the empirical permissible variation of 95% (Tables 3.10 and 3.11).
2. In addition, the period of death is computed using the lower and upper brackets of the evaluated ranges of ambient temperature and corrective

factor, giving the lower and the upper limit of the period of death.

If the second method results in a wider range of the period than the first method, it is used as the final result (Fig. 3.38). There were some such cases in the mentioned field study[45] (e.g. cases 42, 49 and 56 in Table 3.15).

When the method must not be used

This method cannot be used, however, under a number of conditions. Having analysed the situation at the scene carefully, it must be decided whether this approach is feasible:

1. Strong radiation. There is no experience in taking solar or other radiation into account. If a body is found with direct sun on its surface, the situation is apparent. If a body is found at a place where the sun is not actually shining, the question of sun radiation must be checked, to establish whether direct sun radiation on the body might have been possible.

   Example: A body was found at night in a closed room lying on the floor near the south-west window. Using the apparent factors – especially the darkness – a death time of early afternoon was given. As at this time the body would have been in direct sun radiation, we did not give any statement concerning the time of death.

   Situations like this are open to inappropriate use of any temperature method. On the other hand, a short period of direct sun radiation on the body just before examination is not a contraindication to the method.

2. Uncertain severe change of cooling conditions. In contrast to methods with multiple temperature measurements at the scene for direct estimation of the individual values of the required constants, the nomogram method with a single measurement of rectal temperature can still be used when even severe changes of the cooling conditions occur for a short period before examination, if they can be reconstructed in relation to time and type (see above). If the changes in the cooling conditions are assumed but are really unknown in extent and direction, the method must not be used. A common situation of this type is a presumed severe change of cooling conditions during the interval between discovering the body and the beginning of the examination by the crime police.

Example: A body of 51 kg was found lying on its back, extended in a room on the floor. It was clothed only with a gown open at the front. Even the crime police could not decide later whether the windows and the doors were originally open, as the body was found 4.5 hours previously. The actual measured room temperature was 12.4°C. The radiator in the room felt warm. The room thermostat showed 21°C and the heating system was found to be working. The rectal temperature was 21°C.

If the windows and doors were open during the whole time interval since death occurred, the mean room temperature would have been similar to the actual measured temperature of about 12°C. A corrective factor of 0.75 for permanently moving air should be applied (51 kg → 38 kg). The death-time interval would have been 12.5 ± 2.8 hours (95%) according to the nomogram. Conversely, supposing the windows and doors had been closed between the moment of death and finding the body 4.5 hours before examination, the mean room temperature until examination would have been close to 21°C; its fall to 12.4°C must have developed only when windows and doors were opened 4.5 hours before. A special corrective factor (still air) would then be out of the question. In this case, no reliable reading from the nomogram could be made because of the 21°C figure of both the ambient and the rectal temperature.

Later on, the death time could have been calculated as 27 hours before examination at the scene in accordance with the following reconstruction. The body cooling had not yet reached the ambient temperature (about 21°C) when the unidentified person found the body and opened the windows and doors. If the rectal temperature was about 24°C at this moment, the mean nomographic death-time would be 23 hours (51 kg; corrective factor 1.0; ambient temperature 21°C). During the following 4.5 hours with changed cooling conditions, the rectal temperature fell to the measured 21°C.

This example demonstrates the advice to 'analyse carefully the factors at the scene' before giving an estimate of death-time. No special knowledge is necessary, but only general physical thinking about the carefully analysed situation at the scene.

3. Unusual cooling conditions. This point is not only a matter of formally selecting a corrective factor (from Table 3.16) for the special cooling conditions, but is also a matter of personal experience. In cases of unusual cooling conditions without any personal experience, the examination at the scene should still be performed. Nevertheless, a statement of the time since death cannot be given from this method (e.g. cases 31 and 45 in Table 3.15). After a test cooling of the dummy, an opinion can be given later on whether the question of death-time becomes of greater importance (see below).

4. Repeated extensive climatic changes. The method must not be used if repeated extensive climatic changes have occurred which do not allow the evaluation of representative mean figures for ambient temperature and corrective factors for the whole period between death and investigation.

5. Transported body. If the place where the body was found is not the same as the place of death, the method must not be used except when both the place of death and the date of transportation of the body are known. This is uncommon, but the circumstances of transportation become apparent later on. Therefore, the examination of the body at the place where it was found should still be made. Under certain circumstances, a restricted statement of the time since death can be given to support the investigation.

It is strongly recommended not to use the method after the removal of the body to the mortuary if there is only reported information about the place where the body was found. On the other hand, there are no arguments against measurement of the rectal temperature and examination of the other methods estimating the time since death after the removal of the body into the mortuary, provided that the forensic investigator has already inspected the scene of crime and the period of the transportation has not taken too much time. Marty and Baer[48] investigated the influence on body cooling of storing bodies in a closed compartment such as a coffin, a closet or a car boot. Whereas storing a body in a closet or a car boot did not affect the cooling rate significantly, bodies stored in a wooden coffin showed a lower cooling rate corresponding to a mean corrective factor of 1.2 (variation 1.0 to 1.3).

6. Suspicion of general hypothermia. See page 74 and Fig. 3.26. Suspicion of malignant hyperthermia (e.g. case 33 in Table 3.15).

SPECIAL PROBLEMS

Besides the questions referred to above, there are some further problems.

High ambient temperature

As discussed in connection with constant A and its uncertain dependence on the ambient temperature, it is emphasized that the nomogram (see Fig. 3.32) and eqn 3.15 for ambient temperatures above 23°C is based on the data from De Saram *et al.*[24] Among our own data of experimental body cooling, there are no cases which cooled in ambient temperatures above 23°C. Among the casework of a multicentre study ($n = 46$)[49] are seven cases where the ambient temperature was above 23°C. In the field study ($n = 72$)[45] reported above (Tables 3.15 and 3.18) are seven cases where the mean ambient temperature was above 23°C (e.g. cases 48 and 66 in Table 3.15) and four further cases where the upper bracket of the range of ambient temperature was above 23°C. The estimated death-times of these cases using the nomogram of Fig. 3.32 or eqn 3.5 with the 1.11 value of constant *A* are in accordance with the true times of death. However, more experience of body cooling in high ambient temperatures has yet to be gained.

Fever at death

In our cooling experiments reported above, we had some cases with fever at death (see Fig. 3.25). The errors due to fever are included in the given permissible variations of 95%, and are greatest for the first postmortal hours, decreasing later (see Table 3.11 and Fig. 3.26). By computation, the temperature at death can be changed from 37.2°C to a higher figure when adequate investigation or autopsy findings suppose fever at death. When using the nomogram form, the difference between the supposed temperature at death and the normal 37.2°C must be subtracted both from the measured rectal temperature and the ambient temperature (e.g. case 33 in Table 3.15).

Longer agony

If there is a long period between the time of fatal injury and death, the estimate of the time since death should be supplemented emphatically by warning the investigators of a possibly longer interval. Stating only the time since death in cases of a possible longer period of agony can lead to a misunderstanding. In addition, the nomographically estimated time of death may be loaded with a greater error because the regulation of body temperature can be markedly disturbed during agony, either due to a central fever or to hypothermia. In the latter case, cooling may develop even more quickly during agony than on a dead body. During agony, the circulation is acting as convectional heat transfer from the centre of the body to the surface. At the same time, the regulation of homeostasis of body temperature by addi-

tional heat production can be reduced. A clear decision of whether a longer period of agony comes into question or not can be made only after autopsy. The preliminary examination of the body at the scene may suggest a very short agony, even if this is not the case. An immediate autopsy after the procedure at the scene is the best way to recognise such a mistake. The stated death-time can be corrected quickly after autopsy before misleading the investigation. Later on, the findings of toxicological (e.g. ratio of metabolites) or histological (e.g. age of wounds, signs of organ shock) examination may provide evidence of a distinct interval between fatal injury and death.

ACCURACY OF CALCULATED TIME SINCE DEATH

In 1990, Albrecht *et al.*[49] published a multicentre study on the accuracy of calculated time since death. The range of accuracy stated previously (see Figs 3.27–3.30) at the outermost circle of the nomogram results from experimental body cooling under controlled conditions in various research institutes.

Representative assessments of accuracy in using the nomogram method at the scene are difficult to obtain because of technical problems. A single forensic pathologist does not deal with sufficient cases to constitute a scientific study. Therefore, a multicentre study was made using 11 forensic pathologists from six forensic institutes in Germany, Austria and Switzerland.[49] Seventy-six cases were examined at the scene. All bodies were later autopsied. The cooling conditions at the scene varied over a wide range corresponding to evaluated corrective factors between 0.3 (bodies found in flowing water) and 2.1 (thick bedspread). Ambient temperatures varied between –6 and 26°C. The differences (nomographically estimated – actual interval of death) were calculated as follows (Fig. 3.41). As the investigated time of death was known with certainty in most cases, the mean figure, the upper and the lower limit of this interval were related to the mean of nomographically estimated time of death. In consequence, three values of error ($dt\,1$, $dt\,2$ and $dt\,3$) of each case entered into the statistical analysis of error. The 76 cases were divided into two groups.

Group I

Forty-six cases with clearly defined points of contact. The standard deviation of the differences between nomographic and actual death-times resulted in

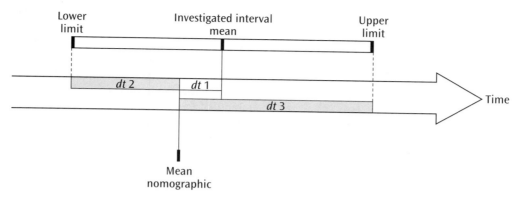

Figure 3.41 *Differences between nomographically calculated time of death and mean* (dt *1*), *lower limit* (dt *2*) *and upper limit* (dt *3*) *of the investigated time of death utilized in the statistic analysis of errors.*[49]

± 1.3 hours, equivalent to permissible variation of 95% of ± 2.6 hours (Figs 3.42 and 3.43). The progress of cooling corresponded in 37 cases to values of $Q > 0.5$, and in nine cases the cooling was more advanced, corresponding to values of $0.5 > Q > 0.2$. There was no trend toward increased errors with advance of cooling, as expected theoretically and from experimental body coolings.

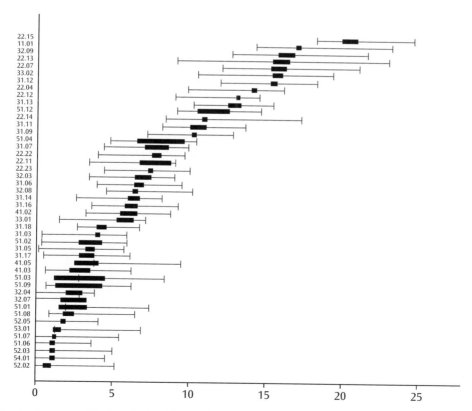

Figure 3.42 ⊢——⊣ = *Nomographically calculated interval according to the permissable variation of 95% given at the nomogram and* ▬▬▬ = *investigated interval of death in group I of casework.*[49]

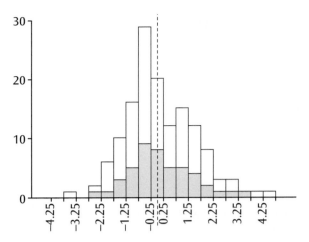

Figure 3.43 *Histogram of errors of all the 46 cases of group I according to* Figs 3.41 *and* 3.42.

In 20 cases the real death-time was less than 4 hours. Among these were five cases in which the nomographic death-time did not agree closely with the actual time, but did not contradict it. These cases could be explained by the problem of stated 37.2°C for *To*, as discussed above. The errors may be avoided by means of examining the mechanical and electrical excitability of muscles (see Chapter 7). Separating the 26 cases with a real death-time above 4 hours, the standard deviation was ± 1 hour – equivalent to a permissible variation of ± 2 hours (Figs 3.44 and 3.45), which is significantly smaller than both the total group I and that suggested by the nomogram. The latter result

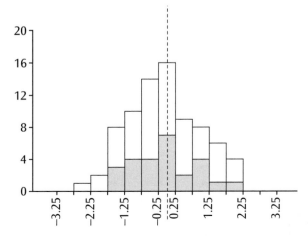

Figure 3.44 *Histogram of errors of that part of the cases of group I having investigated death-times above 4 hours (26 cases; compare with* Fig. 3.45).[49]

seems to indicate lower errors in casework than in experimental body coolings. This rather surprising result could be explained by the previously discussed 'preanalytic' error inherent in experimental body cooling but usually absent in casework (see page 74). Nevertheless, the results of this group confirm the reliability of the nomogram method within the 95% permissible variation.

Group II

An additional 30 cases with uncertain corrective factors. The nomographic death-time interval does not agree with the real investigated interval in five cases, demonstrating that an estimate of the death-time should not be given at all where points of contact are unsure (Fig. 3.46).

In 1999, Henssge *et al.*[45] published a single-centre field study on the experiences with a compound method for estimating the time since death at the scene in 72 consecutive cases. The computer-assisted[42] nomogram method was used as the primary method (examples in Table 3.15 and 3.18) followed by non-temperature-based methods[50] (see Chapter 7).

The reliability of the estimated period since death by the temperature-based nomogram method could be considered in 60 cases where the period of death could be determined by the police investigations with certainty. In all these cases the estimated period since death was consistent with the investigated period. In 50 cases the estimated period since death corresponded completely to the investigated period, and partially in 10 cases. In the latter 10 cases, death could have occurred within the overlapping range between the estimate and the investigated period.

In each of four cases two bodies were found at the same scene, and the question of the sequence of deaths arose. These paired cases (Table 3.18) provide evidence for the degree of differentiation that is achieved with the nomogram method. Despite the different rectal temperatures, congruent periods of death resulted because of different cooling conditions and body weights (cases 6/7; 36/37; and 46/47). In the paired cases 36/37 and 46/47, the police investigation resulted in a nearly simultaneous death of the two persons. In the paired case 6/7, the police investigation could not verify the times of death. In the paired case 70/71, the time of the wife's death could be exactly verified by the investigation, but the time of the man's death remained unclear. In contrast to the other three paired cases, the different cooling conditions and body

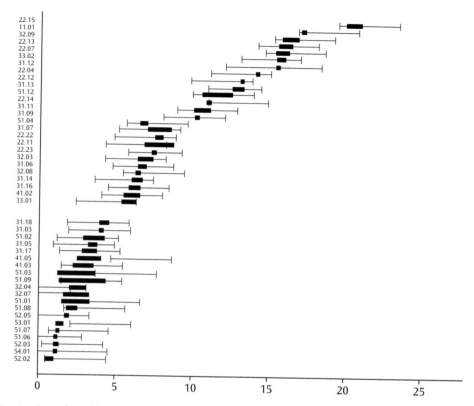

Figure 3.45 ⊢──⊣ = *Investigated interval of death and* ▬▬▬ = *nomographically calculated time of death but with interval according to the permissible variation of 95% of that part of casework having investigated death-times above 4 hours (see Fig. 3.44). The calculated interval does not agree with the investigated interval in case numbers 41.05, 51.01 and 53.01.*

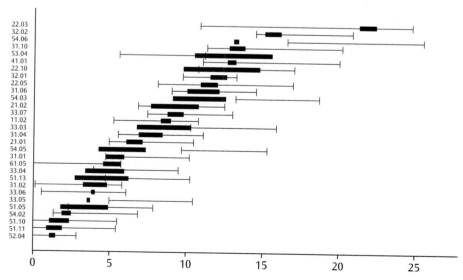

Figure 3.46 *Nomographically calculated and investigated interval of death of group II including 30 cases with recognizable unsure point of contact.*

weights did not compensate the different rectal temperatures, with the result that different periods since death were calculated at the 95% level of permissible variation.

RECONSTRUCTION OF BODY COOLING

When a body is found under special cooling conditions where there is no experience of a corrective factor, a test cooling of a 37°C heated dummy at the place and under the special conditions where the body was found can provide evidence of the true corrective factor. Before a dummy can be used for such a reconstruction, its cooling under the chosen standard conditions must be investigated by several test coolings. As a result of these tests (see Fig. 3.2), the weight of the body can be calculated (eqn 3.3), and this is replaced by the dummy. This weight stands for the chosen standard conditions of cooling. It acts as the real body weight (*bw*) in calculating the corrective factor according to eqn 3.4. The weight resulting from the test cooling under the special conditions at the place where the body was actually found acts as *bw calc* in eqn 3.4.

The additional measurement of heat flow and temperatures on the surfaces of body, especially on the supporting surface, may assist the detection of special influencing factors of the body cooling (see Figs 3.19–3.21), including the influence of heat radiation.

Besides additional measurements concerning the body cooling in special cases, it is recommended in all cases to apply other, simple methods in addition to the nomogram method[50]; these are described in Chapter 7.

REFERENCES

1 Henssge C. Rectal temperature time of death nomogram: dependence of corrective factors on the body weight under stronger thermic insulation conditions. *Forensic Sci. Int.* 1992; **54**: 51–6.

2 Henssge C, Hahn S, Madea B. Praktische Erfahrungen mit einem Abkühlungsdummy (German, English summary). *Beitr. Gerichtl. Med* 1986; **XLIV**: 123–6.

3 Henssge C, Madea B, Schaar U, Pitzken C. Die Abkühlung eines Dummy unter verschiedenen Bedingungen im Vergleich zur Leichenabkühlung (German, English summary). *Beitr. Gerichtl. Med* 1987; **XLV**: 145–9.

4 Knörle T. *Normierungsvarianten für die Wärmeflußmessung an einem Kunstkörper* (German). University of Köln: MD Thesis, 1991.

5 Malt M. *Das Abkühlverhalten eines Kunstkörpers unter Berücksichtigung seines Wärmeflußes* (German). University of Köln: MD Thesis, 1991.

6 Stadtmüller K. *Zur Todeszeitbestimmung aus der Leichenabkühlung: Die Normierung der Abkühlgeschwindigkeit unterschiedlicher Körper auf verschiedene äussere Bedingungen* (German). University of Köln: MD Thesis, 1991.

7 Unland M. *Ein Modell zur Bestimmung der Todeszeit aus dem Wärmefluß* (German). University of Köln: MD Thesis, 1991.

8 Mall G, Hubig M, Beier G, Eisenmenger W. Energy loss due to radiation in postmortem cooling. Part A: Quantitative estimation of radiation using the Stefan-Boltzmann Law. *Int. J. Legal. Med.* 1998; **111**: 299–304.

9 Mall G, Hubig M, Beier G, Büttner A, Eisenmenger W. Energy loss due to radiation in postmortem cooling. Part B: Energy balance with respect to radiation. *Int. J. Legal. Med.* 1999; **112**: 233–40.

10 Henssge C, Frekers R, Reinhardt S, Beckmann E-R. Determination of time of death on the basis of simultaneous measurement of brain and rectal temperature (German, English summary). *Z. Rechtsmed.* 1984; **93**: 123–33.

11 Brinkmann B, May D, Riemann U. Post mortem temperature equilibration of the structures of the head (German, English summary). *Z. Rechtsmed.* 1976; **78**: 69–82.

12 Brinkmann B, Menzel G, Riemann U. Environmental influences to postmortem temperature curves (German, English summary). *Z. Rechtsmed.* 1978; **81**: 207–16.

13 Henssge C, Beckmann E-R, Wischhusen F, Brinkmann B. Determination of time of death by measuring central brain temperature (German, English summary). *Z. Rechtsmed.* 1984; **93**: 1–22.

14 Ratermann J. *Postmortale Hirntemperaturmessungen zur Todeszeitbestimmung – Untersuchungen zur Insertionstechnik der Temperaturmeßsonden* (German). University of Münster: MD Thesis, 1986.

15 Joseph A, Schickele E. A general method for assessing factors controlling postmortem cooling. *J. Forensic Sci.* 1970; **15**: 364–91.

16 Marshall TK, Hoare FE. I Estimating the time of death. The rectal cooling after death and its mathematical expression. II The use of the cooling formula in the study of post mortem body cooling. III The use of the body temperature in estimating the time of death. *J. Forensic Sci.* 1962; **7**: 56–81, 189–210, 211–21.

17 Hiraiwa K, Kudo T, Kuroda F, Ohno Y, Sebetan IM, Oshida S. Estimation of postmortem interval from rectal

temperature by use of computer-relationship between the rectal and skin cooling curves. *Med. Sci. Law* 1981; **21**: 4–9.

18 Hiraiwa K, Ohno Y, Kuroda F, Sebetan IM, Oshida S. Estimation of postmortem interval from rectal temperature by use of computer. *Med. Sci. Law* 1980; **20**: 115–25.

19 Brown A, Marshall TK. Body temperature as a means of estimating the time of death. *Forensic Sci.* 1974; **4**: 125–33.

20 Rainy H. On the cooling of dead bodies as indicating the length of time that has elapsed since death. *Glasgow Med. J.* (new series) 1868; **1**: 323–30.

21 James WRL, Knight BH. Errors in estimating time since death. *Med. Sci. Law* 1965; **5**: 111–16.

22 Prokop O. Die Abkühlung der Leiche. In: *Forensische Medizin* (German). (Prokop O, Gohler W, eds.). Berlin: Verlag Volk und Gesundheit, 1975.

23 Schwarz F, Heidenwolf H. Le refroidissement post mortem. Sa signification quant à l'heure du décès. *Intern. Polizeiliche Revue* 1953; **8**: 339–44.

24 De Saram GSW, Webster G, Kathirgamatamby N. Post-mortem temperature and the time of death. *J. Crim. Law Criminol.* 1955; **46**: 562–77.

25 Fiddes FS, Patten TD. A percentage method for representing the fall in body temperature after death. Its use in estimating the time of death. *J. Forensic Med.* 1958; **5**: 2–15.

26 Green MA, Wright JC. Postmortem interval estimation from body temperature data only. *Forensic Sci. Int.* 1985; **28**: 35–46.

27 Green MA, Wright JC. The theoretical aspects of the time-dependent Z equation as a means of postmortem interval estimation using body temperature data only. *Forensic Sci. Int.* 1985; **28**: 53–62.

28 Henssge C, Madea B. *Methodenzur Bestimmung der Todeszeit an der Leiche.* Lübeck: Schmidt-Römhild-Verlag, 1988.

29 Koppes-Koenen KM. *Untersuchungen zum parameterfreien Verfahren der Todeszeitbesimmung aus Körpertemperaturen von Green und Wright* (German). University of Köln: MD Thesis, 1991.

30 Gruner K. *Todeszeitbesimmung aus der Rektaltemperatur* (German). Medical diploma, Humboldt-Universität, Berlin, 1985.

31 Henssge C. Precision of estimating the time of death by mathematical expression of rectal body cooling (German, English summary). *Z. Rechtsmed.* 1979; **83**: 49–67.

32 Sellier K. Determination of the time of death by extrapolation of the temperature decrease curve. *Acta Med. Soc.* 1958; **11**: 279–302.

33 Stipanits E, Henssge C. Präzisionsvergleich von Todeszeitrückrechnungen ohne und mit Berücksichtigung von Einflußfaktoren (German, English summary). *Beitr. Gerichtl. Med.* 1985; **XLIII**: 323–9.

34 Henssge C. Estimation of death-time by computing the rectal body cooling under various cooling conditions (German, English summary). *Z. Rechtsmed.* 1981; **87**: 147–78.

35 Mueller B. Das Verhalten der Mastdarmtemperatur der Leiche unter verschiedenen äusseren Bedingungen. *Dtsch. Z. ges Gerichtl. Med.* 1938; **29**: 158–62.

36 Wessel H. *Leichenabkühlung bei Bettlagerung* (German). University of Münster: MD Thesis, 1989.

37 Henssge C, Brinkmann B. Todeszeitbestimmung aus der Rektaltemperatur. *Arch. Kriminol.* 1984; **174**: 96–112.

38 Henssge C, Brinkmann B, Püschel K. Determination of time of death by measuring the rectal temperature in corpses suspended in water (German, English summary). *Z. Rechtsmed.* 1984; **92**: 255–76.

39 Grober, Erk, Grigull. *Wärmeübertragung* (German). Berlin: Springer, 1957.

40 Shapiro HA. The post-mortem temperature plateau. *J. Forensic Med.* 1965; **12**: 137–41.

41 Altgassen X. Untersuchungen zum 'postmortalen Temperaturplateau' an Abkühlkurven von Kunstkörpern (German). MD Thesis, Köln, 1992.

42 Henssge C. Homepage with program version of demonstration. http://home.t-online.de/home/Christoph.Henssge/t-zeit.htm

43 Henssge C. Temperatur-Todeszeit-Nomogramm für Bezugsstandardbedingungen der Leichenlagerung. *Kriminal. Forens. Wiss.* 1982; **46**: 109–15.

44 Lyle HP, Cleveland FP. Determination of the time of death by body heat loss. *J. Forensic Sci.* 1956; **1**: 11–23.

45 Henssge C, Althaus L, Bolt J, Freislederer A, Henssge CA, Hoppe B, Schneider V. Experiences with a compound method for estimating the time since death. I. Rectal temperature nomogram for time since death. *Int. J. Legal. Med.* 1999; **113**: 303–19.

46 Henssge C. Death time estimation in case work – I. The rectal temperature time of death nomogram. *Forensic Sci. Int.* 1988; **38**: 209–36.

47 Althaus L, Henssge C. Rectal temperature time of death nomogram: sudden change of ambient temperature. *Forensic Sci. Int.* 1999; **99**: 171–8.

48 Marty W, Baer W. Cooling of cadavers in a coffin (German, English summary). *Rechtsmedizin* 1993; **3**: 51–3.

49 Albrecht A, Gerling I, Henssge C, Hochmeister M, Kleiber M, Madea B, Oehmichen M, Pollak St, Püschel K, Seifert D, Teige K. Zur Anwendung des Rektaltemperatur-Todeszeit-Nomogramms am Leichenfundort (German, English summary). *Z. Rechtsmed.* 1990; **103**: 257–78.

50 Henssge C, Althaus L, Bolt J, Freislederer A, Henssge CA, Hoppe B, Schneider V. Experiences with a compound method for estimating the time since death. II. Integration of non-temperature-based methods. *Int. J. Legal. Med.* 1999; **113**: 320–1.

51 Lundquist F. Physical and chemical methods for the estimation of the time of death. *Acta Med. Leg. Soc.* 1956; **9** (N. spec.): 205–13.

4

Eye changes after death

BURKHARD MADEA AND CLAUS HENSSGE

ELECTROLYTE CONCENTRATIONS IN VITREOUS HUMOUR

Autolysis starts with the cessation of energy metabolism in the cell and causes a dissolution of the chemical, physical and morphological integrity of the body. Cessation of active membrane transport and loss of selective membrane permeability are direct consequences of the energy breakdown. With the loss of selective membrane permeability, diffusion of ions according to their concentration gradients will start. The time course of the autolytic processes is determined by many factors:

- Local anatomical factors (gallbladder, oesophagus, stomach, duodenum).
- Tissue- and cell-specific peculiarities.
- Biochemical factors (rate of glycolysis).
- Further ante- and postmortem factors influencing the 'milieu interieur', especially temperature and pH.

As different tissues – and even the same tissues – at different topographical locations within the body have varying energy depots and rates of glycolysis, the duration of supravital activity varies considerably. As a result, the starting point, as well as the time course (velocity of autolytic processes between different tissues, the same tissues at different locations of the body as well as interindividually between different persons) differs widely.

Therefore, the following conclusions can be drawn concerning autolytic processes dependent on the time since death. Without strict differentiation of the structure investigated, the location of collection of specimen and temperature and antemortem factors (especially those which may affect postmortem pH), the range of scatter of the autolytic parameter investigated will be great, and will rise considerably with increasing postmortem interval. This is true for most investigations dealing with autolytic processes and time since death. They were reviewed by Schleyer[1–3] and Coe[4–10] and will therefore not be addressed here again.

Loss of selective membrane permeability

The equalization of the concentration difference of ions in different compartments begins during and after the supravital period.

The equalization of concentration differences after loss of selective membrane permeability follows Fick's first law of diffusion:

$$\overset{\circ}{m} = D \times \frac{F}{d} \times (C1 - C2) = D \times \frac{F}{d} \times c$$

where $\overset{\circ}{m}$ = the diffusion stream; D = the diffusion coefficient, dependent on the medium and the particles diffusing; c = the concentration difference; F = the surface of the diffusion medium; d = the diameter; and $C1$, $C2$ = concentration in compartments 1 and 2.

Due to its isolated topography, compared with blood and cerebrospinal fluid (CSF), and because of resistance to microbiological contamination with bacterial degradation[11] and biochemical structure, [12–14] vitreous humour is a very suitable medium for postmortem concentration studies.

The most favoured parameter studied is the vitreous potassium, which diffuses postmortem from the retina (and to lesser extent from the lens) into the vitreous body.[15] Animal experiments[15] have shown that supravital metabolism may be maintained for 15 minutes at 37°C. Even during life, there are concentration gradients within and between the intraocular fluid compartments[15,16] (Fig. 4.1), with a K^+ inflow from the lens and an outflow into retinal vessels. In dogs and rabbits, the highest intraocular fluid concentration of potassium was found in the posterior chamber and in cats in the anterior segment of the vitreous. The latter finding can be explained only by

an active K^+ transport across the lens.[16] The K^+ outflow from vitreous to retinal vessels seems to be purely diffusion, since the K^+ concentration of the posterior vitreous is higher than that of the plasma dialysate. Postmortem, the K^+ gradient at the vitreous–retina interface will reverse, with the lowest concentrations probably at the centre of the globe until diffusion equilibrium is achieved.

A striking finding was reported by Pau.[17] While the potassium content of the vitreous body was estimated to be 18–19 mg/dl, Pau noted that the vitreous layer adjacent to the retina contained about 100 mg/dl, which means that the whole vitreous behaves like a body fluid, but the vitreous layer as a body tissue. Whether this higher K^+ concentration of the layer is due to electrochemical binding to the chemical substrate (tropocollagen, hyaluronic acid) is still unknown. These two findings (vitreous potassium gradients and higher concentrations of the layer) already play an important role in the removal of vitreous humour and further preanalytical procedures.

The recommendations of Coe[18] concerning vitreous sample acquisition should be strictly adhered to:

'Vitreous humour should be obtained by means of needle and small syringe with suction applied gradually. The use of Vacutainer™ tubes with their strong initial suction commonly causes fragments of retina or other tissues to contaminate the specimen and such particulate matter will distort biochemical values. With care, over 1 ml of vitreous humour can usually be aspirated from each eye, even in newborn infants. Centrifugation with the use of the supernatant portion prevents clogging of fine tubing used in most current analytical instruments. All the vitreous that can be extracted should be withdrawn as there is variation in the concentration of many solutes between the vitreous humour next to the retina and that obtained from the centre of the globe.'

Only crystal-clear, colourless vitreous humour should be used for analysis. With the onset of decomposition the fluid becomes cloudy and brownish in colour.

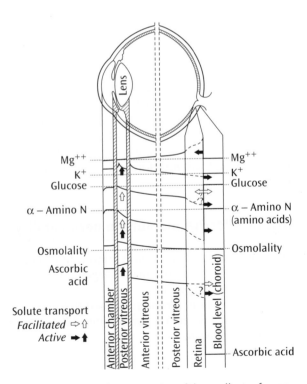

Figure 4.1 *Schematic presentation of the gradients of some solute concentrations and total osmolality in the intraocular fluid system of typical mammalian eye. The blood levels are given by the dotted line and by the value given for the choroid.*[16]

Short review of the literature on vitreous potassium

The relationship between the rise of potassium concentration in the vitreous humour and the time

Table 4.1 *Summary of investigations on vitreous potassium*

Reference	PMI	n	Intercept (K⁺ mmol/l)	Slope (K⁺ mmol/l per hour)	Correlation coeff. (r)	95% limits of confidence	Random sample	Comment
Jaffe[53]	Up to 125 hpm	31					17–81 years; no cases with uraemia or electrolyte imbalances	K⁺ concentration related to logarithm of time; no significant differences between refrigerated bodies and those kept at room temperature
Adelson et al.[22]	24 h	209	5.36 / I 5.27 / II 5.72	0.17 / 0.16 / 0.18		±10 h / ±5.75 h / ±12 h	I Agonal event < 6 h / II Agonal event > 6 h	Straight line relationship between vitreous potassium and PMI
Sturner[19] Sturner and Ganther[21]	Up to 108 h	54	5.48	0.14	0.987	±9.5 h	Coroner cases	PMI = 7.14 × K⁺ −39.1
Hughes[24]	Up to 117 h	135				±20 h	55 coroner cases / 80 hospital deaths	Rise of potassium could not be correlated with sufficient consistency with PMI
Hansson et al.[23]	3–310 h	203	8	0.17		±40 h		In 180 cases with a PMI up to 120 hpm linear rise of vitreous potassium
Leahy and Farber[31]	30 h	52					Hospital patients. Patients dead on arrival	Vitreous potassium concentrations appear to rise erratically after death
Lie[54]	2–95 h	88	5.48	0.14		±3.6 h (1 s.d.)	Hospital cases	Very good agreement with Sturner; slope, intercept and s.d. according to Henry and Smith[30] standard deviation calculated from author's data as variance from Sturner and Ganthers line of best fit'
Marchenko[32]	6–48 h	300				Death-time estimation possible within 3–6 hours	Age 29–70 years	Estimation of time since death possible within ±3 h
Coe[4]	100 hpm	160	I 4.99 / II 6.19	0.332 / 0.1625		±12 hours in the first day after death	Hospital patients with normal electrolytes within 6 h of death and medical examiner cases	I PMI < 6 h / II PMI > 6 h / Individual slope may vary between 0.085 and 0.45 mmol/l
Krause et al.[26]	230 h	262			0.7	Range of scatter between 9 and 107 h for K⁺ values between 5 and 28 mmol/l		$K^+ = 2.96 + 1.65\sqrt{h}$ $h = \left[\dfrac{K - 2.96}{1.65}\right]^2$ Exponential rise of potassium over the PMI
Stegmaier[27]	82 h	98				±12		
Adjutanis and Coutselinis[33]	12 h	120	3.4 (taken from literature)	0.55 for the first 12 hours		ca. ±3.3		Timed bilateral withdrawal (interval 3 h) reveals a rise in precision of death-time estimation from ±3.3 to ±2.2 h
Komura and Oshiro[36]	≈ 30 h	90			0.78–0.92 (according to ambient temperature)			Linear relationship between vitreous potassium and PMI, slope being steeper in ambient temperature of 26–29°C than in 13–17°C

Reference	n	Intercept (K+ mmol/l)	Slope (K+ mmol/per hour)	Correlation coeff. (r)	95% limits of confidence	Random sample	PMI	Comment
Foerch et al.[55]	> 50							Linear correlation between vitreous K+ and PMI
Blumenfeld et al.[52]	127			0.63	±26 h	127 children, age 1 hour–13 years	11–77 h	K+ increases with increasing PMI in an essentially linear fashion
Forman and Butts[56]	82	4.8	0.21	0.787				Linear relationship between potassium level and PMI; $y = 4.75 \times X = 22.8$
Schoning and Strafuss[37–39]	60 (dogs)					Mongrel dogs	48 h	Rise of K+ temperature dependent
Choo-Kang et al.[57]	105	9.67	0.09	0.85				
Balasooriya et al.[48]	59							Comparing vitreous potassium values of both eyes 18.6% of the results varied by more than 10% from the mean
Farmer et al.[58]		238 mg/l	4.752	0.98			24–120 h	
Stephens and Richards[28]	1427	6.324	0.238		±20 h	Newborn–90 years	35 h	
Madea et al.[34]	I 170 II 138 III 107	5.99 5.88 5.48	0.203 0.188 0.186	0.86 0.89 0.91	±34 h ±22 h ±20 h	I Entire sample (clinical and forensic pathology) II Urea < 100 mg/dl III Urea < 100 mg/dl and terminal episode < 6 h	130 h	
Sparks et al.[59]	91			0.87	±10.5 within the first day		≈ 60 h	Concomitantly the levels of 3-methoxy-tyramine (3-MT) were studied in the putamen of the brain; combining K+ and α3-MT determinations the accuracy of predicting PMI may be raised to ±8 h for individuals not dying from organic heart disease
Schmidt[60]		5.35	0.17	0.83	±24.8	Sudden natural and traumatic death (Forensic Pathology)	88.5 h	
Montaldo et al.[29]	289	6.805 6.1–6.99	0.1652 0.15–0.20		±15 ±8 to ±23	Violent or unsuspected death	≈ 80 h	K+ over the PMI in the entire sample and in various subgroups was analysed; subgroups were formed according to age, sex, type of death, autopsy findings, climatic conditions (see Table 4.3)
Gamero et al.[30]	60					Coroner cases	24 h	Best correlation between potassium and PMI in cases dying from acute trauma with a PMI < 17 h
Rognum et al.[42]	87	5.8	0.17 5°C 0.20 10°C 0.25 15°C 0.30 23°C				120 h	Repeated sampling of vitreous humour (twice each eye); the higher the environmental temperature the steeper the slope of vitreous potassium

since death has been established by several authors (see the excellent historical review by Coe[18] and Table 4.1). The most exciting results were presented by Sturner, [19,21] on a random sample of 54 bodies observed up to 100 hours postmortem, the 95% limits of confidence of the potassium concentration were only ± 9.5 hours.

The linear rise of vitreous potassium and the postmortem interval up to 104 hours postmortem was described by the following regression:

$$[K^+] = 5.476 + 0.14\ h, \text{ or } h = 7.14\ [K^+] - 39.1$$

Follow-up investigations[4,22–32] (Table 4.1) could not confirm these 95% limits of confidence and revealed – even in the group of sudden or traumatic deaths – a much wider range of scatter. Figure 4.2, for example, shows the range of scatter of the values found by Hughes[24] with regression line and 95% limits of confidence given by Sturner.[19]

Figure 4.3 shows the values found by Coe[4] – only persons with normal electrolytes 6 hours prior to death are included – and the regression line and 95% limits of confidence given by Sturner.[19] In both instances, the values found do not fit into the 95% limits of confidence given by Sturner.[19] However, one of the fundamental results of Sturner's investigation is that there are different 95% limits of confidence in the group of sudden/or traumatic deaths and hospital deaths. Further important results have been presented by Adelson et al.,[22] who were able to show that the duration of terminal episode also has a great influence

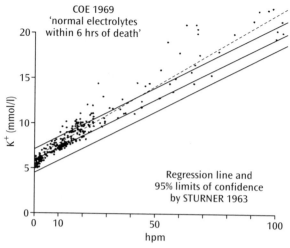

Figure 4.3 *Vitreous potassium values of normal individuals plotted against time since death with a regression line of all values having a postmortem interval above 6 hours (– – – –)[4] and regression line and 95% limits of confidence (———).[19]*

on the range of scatter of potassium concentration over the postmortem interval.

In cases where the terminal episode was less than 6 hours, the scatter was much smaller than in cases over 6 hours. The great obstacle in using potassium concentration in vitreous humour as an aid in estimating the time since death are the different 95% limits of confidence given by different authors. In a postmortem interval of up to roughly 100 hours they vary between ± 9.5 hours and ± 40 hours: in the early postmortem interval of up to 24 hours they vary from ± 6 hours to 12 hours (Fig. 4.4).

95% limits of confidence

	PMI (h)	95% ± h
Sturner (1963)	104	9.5
Stegmaier (1971)	85	16
Hughes (1965)	100	20
Hansson (1966)	120	40
Coe (1969)	24	12
Adelson (1963)	24	10
	12 terminal episodes > 6 h	
	6 terminal episodes < 6 h	

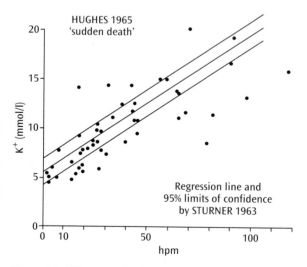

Figure 4.2 *Fifty cases of sudden death published by Hughes[24] with regression line and 95% limits of confidence by Sturner.[19]*

Figure 4.4 *Potassium in vitreous humour. Different 95% limits of confidence quoted in the literature for the early and later postmortem interval (PMI).*

The statistical parameters of the regression line vary correspondingly: (1) the potassium concentration at the moment of death as the intercept of regression lines between 5 and 8 mmol/l; and (2) the rise of potassium concentration per hour between 0.1 and 0.238 mmol/l × hour (Table 4.2).

The slope given by Adjutantis and Coutselinis[33] is as steep as 0.55 mmol/l per hour. Coe[4] found the slope in the first 6 hours to be 0.332 mmol/l per hour, which was much steeper than for the whole investigated period (0.1625 mmol/l per hour). In more than 100 individuals, sampling of the two eyes was made at different times and the slopes for individual pairs ranged from 0.085 to 0.450 mmol/l per hour (Coe[4,18]). Differing individual slopes have also been reported by Madea et al.[34] (Fig. 4.5).

Adjutantis and Coutselinis[33] confirmed the findings of an interindividual variation of the slope of potas-

Table 4.2 Differing statistical parameters of the regression line as quoted in the literature

Reference	n	Intercept (mmol/l)	Slope (mmol/l per hour)
Sturner[19]	54	5.960*	0.132*
		5.600	0.140
Adelson et al.[22]	209	5.360	0.170
Hansson et al.[23]	108	8.000	0.170
Lie[54]	88		0.140
Coe[4]	160	4.990	0.332 (first 6 h)
		6.190	0.1625 (over 6 h)
Adjutantis and Coutselinis[33]			0.550 (for the first 12 h)
Stephens and Richards[28]	1427	6.342	0.238
Madea et al.[34]	170	5.880	0.190

*The authors' own calculations on Sturner's material with differences to Coe's statement.[18] In cases with vitreous potassium of both eyes, the mean value was used for regression analysis. The slope varies between 0.132 and 0.238 mmol/l per hour, a, intercept; b, slope.

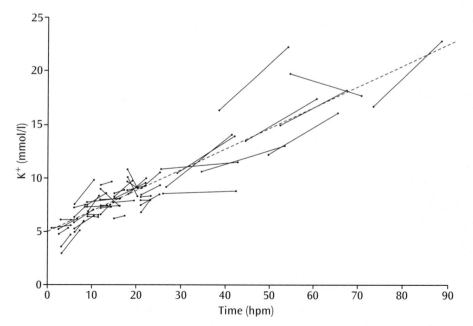

Figure 4.5 Potassium values of 53 cases of both eyes; vitreous humour of both eyes withdrawn at different time intervals after death (intervals between aspiration 2–3 hours, 4–5 hours and 12–24 hours). The 'rise' of potassium concentration of vitreous humour obtained at different time intervals is within the normal range of scatter of values obtained at identical times after death.

sium concentration over the postmortem interval (PMI), and recommended a timed removal of vitreous humour of both eyes at an interval of 3 hours and calculation of the time since death along the individual slope on a 'normal value' of potassium concentration at the moment of death (3.4 mmol/l). Death-time estimation in the first 12 hours would be possible to within an accuracy of ± 1.1 hour.

The reasons for these confusing results concerning regression parameters and the precise estimation of death-time are not clear, as all authors claim to have considered the same careful sample-taking and pre-treatment of samples before analysis.

Factors influencing the postmortem rise of vitreous potassium

Some reasons for the different regression parameters, especially the slope, have been identified:

- The duration of the terminal episode.[22,34]
- The composition of the random sample of deaths: hospital cases, coroner cases (Table 4.3).[19,29,30,34]
- A much steeper slope in cases with raised urea values.[34,35]
- Ambient temperature (Fig. 4.6).[9,15,36–42]*
- Possible influence of alcohol at the moment of death.[43]
- Distribution of cases of the PMI.
- Instrumentation used to measure the concentration (Fig. 4.7).[44]
- Linear relationship between vitreous potassium and PMI. This is obviously not a simple straight line but is biphasic, with a steeper slope in the first 6 hours than for prolonged times.[4]
- Age. The level of vitreous potassium rises much more rapidly in infants than it does in adults,[18] possibly because of smaller diameter of the infant vitreous globe.

Table 4.3 *Regression parameters and 95% limits of confidence in the entire sample and various subgroups according to the mode and cause of death*[29]

	n	Intercept K⁺ (mmol/l)	Slope (mmol/l per hour)	95% limits of confidence
Total number	289	6.805	0.1652	15
≤ 60 years	176	6.677	0.1657	14
> 60 years	113	6.636	0.1663	16
Sudden death	138	6.683	0.1652	16
Violent death	151	6.661	0.1666	16
Sudden death ≤ 60 years	29	6.609	0.1727	14
Sudden death > 60 years	42	6.183	0.1722	17
Violent death ≤ 60 years	111	6.801	0.1656	13
Violent death > 60 years	40	6.663	0.1665	16
Sudden cardiac death ≤ 60 years	36	6.867	0.1803	17
Sudden cardiac death > 60 years	31	6.383	0.1835	23
Violent asphyxial death	26	6.470	0.1689	12
Other violent death	125	6.692	0.1653	16
Death in winter	60	6.989	0.1626	16
Death in summer	74	6.567	0.1715	11
Violent death ≤ 60 years in winter	25	6.999	0.1500	21
Violent death ≤ 60 years in summer	34	6.100	0.2015	8

* From our own unpublished results: 24 bodies were brought, within 3 hours of death, into climate chambers with constant temperatures of 5 and 20°C. Twelve bodies were positioned in both temperatures for up to 40 hours before removal of the vitreous humour. From the 24 bodies, 32 vitreous specimens were obtained. In the 5°C group the intercept is 8.27 mmol/l and the slope 0.04 mmo/l per hour; in the 20°C group the intercept is 5.79 mmol/l and the slope 0.19 mmo/l per hour. Of course, the two temperature classes are too small to serve as reference samples. For this it would be necessary to have pairs of bodies matched for age, mode of death, cause of death, etc., which, immediately after death, were placed in different environmental temperatures and kept for a prolonged time in different temperatures.

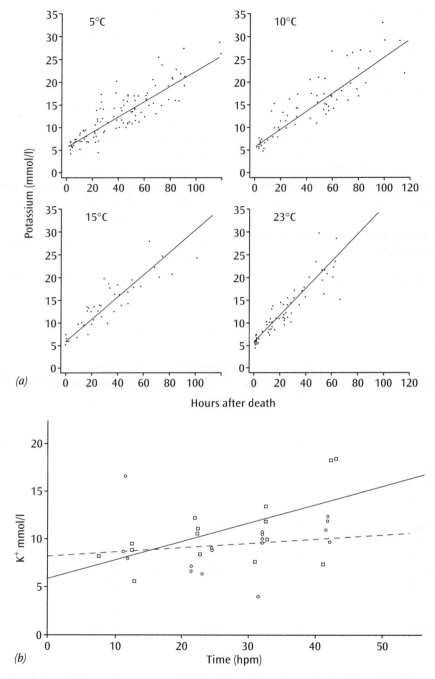

Figure 4.6 (a) *Scatter of plots of vitreous humour potassium levels in subjects kept at 5, 10, 15 and 23°C after death. The median slopes being 0.17 (5°C), 0.20 (10°C), 0.25 (15°C) and 0.30 (23°C) mmol/l per hour). The median slopes are indicated by lines.*[41] *(b) 32 K+ values from 24 bodies brought within 3 hours of death into ambient temperatures of 5°C (□) and 20°C (○).*

Our own investigations on vitreous potassium were based on the following hypothesis. One reason for the varying range of scatter in the different studies may be due to electrolyte imbalances at the moment of death. Unlike experimental studies, in case work information about the electrolyte status prior to the death is

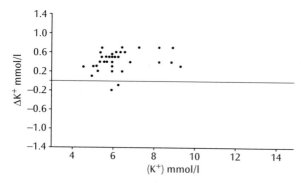

Figure 4.7 *Differences of potassium concentration (K⁺) determined with ion-specific electrodes and flame photometry (ion-specific electrodes minus flame photometry) over the potassium concentration determined with ion-specific electrodes (calculation on the material of Coe and Apple[44]). Determination with ion-specific electrodes reveals slightly higher values than with flame photometry.*

Search for an inner standard of electrolyte homeostasis at the moment of death

MATERIALS AND METHODS

Vitreous humour was sampled from 270 consecutive cases with an accurately known time of death.[34,35,45]

In the forensic case group ($n = 187$), the sudden deaths were mainly due to coronary artery disease, head injury, traffic accidents, fall from height, etc.

In contrast, in the pathology group ($n = 83$), death occurred after chronic lingering disease, i.e. cancer, infectious diseases, renal failure, cardiac failure after myocardial infarction (Table 4.4; Figs 4.8 and 4.9).

After admittance to the mortuary, most of the bodies were kept at +15°C, but some at +5°C. In all cases vitreous humour from both eyes was completely aspirated at the same time using a 10-ml syringe and a 20-gauge needle. Any specimens that were not crystal-clear were rejected. Most of the samples were frozen at −70°C until determinations could be performed. After thawing, the samples were centrifuged for 10 minutes at 3000 r.p.m. according to Adjutantis and Coutselinis.[33] The supernatant was used for determinations. In all cases there was enough material for the following parameters to be measured: potassium, sodium, chloride, urea, calcium. In some cases, creatinine was also determined. Sodium, potassium,

lacking. Therefore for investigations on vitreous humour it would be valuable to perform measurements of different parameters, of which some act as an inner standard. This should give information about homeostasis of electrolytes – mainly potassium – at the moment of death. Such an inner standard should have a small standard range in life, be stable postmortem, and have a close relationship to electrolyte metabolism.

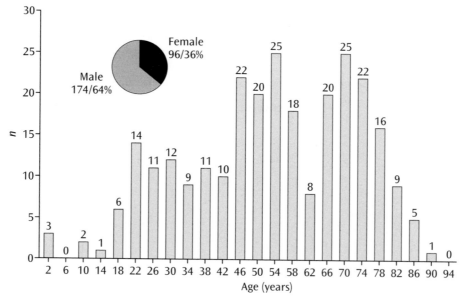

Figure 4.8 *Distribution of the authors' random sample with regard to sex and age.*

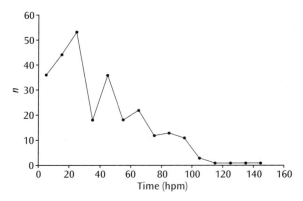

Figure 4.9 *Distribution of the postmortem interval of the authors' random sample (n = 270).*

chloride and calcium were determined using ion-sensitive electrodes. As the linearity of the potassium electrode of the Hitachi 705 system used in this investigation was confined to 10.9 mmol/l, most samples had to be measured once more after correct dilution with ion-free water.

Urea was determined using an enzymatic method according to Gutman and Bergmeyer.[46] The presence of ammonia did not affect the results. Creatinine was measured using the kinetic (Jaffe) method.[47] In all instances, right and left eye aspirates were analysed independently.

RESULTS AND DISCUSSION

Differences between each eye/timed bilateral withdrawal

As the left and right eye aspirates were determined independently, some remarks will be made on the differences between each eye. There were deviations of up to 10% in the single values from the mean value, even in the early postmortem interval (Fig. 4.10). These percentage deviations of the single values of each eye from the mean value are not related to the time since, or the mode of, death. These findings are in good accordance with those of Stegmaier,[27] but they are not as marked as those reported by Balasooriya *et al.*[48] (Table 4.5). We have also obtained similar differences between each eye for sodium, chloride and calcium.[35] As we used the same pretreatment of samples as Adjutantis and Coutselinis[33] before analysis, these differences of potassium concentration between the eyes do not allow us to use the method of Adjutantis and Coutselinis, which consists of determining the individual slope up to 12 hours postmortem after aspiration of vitreous humour of both eyes at different time intervals in order to obtain a more precise estimation of time since death. Another argument against their method is that the potassium values of vitreous humour in both eyes obtained at different times after death (3 to 4 hours apart) are within the normal range of scatter of values obtained at identical times after death (see Fig. 4.5). Correspondingly, Schleyer[48] mentioned that he could not confirm the results of Adjutantis and Coutselinis using their formula.

Urea as an internal standard

While there are differences in single potassium values taken at identical times, the statistical parameters of potassium concentration over time since death for each eye do not differ from those of the mean value for both eyes: the regression lines are identical. Therefore,

Table 4.4 *Composition of the random sample (n = 270) with regard to the cause of death*

	Forensic pathology	Clinical pathology	Total
Neoplasms	3	32	35
Accidents	47	3	50
Fall from height	21		21
Hanging	5		5
Myocardial infarction	71	21	92
Pulmonary thromboembolism	1	2	3
Cerebral infarction/cerebral bleeding		5	5
Liver or renal failure	3	7	10
Gunshot	7		7
Intoxication	8		8
Burns	4		4
Other	17	13	30
Total	187	83	270

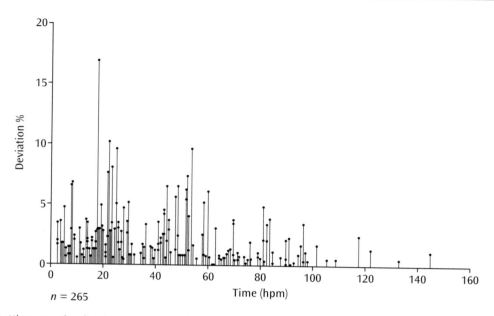

Figure 4.10 *Histogram showing the percentage deviation of the single potassium values of each eye from the mean value of both eyes.*

Table 4.5 *Percentage difference in results of K^+, Na^+ and urea in each eye expressed as a percentage of the mean result*

Potassium difference	< 4%	4–10%	> 10%
n	29 (240)	19 (23)	11 (2)
%	49.2 (90.5)	32.2 (8.7)	18.6 (0.8)
Sodium difference	< 2%	2–5%	> 5%
n	35 (173)	18 (56)	6 (36)
%	59 (65)	31 (21.1)	10 (13.5)
Urea difference	< 6%	6–12%	> 12%
n	27 (217)	11 (27)	9 (20)
%	57 (82.2)	23 (10.2)	19 (7.6)

Data from Balasooriya et al.[48] Authors' data in brackets.

for further statistical analysis, only the mean values of both eyes were used.

Figure 4.11 shows the potassium values of 270 cases (mean values of both eyes) plotted against time after death. There is a linear relationship between potassium concentration and time after death up to 120 hours. The slope is 0.20 mmol/l per hour; the intercept 6.10 mmol per hour.

The 95% limits of confidence in this entire group – which consists of both sudden traumatic and hospital deaths – are ± 25.51 hours up to 120 hours postmortem (Table 4.6).

The first step to reduce these 95% limits of confidence was to look at which of the other parameters could be indicative of antemortem imbalance of metabolism. Sodium, calcium, chloride, urea and creatinine are stable in the postmortem interval for up to 120 hours after death (Figs 4.12–4.14). Figures 4.15a and 4.15c show a marked increase of urea in many cases, indicative of antemortem urea retention. That these high urea values are due to antemortem retention and not to postmortem changes has been shown by Coe,[4] who compared urea values obtained from each eye at different time intervals after death.

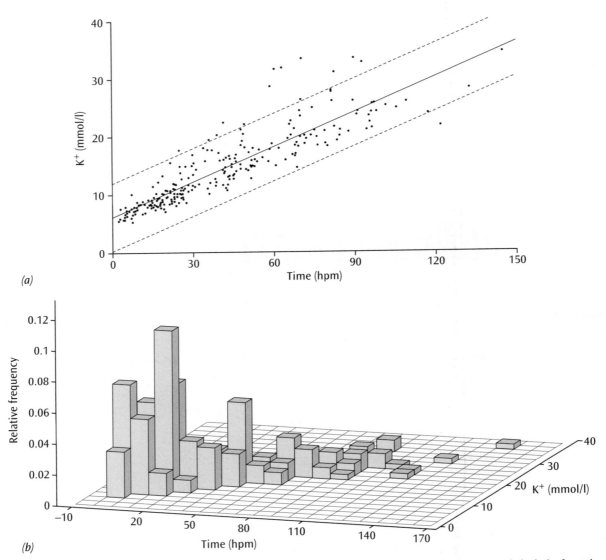

Figure 4.11 (a) *Potassium value (mean value) of 270 cases plotted against time since death. This entire sample includes forensic and hospital cases.* (b) *Two-dimensional distribution of K⁺ values and PMI.*

Table 4.6 *Urea as internal standard. Statistical parameters of the entire sample and the subgroups*

		Urea as internal standard			
		Urea < 100 mg/dl	Change (%)	Urea < 70 mg/dl	Change (%)
n	270 (170)	228 (138)	−15.5	206	23.7
Intercept	6.10 (5.99)	6.02 (5.88)	−1.3	5.92	−2.9
Slope	0.20 (0.2033)	0.18 (0.1877)	−10	0.18	−10.0
Correlation coefficient	0.89 (0.86)	0.91 (0.89)	+2.2	0.93	+4.5
Variance s^2_{yx}	8.57	5.09	−40.6	4.09	−47.7
Standard deviation s_{yx}	2.93 (3.42)	2.25 (2.62)	−23.2	2.02	−31.0
95% limits of confidence (h)	±25.51 h (±34)	±21.78 h (±22)	−14.6	±20.4 h	−21.3

The data in parentheses are from Madea *et al.*[34]

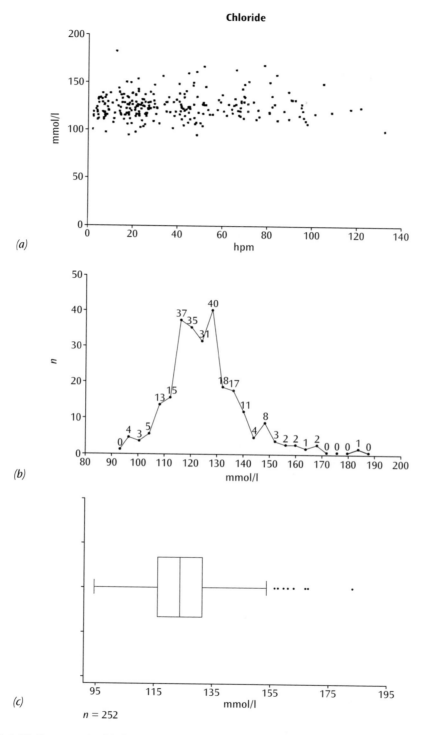

Figures 4.12–4.16 *Concentration* (a), *frequency distribution* (b) *of concentration and box plots* (c) *of chloride (figure 4.12), sodium (figure 4.13), calcium (figure 4.14), urea (figure 4.15) and creatinine (figure 4.16) concentration. The rectangular box contains 50% of all values found, marked by the upper and lower quartile. The box is divided by the median in two parts. The lines on the right and the left of the box correspond to the 90% confidence interval and the median. The distribution becomes evident from the box plots.*

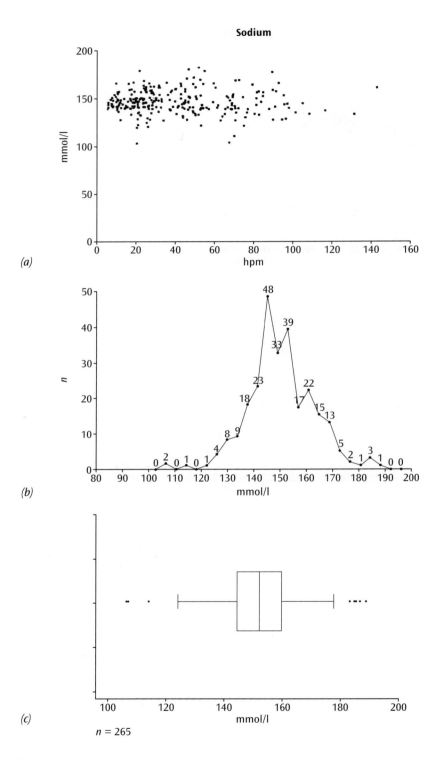

Figure 4.13

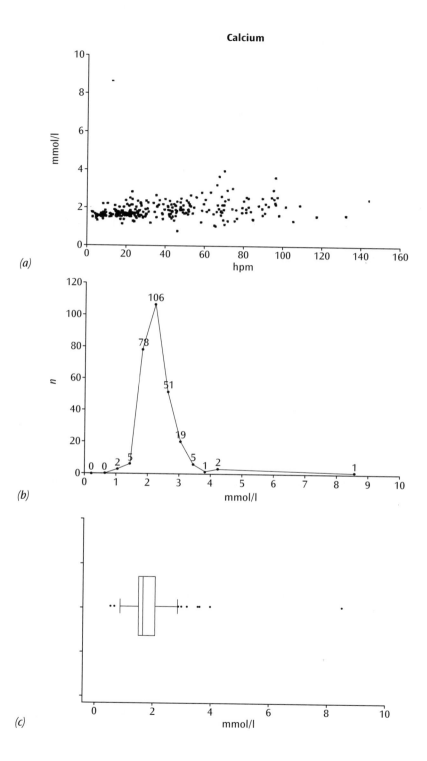

Figure 4.14

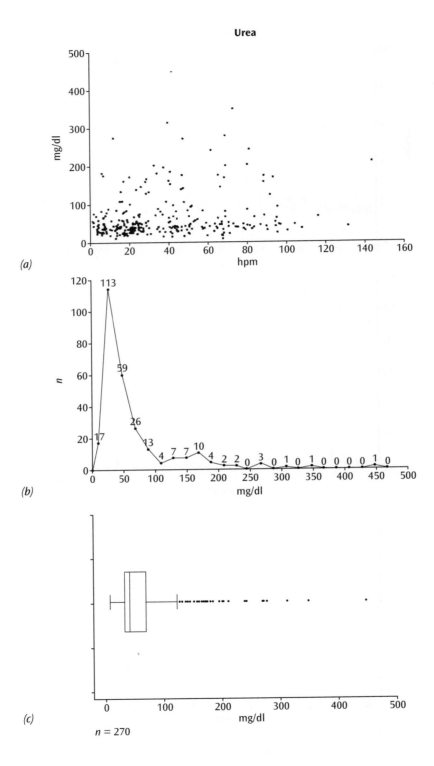

Urea

(a)

(b)

(c)

$n = 270$

Figure 4.15

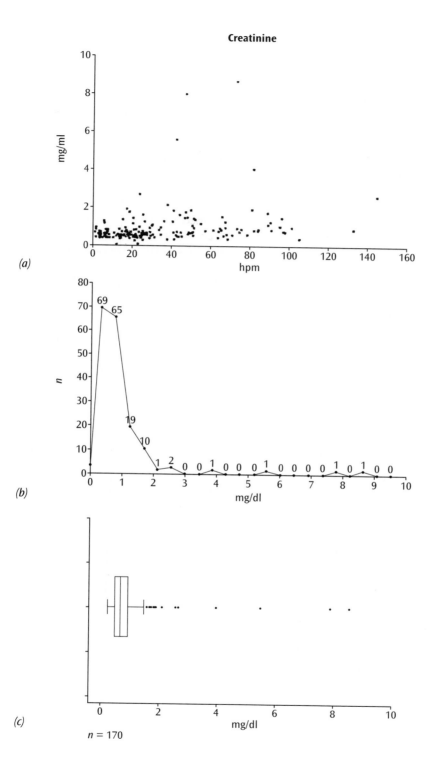

Figure 4.16

The difference in the values did not exceed 5 mg/dl, even in the cases with very long intervals between two samples. Thus, vitreous urea nitrogen (VUN) can be used as an internal standard, being stable postmortem and having a close relationship to electrolyte metabolism. In the next step, all cases having a VUN above 100 mg/dl were excluded from the entire group of potassium values in order to check whether, in this diminished random sample, there is a closer connection between potassium concentration and time since death. In 42 cases of the entire group there was vitreous urea nitrogen above 100 mg/dl (Table 4.6).

In the diminished group ($n = 228$), the intercept was 6.02 mmol/l and the slope 0.18 mmol/l per hour. The 95% limits of confidence up to 120 hours postmortem were reduced from ± 25.51 to ± 21.78 hours (Fig. 4.15).

The difference in the 95% limits of confidence of the entire group and the diminished sample is significant. All patients with a urea level above 100 mg/dl had suffered from chronic diseases. The different 95% limits of confidence in the entire group and the diminished group are in general in good accordance with Sturner's report,[19] which found that coroner cases of sudden and traumatic death have a better corre-lation between potassium concentration and time since death than hospital cases.

In a third step, we excluded all cases with urea values <70 mg/dl (Table 4.6; Fig. 4.16). However, the improvement in accuracy was not significant compared with the first step of elimination.

Creatinine as an internal standard

The value of creatinine as an internal standard was also checked. Creatinine and vitreous potassium were determined in 170 cases. Different creatinine values were chosen as a limiting value (Table 4.7). The comparison of urea and creatinine as an internal standard revealed that urea is the more sensitive (Table 4.7). The combination of limiting values for urea <70 mg/dl and creatinine <1 mg/dl reveals the most precise death-time estimation with 95% limits of confidence of ± 15 hours in the time interval up to 120 hours postmortem. Considering from our random sample only sudden traumatic deaths ($n = 71$), and excluding all cases with urea >70 mg/dl, reveals a significant reduction in the 95% limits of confidence from ± 22.34 to ± 17 hours (Table 4.8; Figs 4.17 and 4.18).

Table 4.7 *Creatinine as internal standard and creatinine compared with urea as internal standard in a random sample of 170 cases*

		Crea < 2 mg/dl	Crea < 1.5 mg/dl	Crea < 1.2 mg/dl	Crea < 1.0 mg/dl
Creatinine as internal standard					
n	170	163	154	142	133
Intercept	6.19	6.20	6.25	6.13	5.99
Slope	0.19	0.18	0.18	0.18	0.18
Correlation coefficient	0.93	0.94	0.94	0.95	0.95
Variance s^2_{yx}	4.39	3.37	3.20	2.79	1.62
Standard deviation s_{yx}	2.10	1.84	1.79	1.67	
95% limits of confidence (h)	±19.89	±18.08	±17.99	±16.94	±16.22

		Urea < 100 mg/dl	Urea < 70 mg/dl	Urea< 70 and Crea < 1 mg/dl
Urea as internal standard compared with creatinine				
n	170	146	135	127
Intercept	6.19	6.06	5.90	5.87
Slope	0.19	0.187	0.18	0.18
Correlation coefficient	0.93	0.95	0.96	0.96
Variance s^2_{yx}	4.39	2.58	2.25	2.22
Standard deviation s_{yx}	2.10	1.60	1.50	1.49
95% limits of confidence (h)	±19.89	±16.33	±15.22	±14.99

Crea = creatinine.

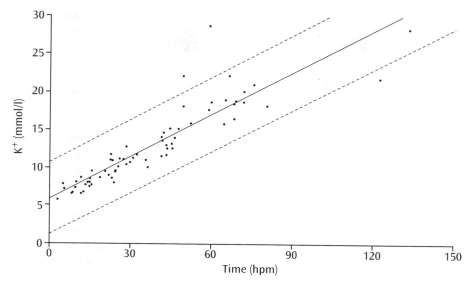

Figure 4.17 *Potassium values in cases of sudden traumatic death (*n = 71*).*

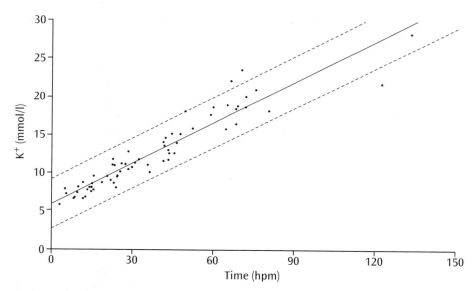

Figure 4.18 *Potassium values in cases of sudden traumatic death, elimination of all cases with urea values > 70 mg/dl. Significant rise in the precision of death-time estimation.*

Table 4.8 *Urea values < 70 mg/dl as internal standard in cases of sudden traumatic death*

	Entire sample	**Urea < 70 mg/dl**
n	71	68
Intercept	6.0	6.0
Slope	0.18	0.177
r	0.90	0.94
s^2_{yx}	5.341	2.528
95%	22.72	17.14

The result of these steps of elimination to obtain a closer relationship between potassium and time since death is that, by these means, a separation in cases with and without severe disturbances of metabolism is possible. Depending on the information obtained from the corpse – no other knowledge about health prior to death should be necessary – one can choose the reference for estimating time since death with different 95% limits of confidence (Tables 4.6–4.8). A limiting value for urea of 100 mg/dl – which has been chosen arbitrarily – seems to be sufficient to separate cases with and without disturbances of metabolism at the moment of death.

Our conclusion that vitreous urea nitrogen is the most suitable internal standard of disturbed homeo-stasis of electrolyte metabolism is confirmed by our augmented study.[34]

Recommendations for further studies

A number of internal and external factors have been identified which govern the postmortem rise of vitreous potassium. The rise of vitreous potassium in different temperature groups must be studied further to have reference material for casework. However, further studies on vitreous potassium, in our opinion, make sense only if the external and internal factors influencing the postmortem increase of K^+ are taken into consideration. For these studies, more case material is necessary to determine not only the effect of influencing factors but also to obtain useful statistical parameters for application in casework.

Rognum et al.[42] recently published a paper on the postmortem increase of vitreous hypoxanthine (Hx) in comparison with vitreous potassium; the vitreous humour was collected by repeated sampling. The scatter of the potassium values was greater than for Hx. However, our own preliminary studies give contrary results, with the scatter of levels for Hx being greater than for potassium.[49] Perhaps by combining both methods and performing multiple linear regres-sion analysis, the estimation of death-time can be improved.

Which formula should be used in casework?

Coe[18] asked in his recent historical review whether vitreous potassium could be considered to have any value for the forensic pathologist at the present time. He recommends the test, and we share his opinion. Vitreous potassium is of only limited value in estimat-ing the time since death in the first 24 hours post-mortem because other methods (body cooling, electrical excitability of skeletal muscle, chemical excitability of the iris) work quite satisfactorily in this postmortem period, but the value of vitreous potas-sium may increase with increasing PMI, especially when the body has lain in a low to moderate environ-

mental temperature. However, Coe proposes as the simplest procedure the well-known equation developed by Sturner:

$$PMI = 7.14 \times K^+ \text{ concentration} - 39.1$$

Although the slope in Sturner's material is the flat-test reported in the literature (see Table 4.2), Coe states that results obtained from this formula are most satisfactory when the ambient temperature in which the body has lain is below 50°F, and emphasizes that results even under these conditions may be quite inexact. The 95% limits of confidence will be much greater than ± 4 hours in the first day, and will increase with increasing PMI. However, clear values for the precision of estimating the time since death (95% limits of confidence) using the Sturner formula are lacking. Madea et al.[45] compared the suitability and precision of death-time estimation using the Sturner formula, compared with their own equation with a much steeper slope (Fig. 4.19). In 100 cases, mostly sudden traumatic or natural death with a short terminal episode and an ambient temperature below 50°F, the time since death was extrapolated using both the Sturner formula:

$$PMI = 7.14 \times K^+ \text{ concentration} - 39.1$$

and our own formula:

$$PMI = 5.26 \times K^+ \text{ concentration} - 30.9$$

From the deviation between real and extrapolated time since death, statistical parameters of precision of death-time estimation were calculated. In a second step, we calculated the time since death for all cases in our random sample ($n = 270$) with a postmortem interval over 30 hours and an urea value below 100 mg/dl ($n = 109$) using Sturner's equation. This random sample is comparable to Sturner's material, in respect of cause and mode of death. Using the Sturner equation there is a systematic deviation between real and extrapolated time since death (Fig. 4.20; Table 4.9). The mean difference between real and extrapo-lated time since death is 15 hours in the group of 100 cases compared with only –0.26 hours using our own equation. In the group of cases with a postmortem interval over 30 hours and with urea values below 100 mg/dl, the mean difference (x) rises to 26 hours and the 95% limits of confidence to ± 41 hours (Fig. 4.21; Table 4.10). This means that they cover nearly the whole investigated postmortem interval. The systematic over-estimation of the time since death using Sturner's equation was expected: the reason is

Table 4.9 *Mean differences ($\bar{x}$), standard deviation (s) and 95% limits of confidence (in hours) between real and extrapolated time since death for 100 independent cases in the postmortem interval from 3 to 100 h postmortem, using Sturner's, and the authors' own, equations for extrapolating the time since death*

	Sturner's equation	Authors' equation
n	100	100
$\bar{x}$	15.35	−0.258
s	±16.43	±0.56
95%	±32.76	±19.06

Table 4.10 *Mean difference ($\bar{x}$), standard deviation (s) and 95% limits of confidence (in hours) between real and extrapolated time since death for 109 cases with a postmortem interval of over 30 h and a vitreous urea value below 100 mg/dl*

	Sturner's equation
n	109
	PMI > 30 h
	Urea < 100 mg/dl
$\bar{x}$	26.68
s	±20.88
95%	±40.92

the flat slope (Fig. 4.19). Nearly all studies with a larger case material reveal a much steeper slope between 0.17 and 0.238 mmol/l per hour. Therefore, when using vitreous potassium to estimate the time since death, equations with a steeper slope than that reported by Sturner should be preferred to avoid systematic over-estimations of the time since death.

Estimating the time since death with a slope of 0.19 mmol/l per hour and an intercept of 5.88 mmol/l (which is almost the same as the intercept calculated from Sturner's material of 5.96 mmol/l) provides an estimation of the time since death with no systematic deviations. The 95% limits of confidence are ± 20 hours up to 100 hours postmortem.

Re-analysis of original data and construction of a local regression model

Lange *et al.*[61] re-analysed the data of six studies on the rise of vitreous potassium[4,19,22,24,27,34] comprising altogether 790 cases. This re-analysis revealed that:

- the relationship between vitreous potassium and PMI is not completely linear; and
- the residual variability of vitreous potassium as a function of PMI is not constant.

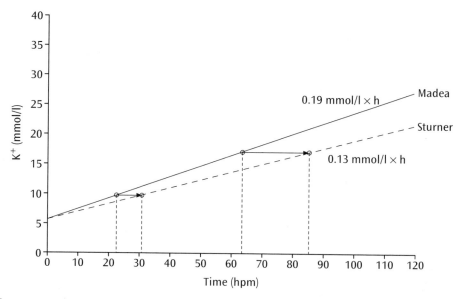

Figure 4.19 *Vitreous potassium over the postmortem interval (in hours). Regression lines of Sturner and of the authors' own material. The intercept of both regression lines is nearly identical but the slope varies between 0.13 mmol/l per hour (Sturner) and 0.19 mmol/l per hour (authors' material). The much flatter slope of Sturner's regression for the same potassium values causes a systematic over-estimation of the time since death compared with the authors' regression. This over-estimation increases with increasing postmortem interval.*

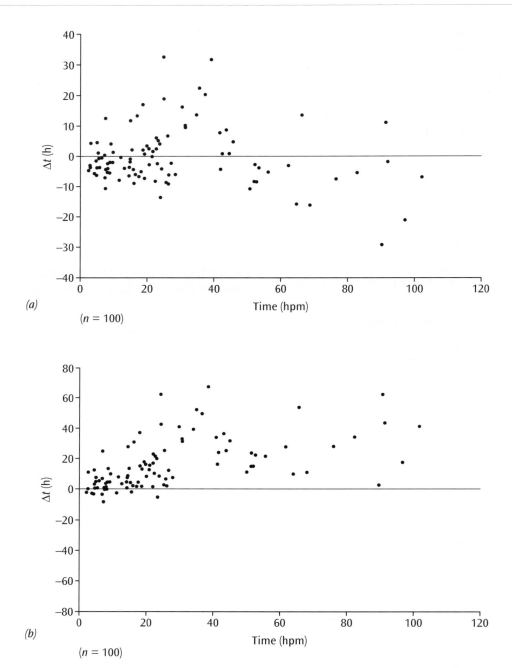

Figure 4.20 *Deviations between extrapolated and real time since death (Δt in hours) over the postmortem interval for 100 independent cases in the postmortem interval from 3 to 100 hpm. Deviations using the authors' formula (a); no systematic deviations. Deviations using the Sturner equation: systematic over-estimation of the time since death (b).*

Therefore, they developed a new approach for modelling vitreous potassium and PMI that accommodates non-linearities and changing residual variability. At first, a local regression model – specifically a loess smooth curve – is fitted separately to the

data from each of the six studies. The data of all six studies were then combined to yield a single loess curve with 95% confidence limits (Fig. 4.22).

The estimated loess curve and confidence limits were then used in an inverse prediction method to

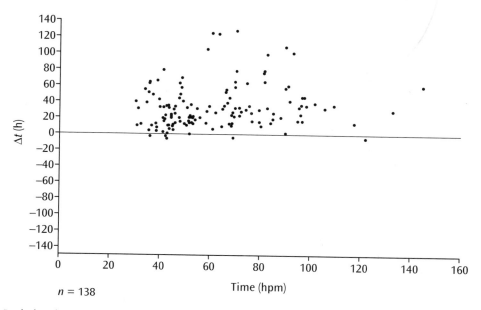

Figure 4.21 *Deviations between real and estimated time since death over the postmortem interval in hours for 109 cases with a postmortem interval over 30 hours and vitreous urea values between 100 mg/dl. Extrapolation of the time since death with Sturner's equation.*

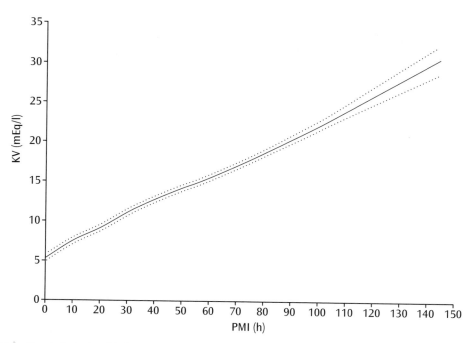

Figure 4.22 *The estimated relationship between vitreous potassium and PMI for six studies, with 95% lower and upper confidence bands. From Lange et al.[61]*

construct low, middle and high PMI estimates at given values of vitreous potassium (Table 4.11).

The reliability of estimated PMI decreases with increasing potassium concentration. However, PMI estimates are more precise over the entire range of vitreous potassium and PMI than those obtained from any single study alone. For potassium values <7 mmol/l, the extent of the lower and upper 95% confidence limits is ± 1 hour. For potassium values >7 mmol/l but <12 mmol/l, the extent of these confidence limits is ± 2 hours. For a potassium value >12 mmol/l and <18 mmol/l the extent is ± 3 hours, while for a value >18 mmol/l the extent is ± 5 hours. For concentrations >18 mmol/l the extent is even greater.

However, due to the much greater variability of the single potassium concentrations of the included studies from the 'single loess curve' with its 95% confidence limits, the reliability of the statistical evaluation remains unclear. Obviously, the 95% confidence limits concern the 'single loess curve', and not the deviations of the single values from the 'single loess curve'. Therefore, application of the proposed method may be very restricted and cannot be recommended for practical casework.

Multiple linear regression analysis

Multiple linear regression analysis uses, besides vitreous potassium, further time-dependent changing vitreous analytes. By using the multiple linear regression formula:

$$PMI = 24.64 + (4.3741 \times K^+) - (0.278 \times Na^+) - (0.065 \times urea) - (1.08 \times \log glucose)$$

95% confidence limits of ± 14 hours could be achieved (Fig. 4.23). Using potassium alone, the 95% confidence limits on the same sample ($n = 85$) were ± 16.2 hours. Therefore, it can be concluded that, by using multiple linear regression analysis, a slight increase can be achieved in the precision of death time estimation.

Table 4.11 *Estimated values of postmortem interval for various increasing values of potassium obtained through combining all 790 cases and the loess procedure*

Measured vitreous potassium concentration (mm/l)	Estimated potassium interval (h)		
	Lower 95% value	Mean value	Upper 95% value
5.9	2	3	4
6.4	3	5	6
7.0	6	7	8
7.5	8	10	12
8.0	11	13	15
8.5	14	16	19
9.1	18	21	22
10.1	23	25	27
11.1	29	30	32
12.1	33	35	38
13.0	39	41	44
13.9	44	47	50
14.9	51	54	57
15.9	58	61	64
17.0	66	69	72
18.3	74	77	81
19.7	81	85	90
21.1	89	94	100
22.6	98	103	111
24.2	106	113	123

From Lange *et al.*[61]

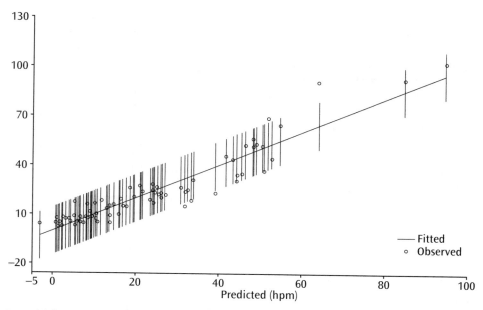

Figure 4.23 *By multiple regression analysis calculated time since death over the real time since death. The vertical lines represent the 95% limits of confidence.*

REFERENCES

1 Schleyer F. *Postmortale klinisch-chemische Diagnostik und Todeszeitbestimmung mit chemischen und physikalischen Methoden.* Stuttgart, Thieme Verlag, 1958.

2 Schleyer F. Determination of the time since death in the early postmortem interval. In: *Methods of Forensic Science*, Vol. II (Lundquist F, ed.). New York: Interscience Publishers, John Wiley and Sons, 1963: 253–93.

3 Schleyer F. Neuere Erkenntnisse über agonale und früh-postmortale chemische Vorgänge in den Körperflüssigkeiten. *Dtsch. Z. ges. Gerichtl. Med.* 1967; **59**: 48–57.

4 Coe JI. Postmortem chemistries on vitreous humour. *Am. J. Path.* 1969; **51**: 741–50.

5 Coe JI. Further thoughts and observations on post-mortem chemistries. *Forensic. Sci. Gaz.* 1973; **5**: 2–6.

6 Coe JI. Postmortem chemistries on blood with particular reference to urea nitrogen, electrolytes and bilirubin. *J. Forensic Sci.* 1974; **19**: 33–42.

7 Coe JI. Postmortem chemistry: Practical consideration and a review of the literature. *J. Forensic Sci.* 1974; **19**: 13–42.

8 Coe JI. Postmortem chemistry of blood, cerebrospinal fluid and vitreous humour. In: *Legal Medicine Annual* (Wecht CH, ed.). New York: Appleton-Century-Crofts, 1976: 53–91.

9 Coe JI. *Definition and Time of Death; Modern Legal Medicine, Psychiatry and Forensic Science.* Philadelphia, FA Davis Company, 1980.

10 Coe JI. Postmortem biochemistry of blood and vitreous humour in pediatric practice. In: *Pediatric Forensic Medicine and Pathology* (Mason JK, ed.). London: Chapman & Hall Medical, 1989: 191–203.

11 Harper DR. A comparative study of the microbiological contamination of postmortem blood and vitreous humour samples taken for ethanol determination. *Forensic Sci. Int.* 1989; **43**: 37–44.

12 Wurster U, Hoffmann K. Glaskörper. In: *Biochemie des Auges* (Hockwin O, ed.). Stuttgart: Enke, 1985: 100–34.

13 Balazs EA, Denlinger JL. The vitreous. In: *The Eye*, Vol. 1a, 3rd edition. Herausgeber: Hugh Dawson, 1984: 533–89.

14 Berman ER, Voaden M. The vitreous body. In: *Biochemistry of the Eye* (Graymore CN, ed.). London: Academic Press, 1970: 373–471.

15 Bito LZ. Intraocular fluid dynamics I: Steady state concentration gradients of magnesium, potassium and calcium in relation to the sites and mechanisms of ocular cation transport processes. *Exp. Eye Res.* 1970; **10**: 102–16.

16 Bito LZ. The physiology and pathophysiology of intraocular fluids. In: *The Ocular and Cerebrospinal Fluids* (Bito LZ, Davson H, Fenstermacher JD, eds.). London: Academic Press, 1977: 273–89.

17 Pau H. Betrachtungen zur Physiologie und Pathologie des Glaskörpers. *Graefes Arch. Ophthalmol.* 1951; **152**: 201–47.

18 Coe JI. Vitreous potassium as a measure of the post-mortem interval: an historical review and critical evaluation. *Forensic Sci. Int.* 1989; **42**: 201–13.

19 Sturner WQ. The vitreous humour; postmortem potassium changes. *Lancet* 1963; **i**: 807–8.

20 Sturner WQ. Die gerichtmedizinische Bedeutung der Glaskörperflüssigkeit. In: *Aktuelle Fragen der gerichtlichen Medizin II.* (Vamosi M, ed.). Wissensch. Beitr. Univ. Halle-Wittenberg, 1965: 57–62.

21 Sturner WQ, Gantner GE. The postmortem interval, a study of potassium in the vitreous humour. *Am. J. Clin. Path.* 1964; **42**: 137–44.

22 Adelson L, Sunshine I, Norman B, Rushford PhD, Marnkoff M. Vitreous potassium concentration as an indicator of postmortem interval. *J. Forensic Sci.* 1963; **8**: 503–14.

23 Hansson LMA, Uotila U, Lindfors R, Laiho K. Potassium content of the vitreous body as an aid in determining the time of death. *J. Forensic Sci.* 1966; **11**: 390–4.

24 Hughes W. Levels of potassium in the vitreous humour after death. *Med. Sci. Law* 1965; **150**: 150–6.

25 Klein A, Klein S. *Todeszeitbestimmung am menschlichen Auge.* Dresden University: MD Thesis, 1978.

26 Krause D, Klein A, Meissner D, Roitzsch E, Herrmann WR. Die Bedeutung der Kaliumkonzentration im Glaskörper menschlicher Augen für die Todeszeitbestimmung. *Zschr. ärztl. Fortbildung* 1971; **65**: 345–8.

27 Stegmaier K. *Untersuchungen über die postmortale Kaliumkonzentration in Glaskörperinhalt und Kammerwasser und ihre Beziehung zur Todeszeit.* Marburg University: MD Thesis, 1971.

28 Stephens RJ, Richards RG. Vitreous humour chemistry: the use of potassium concentration for the prediction of the postmortem interval. *J. Forensic Sci.* 1987; **32**: 503–9.

29 Montalo B, Umani Ronchi G, Marchiori A, Forgeschi M, Barbato M. La determinatione della concentrazione del potassio nel'umor vitreo: verifica di un methodo strumentale tanatocronologico. *Riv. Ital. Med. Leg.* 1989; **11**: 180–99.

30 Gamero JJ, Romero JL, Arufe MI, Vizcaya MA. Incremento de la concentracion de potassio en humour vitreo en funcion del tiempo postmortem. *Riv. Ital. Med. Leg.* 1990; **12**: 785–801.

31 Leahy MS, Farber R. Postmortem chemistry of human vitreous humour. *J. Forensic Sci.* 1967; **12**: 214–22.

32 Martchenko HP. Veränderungen des Kaliumgehaltes der Glaskörperflüssigkeit in Abhängigkeit von der Todeszeit. Ref 7. *Gerichtl. Med.* 1966; **61**: 295.

33 Adjutantis G, Coutselinis A. Estimation of the time of death by potassium levels in the vitreous humour. *Forensic Sci. Int.* 1972; **1**: 55–60.

34 Madea B, Henssge C, Honig W, Gerbracht A. References for determining the time of death by potassium in vitreous humour. *Forensic Sci. Int.* 1989; **8**: 231–43.

35 Madea B, Henssge C, Staak M. Postmortaler Kaliumanstieg in Glaskörperflüssigkeit: Welche Parameter sind als Indikatoren einer vitalen agonalen Elektrolytdysregulation geeignet? *Z. Rechtsmed.* 1986; **97**: 259–68.

36 Komura S, Oshiro S. Potassium levels in the aqueous and vitreous humour after death. *Tohoku J. Exp. Med.* 1977; **122**: 65–8.

37 Schoning O, Strafuss AC. Determining time of death of a dog by analysing blood, cerebrospinal fluid and vitreous humour collected postmortem. *Am. J. Vet. Res.* 1980; **41**: 955–7.

38 Schoning P, Strafuss AC. Postmortem biochemical changes in canine cerebrospinal fluid. *J. Forensic Sci.* 1980; **25**: 60–6.

39 Schoning P, Strafuss AC. Postmortem biochemical changes in canine vitreous humour. *J. Forensic Sci.* 1980; **25**: 53–9.

40 Bray M. The eye as a chemical indicator of environmental temperature at the time of death. *J. Forensic Sci.* 1984; **29**: 396–403.

41 Bray M. The effect of chilling, freezing and rewarming on the postmortem chemistry of vitreous humour. *J. Forensic Sci.* 1984; **29**: 404–11.

42 Rognum TO, Hauge S, Oyasaeter S, Saugstrad OD. A new biochemical method for estimation of postmortem time. *Forensic Sci. Int.* 1991; **51**: 139–46.

43 Sturner WQ, Dowdey ABC, Putman RS, Dempsey JL. Osmolality and other chemical determinations in postmortem human vitreous humour. *J. Forensic Sci.* 1972; **18**: 387–93.

44 Coe JI. Variations in vitreous humour chemical values as a result of instrumentation. *J. Forensic. Sci.* 1985; **30**: 828–35.

45 Madea B, Herrmann N, Henssge C. Precision of estimating the time since death by vitreous potassium – comparison of two different equations. *Forensic Sci. Int.* 1990; **46**: 277–84.

46 Gutman I, Bergmeyer HU. *Methods of Enzymatic Analysis, Vol. IV,* 2nd edition. New York: Academic Press, 1974: 1794.

47 Bartels H, Böhmer M, Heirli C. Serum-Kreatinin-Bestimmung ohne Enteiweissung. *Clin. Chim. Acta* 1972; **37**: 193–7.

48 Balasooriya BAW, Hill CAS, Williams AR. The biochemistry of vitreous humour. A comparative study of the potassium, sodium and urate concentration in the eyes at identical time intervals after death. *Forensic Sci. Int.* 1984; **26**: 85–91.

49 Schleyer F. Wie zuverlässig ist die Kaliumbestimmung im Glaskörperinhalt als Mittel zur Todeszeitschätzung? *Z. Rechtsmed.* 1973; **71**: 281–8.

50 Henry JB, Smith FA. Estimation of the postmortem interval by chemical means. *Am. J. Forensic Med. Path.* 1980; **1**: 341–7.

51 Madea B, Käferstein H, Hermann N, Sticht G. Hypoxanthine in vitreous humour and cerebrospinal fluid – a marker of postmortem interval and prolonged (vital) hypoxia? Remarks also as hypoxanthine in SIDS. *Forensic Sci. Int.* 1994; **65**: 19–31.

52 Blumenfeld TA, Mantell CH, Catherman RL, Blanc WA. Postmortem vitreous humour chemistry in sudden infant death syndrome and in other causes of death in childhood. *Am. J. Clin. Path.* 1979; **71**: 219–23.

53 Jaffe FA. Chemical postmortem changes in the intraocular fluid. *J. Forensic Sci.* 1962; **7**: 231–7.

54 Lie JT. Changes of potassium concentration in vitreous humour after death. *Am. J. Med. Sci.* 1967; **254**: 136–42.

55 Foerch JS, Forman DT, Vye MV. Measurement of potassium in vitreous humour as an indication of the postmortem interval. *Am. J. Clin. Path.* 1979; **72**: 651–62.

56 Forman DT, Butts J. Electrolytes of the vitreous humour as a measure of the postmortem interval. *Clin. Chem.* 1980; **26**: 1024.

57 Choo-Kang E, McKoy C, Escoffrey C. Vitreous humour analytes in assessing the postmortem interval and the antemortem clinical status. *Wiss. Med. J.* 1983; **32**: 23–6.

58 Farmer JG, Benomran F, Watson AA, Harland WA. Magnesium, potassium, sodium and calcium in postmortem vitreous humour from humans. *Forensic Sci. Int.* 1985; **27**: 1–13.

59 Sparks DL, Oeltgen PR, Kryscio RJ, Hunsaker JC, III. Comparison of chemical methods for determining the postmortem interval. *J. Forensic Sci.* 1989; **34**: 197–206.

60 Schmidt V. Postmortale Elektrolytbestimmungen in Glaskörperflüssigkeiten und Liquor zur Todeszeitbestimmung. Med Diss, Hamburg, 1988.

61 Lange N, Swearer ST, Sturner WQ. Human postmortem interval estimation from vitreous potassium: an analysis of original data from six different studies. *Forensic Sci. Int.* 1994; **66**: 159–74.

HYPOXANTHINE ('Hx')

Elevated Hx-values due to tissue hypoxia have been demonstrated by several authors in different body fluids (plasma, urine, CSF, fetal scalp blood)[1–17] These elevated Hx-values are thought to be a good marker of hypoxia, mainly in paediatric cases.[3,4,6–9,12,16,17] The increase of Hx during hypoxia was thought to be due to the following three mechanisms:

1. An increased concentration of cellular AMP.
2. A decreased transformation of Hx into uric acid.
3. Inhibition of xanthine oxidase (Fig. 4.24).

In 1957, Praetorius *et al.*[12] reported a postmortem rise of Hx in CSF, and there are some reports on postmortem elevation in skeletal muscle as an aid in estimating the time since death. A recent study[13] on a new biochemical method for estimation of postmortem time on 87 cases revealed:

- a linear rise of Hx in vitreous humour in the postmortem interval up to 120 hours postmortem (HPM);
- a dependence of the slope of rise of vitreous Hx on temperature (the higher the ambient temperature, the steeper the slope);
- a strong correlation between vitreous Hx and vitreous potassium values; and
- a smaller range of scatter of the vitreous hypoxanthine than the vitreous potassium values.

These results are based on 368 vitreous samples taken from 87 cases; two samples were taken from each eye, and four values per case were obtained.

The authors suggested further investigations on vitreous Hx in comparison with vitreous K^+. These are indeed necessary as there are no statistical parameters on the precision of death-time estimation by vitreous Hx compared with vitreous K^+.

Materials and methods

Our own investigations[5] were performed on 92 bodies with a known time since death. Each globe was punctured only once, and the whole vitreous humour was withdrawn. Each sample was analysed independently. In these 92 cases, the vitreous humour of both eyes was withdrawn at the same time postmortem.

In an additional 43 cases, vitreous humour of both eyes was withdrawn at timed intervals, ranging from 2 to 20 hours after death. The CSF samples were

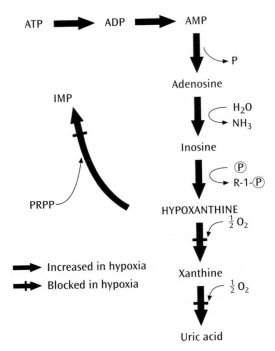

Figure 4.24 *Cellular mechanisms for the increase in hypoxanthine concentration during hypoxia. (From Saugstad.[16])*

obtained by single puncture of the cisterna cerebellomedullaris.

The cases used for this study were all adults who had died either from sudden natural causes with a brief terminal episode, or from traumatic causes with a brief terminal episode.

The potassium concentration was determined using ion-selective electrodes, and the Hx concentration using a HPLC-method analogous to that of Rognum *et al.*[13]

Results and discussion

VITREOUS HUMOUR

The vitreous samples of both eyes taken at the same time postmortem showed a good correspondence of Hx and K^+ values. For statistical analysis, the mean values of the K^+ and Hx concentrations of both eyes were used.

Hx increased in a linear fashion over the PMI, the linear rise beginning immediately postmortem rather than after a certain 'stable interval' of some 48 to 72 hours as originally described[17] (Fig. 4.25). This immediate postmortem rise of Hx concentration is in good accordance with experimental animal findings of Gardiner *et al.*[2] and the recent findings of Rognum and co-workers.[13]

The K^+ concentration increases linearly, as has long been known (Fig. 4.26), and has a much stronger correlation with the time since death than the Hx concentration (correlation coefficient $r = 0.925$ for K^+ compared with $r = 0.714$ for Hx), the 95% confidence limits are ± 17 hours for vitreous potassium and ± 32 hours for vitreous Hx (Table 4.12).

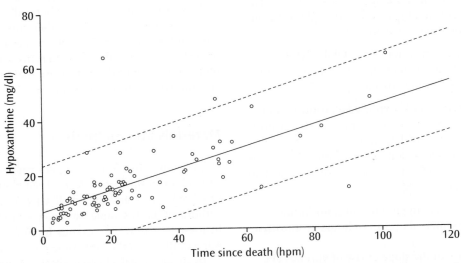

Figure 4.25 *Hypoxanthine (Hx) concentration in vitreous humour over the time since death (hours postmortem, hpm), with 95% confidence limits.*

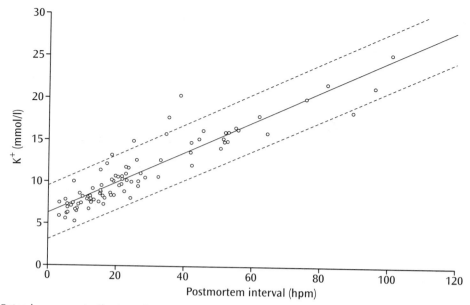

Figure 4.26 *Potassium concentration over the postmortem interval (hpm), with 95% confidence limits.*

The conclusion of Rognum *et al.*[13] that the scatter of levels is greater for potassium than for Hx, cannot be confirmed on our own material.

In cases with timed bilateral withdrawal of vitreous humour (interval from 2 to 20 hours), there are great interindividual differences in the rise of Hx concentrations. As is already known for vitreous potassium, there may be greater differences between the concentration in both eyes, even when samples are withdrawn at the same time. This is also true for the Hx concentration. Indeed, if there are greater differences between both eyes, the later sample may have an even lower Hx concentration than the earlier.

The differences between the results from our study[5]

Table 4.12 *Statistical parameters on the precision of estimating postmortem interval by vitreous hypoxanthine (Hx) and K[+]*

	Hx	Potassium
n	92	92
r	0.7138	0.925
a	3.6991	6.3177
b	1.293	0.179
95%	±30.1	±16.3

n, number of cases; *r*, correlation coefficient; *a, b*, regression parameters for slope and intercept; *95%*, 95% confidence limits in hours.

and those of Rognum and co-workers[13] on vitreous Hx and K[+] are apparent. However, as we have used similar methods and the random samples consisted of comparable cases, an explanation for this discrepancy is not straightforward. One reason may be seen in the repeated sample-taking with disturbance of the vitreous concentration gradient. During life there are, in mammalian eyes, concentration gradients for several parameters between different intraocular fluid compartments. After death, new gradients are established, mainly between the retina and the centre of the globe. Therefore, for biochemical analysis it is mandatory to aspirate the whole of the vitreous humour. Repeated sample-taking will disturb the diffusion gradient and establish a drainage effect, as has already been described by Schourup[18] and Dotzauer and Naeve[1] in their studies on CSF.[1,18]

Rognum and Saugstad[14] seemed to be aware of this drainage effect in another study on vitreous Hx-values in sudden infant death syndrome (SIDS) cases. Although each globe was punctured twice, the Hx-values of the second sample were found to be too high. These authors reported that, 'Multiple sampling during hypoxaemia was attempted, but this procedure led to artificially high values of hypoxanthine compared with control values from the left eye ... and the procedure had to be abandoned'.[10] These authors added that, 'Furthermore, in the group in which sampling was started early after death, there was a slight tendency for the Hx increase to be greater at the second sampling within the same eye. This increase could be attributable to a certain degree of tissue mutilation during the sample procedure'.

A second possible reason for the different results may be the fact that Hx not only increases postmortem in vitreous humour and CSF due to irreversible circulatory arrest, anoxaemia and diffusion, but also that already during vital hypoxia, 'there is an accelerated catabolism of adenosine monophosphate to hypoxanthine which accumulates in tissue and body fluids.'

In 1975, increased levels of plasma Hx were reported in newborn infants with clinical signs of intrauterine hypoxia during labour, compared with newborn infants after normal delivery. These increased values were interpreted as being due to hypoxia, and the Hx accumulation in plasma was seen as a sensitive parameter of hypoxia.

The increase in Hx levels in different body fluids has been confirmed by several groups. The vital elevation due to hypoxia is a factor of about 2.5 to 5, but is seldom 10 or more. Compared with this vital elevation, the postmortem rise has a 66-fold increase,[2] which is much more marked. However, if hypoxia during life causes a marked increase in vitreous Hx, this of course may result in a greater scatter of postmortem Hx values than of potassium values.

The postmortem rise of vitreous K^+ is mainly due to diffusion from the retina into the centre of the globe, while Hx is a postmortem degradation product of adenine nucleotide metabolism. Hx is formed by the action of several enzymatic reactions (see Fig. 4.24) and then diffuses along the concentration gradient. In theory, it might be expected that a parameter such as a postmortem increase which is solely due to diffusion would correlate much more strongly with time since death than would a parameter that increases due to vital/postmortem degradation and diffusion.

In CSF, there is an exponential rise in Hx concentration, with the steepest slope during the first 15 hours postmortem (Fig. 4.27). This steep rise during the early PMI is apparent from the results of Praetorius et al.,[12] who found a more than 100-fold increase in Hx and xanthine values in CSF during the time interval up to 36 hours postmortem.

Manzke et al.[24] observed no significant differences in the oxypurine concentration of CSF samples during the first three days postmortem (the samples were reserved during autopsy), but these authors clearly obtained their samples too late. Immediately after death, a rapid and marked rise of Hx in CSF occurs, and an equilibration seems to be achieved after about 20 hours. An exponential rise has also been reported in CSF potassium levels. Among several other components of CSF examined by Schourup,[18] the steepest rise occurs within the first few hours postmortem, and equilibration is achieved after about 15 hours.

The mean normal value for CSF Hx in newborn

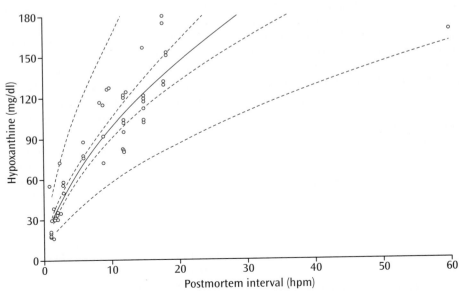

Figure 4.27 *Increase of hypoxanthine (Hx) in cerebrospinal fluid (CSF) over various postmortem intervals. An equilibration is achieved after 15–20 hours postmortem (hpm).*

infants was found to be 3.6 (range: 1.8–5.5) μmol/l, while that in adults was 1.8 (range: 0.6–5.1) μmol/l.[3,4]

Compared with the rise in Hx in CSF that occurs as a consequence of hypoxia, the postmortem rise and the postmortem Hx levels are much more marked. Neither CSF potassium nor CSF Hx concentrations can be recommended for practical use in death time estimation as the 95% confidence limits are wide, and also increase with increasing PMI. Other methods function satisfactorily during this early PMI, for up to 20 hours.

REFERENCES

1 Dotzauer G, Naeve W. Vergleichende Untersuchungen über den Natrium- und Kaliumgehalt im Serum wie im Liquor postmortem. *Dtsch. Z. Gerichtl. Med.* 1960; **49**: 406–19.

2 Gardiner EE, Newberry RC, Keng JY. Postmortem time and storage temperature affect the concentrations of hypoxanthine, other purines, pyrimidines, and nucleosides in avian and porcine vitreous humor. *Pediatr. Res.* 1989; **26**: 639–42.

3 Harkness RA, Lund RJ. Cerebrospinal fluid concentrations of hypoxanthine, xanthine, uridine and inosine: high concentrations of the ATP metabolite, hypoxanthine, after hypoxia. *J. Clin. Pathol.* 1983; **36**: 1–8.

4 Harkness RA. Review: hypoxanthine, xanthine and uridine in body fluids. Indicators of ATP depletion. *J. Chromatogr.* 1988; **429**: 255–78.

5 Madea B, Käferstein H, Herrman N, Sticht G. Hypoxanthine in vitreous humor and cerebrospinal fluid – marker of postmortem interval and prolonged (vital) hypoxia? *Forensic Sci. Int.* 1994; **65**: 19–31.

6 Manzke H, Staemmler W. Oxypurine concentration in the CSF in children with different diseases of the nervous systems. *Neuropediatrics* 1981; **12**: 209–14.

7 Manzke H, Dörner K, Grünitz J. Urinary hypoxanthine, xanthine and uric acid excretion in newborn infants with perinatal complications. *Acta Paediatr. Scand.* 1977; **66**: 713–17.

8 Manzke H, Krämer M, Dörner K. Postmortem oxypurine concentrations in the CSF. In: *Purine and Pyrimidine Metabolism in Man. V. Festschrift for JE Seegmiller.* Nyhan WL, Thompson LF, Watts RWE (eds.). Plenum Press, New York, 1986; 587–91.

9 Meberg A, Saugstad OD. Hypoxanthine in cerebrospinal fluid in children. *Scand. J. Clin. Lab. Invest.* 1978; **38**: 437–40.

10 Poulsen JP, Rognum TO, Oyyasaeter S, Saugstad OD. Changes in oxypurine concentrations in vitreous humor of pigs during hypoxemia and postmortem. *Pediatr. Res.* 1990; **28**: 482–4.

11 Poulsen JP, Oyasaeter S, Rognum TO, Saugstad OD. Hypoxanthine, xanthine, and uric acid concentrations in the cerebrospinal fluid, plasma, and urine of hypoxemic pigs. *Pediatr. Res.* 1990; **28**: 477–81.

12 Praetorius E, Poulsen H, Dupont H. Uric acid, xanthine and hypoxanthine in the cerebrospinal fluid. *Scand. J. Clin. Lab. Invest.* 1957; **9**: 133–7.

13 Rognum TO, Hauge S, Oyasaeter S, Saugstad OD. A new biochemical method for estimation of postmortem time. *Forensic Sci. Int.* 1991; **51**: 139–46.

14 Rognum TO, Saugstad OD. Hypoxanthine levels in vitreous humor: evidence of hypoxia in most infants who died of Sudden Infant Death Syndrome. *Pediatrics* 1991; **87**: 306–10.

15 Rognum TO, Saugstad OD, Oyasaeter S, Olaysen B. Elevated levels of hypoxanthine in vitreous humor indicate prolonged cerebral hypoxia in victims of Sudden Infant Death Syndrome. *Pediatrics* 1988; **82**: 615–18.

16 Saugstad OD. Hypoxanthine as a measurement of hypoxia. *Pediatr. Res.* 1975; **9**: 158–61.

17 Saugstad OD, Olaisen B. Postmortem hypoxanthine levels in the vitreous humor. An introductory report. *Forensic Sci. Int.* 1978; **12**: 33–6.

18 Schourup K. Dodstidsbestemmelse pa grundlag of postmortelle cisternevaedskevorandringer og detpostmortelle temperaturfald. English Summary: Determination of the time since death. *Med. Diss. Kopenhagen, Danks Vindenskabs. Kobenhavn.*, 1950.

5

Muscle and tissue changes after death

BURKHARD MADEA, THOMAS KROMPECHER, BERNARD KNIGHT AND LEONARD NOKES

INTRODUCTION

As far as we know, the last review in the English literature on determination of the time since death in the early postmortem interval (dealing also in detail with supravital reactions) was published by Schleyer in 1963 in Volume II of Lundquist's *Methods of Forensic Science*. Since then, much work has been carried out on supravital reactions, and some progress has been made. This, and the fact that many scientific papers in this field have been published in German, may justify a new review on supravital reactions in English. Those supravital reactions which are of practical value in casework (mechanical excitability of skeletal muscle,

electrical excitability of skeletal muscle with a subjective grading of muscular contraction, chemical excitability of the iris) will be mentioned briefly again in Chapter 7.

The objective of this chapter is to present some basic considerations on supravitality, review the work on mechanical and electrical excitability of skeletal muscle and present some recent longitudinal studies on electrical excitability which have, until now, no practical value in casework but may be of some heuristic interest and may form the basis for future work on influencing factors. A complete summary on supravital reactions was published in German in 1988 by Henssge and Madea.[1]

Supravitality in tissues

BURKHARD MADEA

DEFINITIONS

Irreversible circulatory arrest is the starting point for a period of survival of some tissues under the condition of global ischaemia; this is called the 'supravital period' or 'intermediary life'.

Investigations on global ischaemia in various organs have been performed mainly with regard to the survival period and resuscitation period (Fig. 5.1).[2–10]

The *latency period* is defined as an undisturbed period characterized by continuing aerobic energy production.

The *survival period* is the interval up to the point after which every aspect of life ceases. During the survival period there is spontaneous activity of organs (e.g. spontaneous but decreasing myocardial contractility), also reagibility (e.g. the response of muscle to stimulation), on excitation (e.g. evoked potentials on acoustic stimulation, nerve action potentials on electrical stimulation of nerves).[11–17]

The *resuscitation period* is the duration of global ischaemia after which the ability to recover expires. The resuscitation period is mainly defined as the interval when complete recovery of morphological, functional and biochemical parameters in the post-ischaemic period is possible. The time required for the complete recovery of these parameters is the 'recovering time'. The latency period is limited by the oxygen reserve as the basis of aerobic energy production characterized biochemically by the exhaustion of creatinine phosphate and a small decrease of ATP. During the resuscitation period, there is a breakdown of ATP to below 60% of the normal value and a steep increase of lactic acid (Fig. 5.2).[10,18]

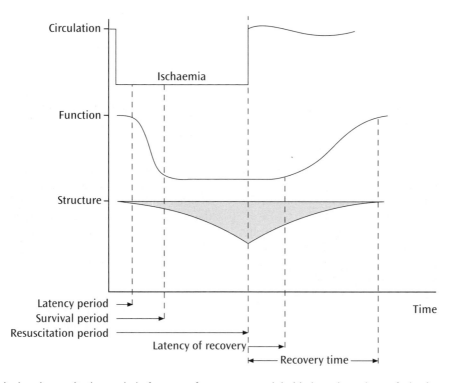

Figure 5.1 *Survival and resuscitation period of organs after temporary global ischaemia and reperfusion.*[9]

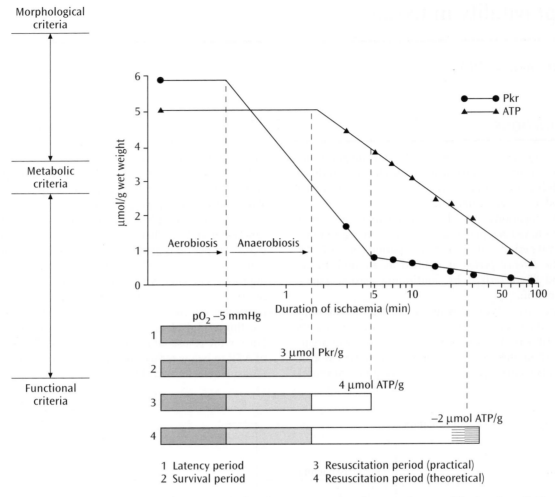

Figure 5.2 *Latency, survival and resuscitation period of the heart compared to the state of energy-rich phosphates.*[18] *Pkr, phosphocreatine.*

Ischaemia, resulting in cessation of nutrition and waste product removal, not only causes reversible consequences – 'effects' – but, after a longer duration, also results in irreversible changes – 'damage'.

The end of the resuscitation period demarcates both these steps of deficiency – reversible effects and irreversible damage.[2,4,5,8]

Although 'survival period' and 'resuscitation period' are terms of great importance in physiology, organ preservation and transplantation because they describe the maximal ischaemic damage which is completely reversible regarding structure and function, Forensic medicine is also interested in the subsequent period – that which is characterized by increasingly irreversible damage to structure and function.

While the definition of the resuscitation period of organs and tissues is based on the complete recovery of different functional and biochemical parameters in the post-ischaemic period, supravitality is mainly defined by reagibility on excitation in the ischaemic period itself, irrespective of whether the damage to function is reversible (Fig. 5.3).

As a result, the data on the duration of the resuscitation period on the one hand, and the supravital period on the other, are not comparable. The resuscitation period of skeletal muscle under normothermic conditions is 2 to 3 hours; supravital reagibility of skeletal muscle may be maintained in some cases for up to 20 hours postmortem.[19–22]

The resuscitation period of the heart under

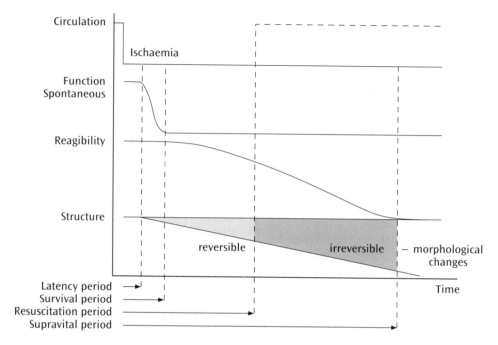

Figure 5.3 *Postmortem course of function (spontaneous function and reagibility) and structure after continuous global ischaemia (compare this with* Fig. 5.1*).*

normothermia is 3.5 to 4 minutes (without cardiac massage in the postischaemic period), but supravital electrical excitability of cardiac muscle, according to Raule *et al.*,[23] is preserved for up to 100 to 120 minutes postmortem.

One difference between the resuscitation and supravital periods is described by the 'reversibility/irreversibility' of damage. Another important difference is that physiologists and experimental surgeons are working on the restoration of the function of organs after ischaemic damage within an intact organ system, whereas forensic medicine is concerned with the function of tissues, since organ functions cannot be restored after irreversible loss of the function of the great systems and their coordination.

Supravitality is compared with the resuscitation period the longer the survival on a morphologically deeper step of organization. On a yet deeper step (the cell) reagibility of the myofibrils may be preserved even longer than in tissues.

Up to 104 days postmortem, muscle cells in frozen muscle pulp may react on ATP administration with a strong contraction, the weak contraction being finished after 5 minutes.[24]

SPONTANEOUS SUPRAVITAL ACTIVITY

These introductory definitions are not only of theoretical value but may also be of great practical importance, for instance in cases where spontaneous supravital activity is in question.

This can be illustrated by a short case history published in *Medicine, Science and the Law.*[25] A 78-year-old woman – cause of death spontaneous cerebral haemorrhage – displayed coordinated motor movements of the right lower limb, especially the right foot, for 2 hours postmortem. These motor movements were thought to be coordinated by the spinal cord, and are seen in analogy to movements of the decapitated chicken. However, this interpretation of the authors requires that, at 2 hours postmortem, spontaneous activity of the spinal cord and peripheral nerves is still preserved. According to all basic investigations on the supravital period and resuscitation period of spinal cord and nerves, spontaneous activity of spinal cord tissue is impossible 2 hours postmortem.[7,11,26, 27]

In my opinion, there was no spontaneous supravital activity; this was the spontaneous activity of a woman still alive but declared dead.

Supravital reagibility

From the definition of supravital reactions – beyond individual death obtainable vital reaction patterns of special tissues on proper excitations – it becomes evident that no fixed postmortem interval can be given for the supravital period.

The supravital period is specific for each tissue; it depends on the tissue-specific metabolism (enzymes, substrates) under the condition of global ischaemia. Within the same tissue, it depends on the topographical localization within the body (different cooling velocity at different sites of the body depending on the diameter). Lastly, the postmortem duration of supravital reagibility depends on the mode of excitation and recording of the reaction (Fig. 5.4). For instance, Popwassilew and Palm[28] reported the maximal duration of electrical excitability of the thenar muscles to be 5.5 hours postmortem, while in my own investigations, with different modes of excitation and by objectifying muscular contraction of thenar muscles, reactions could be obtained up to 13–15 hours postmortem (see page 173).

SUPRAVITAL METABOLISM

The basis of supravital reactions is the vital metabolism which, after death, runs down until substrates (e.g. glycogen) are exhausted or (and just as important) until

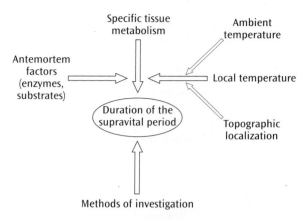

Figure 5.4 *Factors determining the time course of supravitality.*

reaction-limiting changes of the milieu interieur cease (for instance, cessation of anaerobic glycolysis at pH 6.3).

Postmortem anaerobic glycolytic metabolism proceeds at a high rate during the first 10 hours postmortem, but afterwards at a low rate. Correspondingly, lactic acid shows the steepest increase within the first 6 to 8 hours postmortem, as has been shown by Schourup[29] in the cerebrospinal fluid (Fig. 5.5). In contrast, the pH shows the steepest decrease in the same time interval (Fig. 5.6),[30] the decrease of the blood in the heart being steeper than

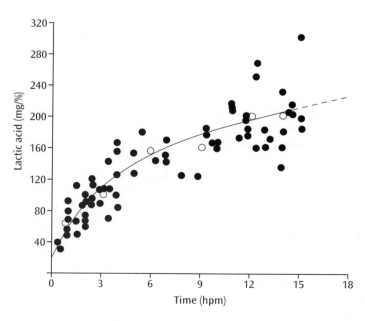

Figure 5.5 *Lactic acid in mg% of cerebrospinal fluid over the postmortem interval.* ● = *single values;* ○ = *mean values.*[29]

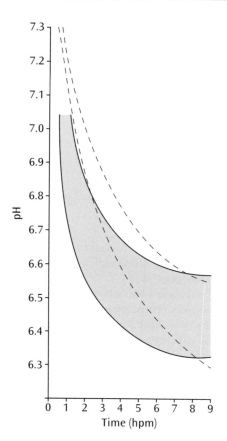

Figure 5.6 *pH of cerebrospinal fluid (---) and heart blood (shaded) in the first 9 hours postmortem.*[31]

that of the blood in the peripheral veins. This can be attributed to the higher glycogen content of heart muscle and to the different cooling velocity of central and peripheral measuring points, as has been shown by Dotzauer and Naeve.[30]

During the first 10 hours postmortem, the pCO_2 shows the steepest increase, as well as the accumulation of lactic acid, as has been shown on vitreous humour by Klein and Klein.[20] After 10 hours postmortem, the pCO_2 is decreasing very slowly by diffusion; after 120 hours postmortem, it has not yet reached its original level.

While blood gases and substrates and metabolites of anaerobic glycolytic metabolism show the most marked changes of concentration within the first 10 hours postmortem, all authors agree that these parameters are of only limited value for determining the time since death, because of great interindividual variability.

The interindividual variability of supravital reactions cannot, of course, be smaller than that of the substrates and metabolites of the basic metabolic processes.[1]

PHYSIOLOGICAL PECULIARITIES OF SUPRAVITAL REAGIBILITY

The smooth iris muscle is reactive to electrical and pharmacological stimulation for a longer period than skeletal muscle. Klein and Klein[20] presented extensive experimental data on death-time estimation using the smooth iris muscle (electrical and pharmacological stimulation). These authors examined 18 different pupillomotoric drugs in different concentrations. The onset of reaction varied between 5 and 30 minutes; the duration of reaction lasted at least 1 hour. The drug concentration had no influence on the duration and strength of reaction. The onset of the reaction was later with increasing postmortem interval, the maximum reaction being reached later; the intensity of reaction (pupil dilatation in mm) decreased with increasing postmortem interval (Table 5.1; Fig. 5.7). The postmortem pharmacological excitability to adrenaline, atropine and cyclopentolate covers three different postmortem intervals; adrenaline and acetylcholine have additionally the longest postmortem efficiency (Table 5.2). For practical use of pharmacological excitability of the iris in casework, see Chapter 7.

The strongest and longest postmortem effect of acetylcholine and noradrenaline, as the natural transmitters of cholinergic and adrenergic fibres, is due to Cannon and Rosenblueth's law of denervation. According to this law, each denervated structure becomes supersensitive for the humoral mediator. This supersensitivity also becomes evident from the concentration of the drugs used in the cadaver experiments, which would cause no or only a small change of pupillary diameter in living people.

The physiological mechanism of supersensitivity of denervated smooth muscle to adrenergic drugs is due to the loss of the main mechanism for the regulation of adrenergic drugs at the receptor – the neuronal

Table 5.1 *Pharmacological excitability of the iris*[20]

Investigation of 5765 eyes of 3979 bodies
Subconjunctival injection instead of injection into the anterior chamber reaction after 5–30 minutes
Duration of reaction at least 1 hour
Concentration of drugs has no influence on the intensity and duration of reaction

Table 5.2 *Pharmacological excitability of the iris. Postmortem duration of excitability after injection of different drugs*

		Number of bodies		
		Postmortem excitability (h)	Subconjunctival (*n*)	Anterior chamber (*n*)
Mydriatica				
Noradrenaline/adrenaline	1.00%	14–46	573	737
Tropicamide	0.25%	5–30	307	320
Atropine/cyclopentolate	1%/0.50%	3–10	131	145
Miotica				
Acetylcholine	5.00%	14–46	586	721

In two cases there was no mydriasis in the interval 3 to 12 hours postmortem.

re-uptake. It is a presynaptic specific supersensitivity (Fig. 5.8).

For acetylcholine, the physiological mechanism of supersensitivity after denervation is the decrease in activity of the cholinesterase.

In discussing Cannon and Rosenblueth's law of denervation, we have seen that denervated structures may be supersensitive to physiological excitations; however, other tissues, with increasing postmortem intervals, need much stronger excitations than vital tissues. While impulses of 0.2 ms duration are a common means of excitation in clinical neurophysiology, skeletal muscle fails to react 2 hours postmortem to a stimulus of such a low duration, while impulses of 1 second duration stimulate muscular contractions (Fig. 5.9) (see page 200).

While muscular contraction on mechanical excitation in the early postmortem interval is characterized by a contraction of the whole muscle, i.e. a propagated excitation, with increasing postmortem interval the contraction will be confined to the place of excitation; there then results a local contraction called 'idiomuscular contraction' or 'idiomuscular pad'.[32–36] This change from propagated excitation to local contraction can also be seen after electrical excitation in both skeletal muscle and smooth muscle.[20]

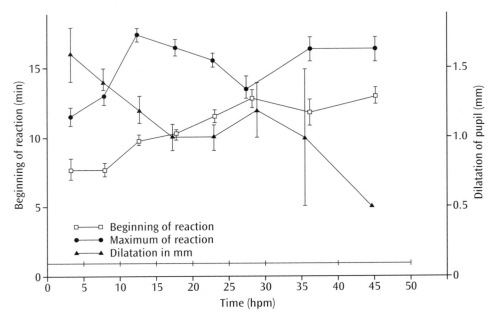

Figure 5.7 *Postmortem excitability of the iris after injection of noradrenaline. x axis = hours postmortem; left y axis = beginning of the reaction after injection (in minutes); right y axis = dilatation of pupil (in mm). For each classified time interval the mean value and 95% confidence limits are given. The figure is designed using original data from Klein and Klein.[20]*

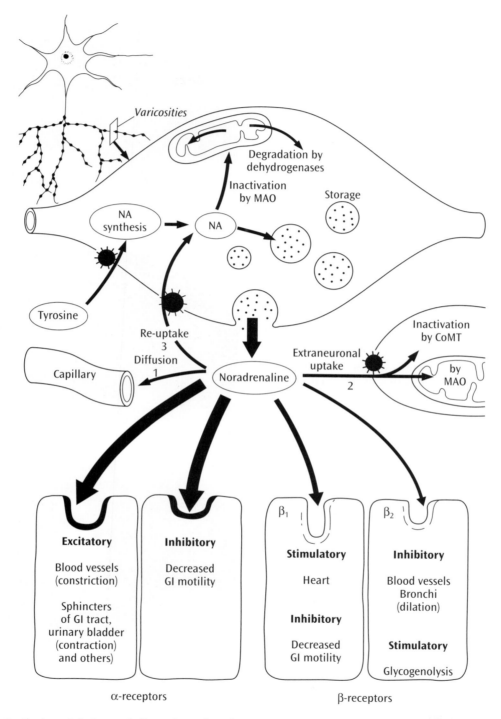

Figure 5.8 *Synthesis, metabolism and effects of noradrenaline (NA). The neuronal re-uptake, (3) is the main mechanism for the regulation of adrenergica at the receptor; it ceases after denervation.*[32] *CoMT, Catechol-O-methyltransferase; MAO, monoamine oxidase.*

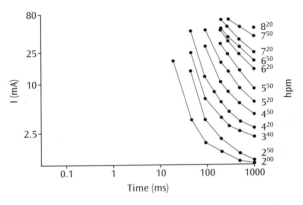

Figure 5.9 *Strength–duration curve. y axis = current intensity I (in ln mA); x axis = duration of stimulus in ms. At the right: time of death in hours and minutes. Using stimuli with a duration of less than 10 ms, at 2 hours postmortem no muscular reaction can be obtained.*

For instance, on electrical excitation, the smooth iris muscle reacts in the early postmortem interval with a miosis (propagated excitation), but in the later postmortem interval there is only a drawing out of muscle fibres into the direction of the electrodes – a local contraction (Fig. 5.10).

These few comments on supravitality can be summarized as follows:

1. Supravitality, especially reagibility on excitation, covers a much longer postmortem period than latency, survival and resuscitation times. Clinically oriented investigations on latency, survival and resuscitation periods may form the only scientifically safe basis for the explanation of spontaneous supravital activity, but do not provide an explanation for the upper margin for vital actions/reactions beyond the end of the resuscitation period. That part of the supravital period beyond the end of the resuscitation period needs further scientific investigation.

2. The correlation of functional and biochemical parameters, which have been performed for the latency, survival and resuscitation periods, should be extended over the whole supravital period. The aim of these investigations would be to improve the precision of death-time estimation using supravital reactions, by narrowing down the great interindividual variability of supravital reagibility by considering complementary parameters of metabolism.

3. With increasing postmortem interval, the

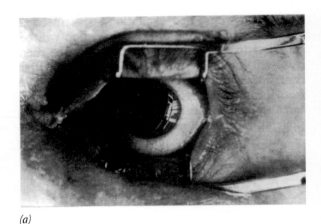

(a)

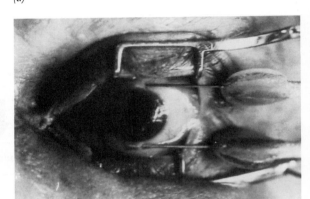

(b)

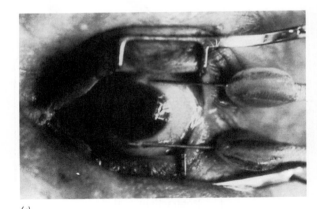

(c)

Figure 5.10 *Electrical excitability of the iris. (a) Pupil before excitation. (b) Miosis after excitation (propagated excitation). (c) Drawing out of the pupil in the direction of the electrodes (local contraction).*[20]

supravital reaction pattern differs not only quantitatively but qualitatively from physiological conditions. Investigations on supravital reagibility should address this, with the aim of extending the investigations over a postmortem period for as long as possible.

REFERENCES

1 Henssge C, Madea B. *Methoden zur Bestimmung der Todeszeit an Leichen.* Lübeck: Schmidt-Römhild, 1988.

2 Opitz E. Physiologie der Erstickung und des Sauerstoffmangels. In: *Lehrbuch der Gerichtlichen Medizin* (Ponsold A, ed.). Stuttgart: Thieme, 1950: 174–218.

3 Opitz E. Der Stoffwechsel des Gehirns und seine Veränderungen bei Kreislaufstillstand. *Verh. Dtsch. Ges. Kreislaufforsch.* 1953; **19**: 26–44.

4 Opitz E, Schneider M. Über die Sauerstoffversorgung des Gehirns und den Mechanismus von Mangelwirkungen. *Ergebn. Physiol.* 1950; **46**: 126–260.

5 Schneider M. Über die Wiederbelebung nach Kreislaufunterbrechung. *Thoraxchir.* 1958; **6**: 95–106.

6 Schneider M. Die Wiederbelebungszeit verschiedener Organe nach Ischämie. *Langenbecks Arch. Klin. Chir.* 1964; **308**: 252–64.

7 Rotter W. Über die postischämische Insuffizienz über-lebender Zellen und Organe, ihre Erholungszeit und die Wiederbelebungszeit nach Kreislaufunterbrechung. *Thoraxchir.* 1958/59; **6**: 107–24.

8 Blasius W. Allgemeine Physiologie des Nervensystems. In: *Lehrbuch der Physiologie des Menschen*, Bd 2, 28 (Rosemann HU, ed.). München: Urban und Schwarzenberg, 1962: 629–62.

9 Isselhard W. Akuter Sauerstoffmangel und Wiederbelebung. *Dtsch. Med. Wschr.* 1965; **90**: 349–55.

10 Bretschneider HJ, Hübner G, Knoll D, Lohr B, Nordbeck H, Spieckermann PG. Myocardial resistance and toler-ance to ischaemia: physiological and biochemical basis. *J. Cardiovasc. Surg.* 1975; **16**: 241–60.

11 Wright EB. A comparative study of the effects of oxygen lack on peripheral nerve. *Am. J. Physiol.* 1946; **147**: 78–89.

12 Gerard RW. The response of nerve to oxygen lack. *Am. J. Physiol.* 1930; **92**: 498–541.

13 Hirsch H, Hohmann V, Kaegler M, Sickel B. Auditory evoked potentials during and after complete ischaemia of the brain. *Adv. Neurosurg.* 1986; **14**: 364–7.

14 Hirsch H, Kaegler M, Hohmann V, Mues B. Latency of recovery and electrical silence of auditory potentials and the electrocorticogram after peracute complete brain ischaemia of 2–30 minutes duration. *Adv. Neurosurg.* 1989; **17**: 254–8.

15 Hirsch H, Hohmann V, Kaegler M, Sickel B. Recovery of auditory evoked potentials after long-term complete brain ischaemia. *Neurosurg. Rev.* 1989; **12** (Suppl. 1): 313–16.

16 Hirsch H. Recovery of the electrocorticogram after incomplete and complete ischaemia of the brain. *Acta. Neurochir.* 1982; **66**: 147–58.

17 Hirsch H, Tesch P. Recovery of the electrocorticogram of canine brains after complete cerebral ischaemia at 37 and 32°C. *Neurosurg. Rev.* 1982; **5**: 49–54.

18 Spieckermann PG. *Überlebens – und Wiederbelebungszeit des Herzens. Anaesth and Resuscit 66.* Berlin: Springer, 1973.

19 Bohn HJ. *Status energiereicher Phosphate und glykolyt-ischer Metabolite in der Extremitälenmuskulatur der Ratte bei Ischämie und in der postischämischen Erholung.* Köln University: MD Thesis, 1974.

20 Klein A, Klein S. *Die Todeszeitbestimmung am menschLichen Auge.* Dresden University: MD Thesis, 1978.

21 Madea B. *Supravitale elektrische Erregbarkeit der Skelettmuskulatur – Längsschnittuntersuchungen zur Objektivierung der muskulären Reaktion an 70 Leichen.* Köln: Habil Schrift, 1989.

22 Madea B, Henssge C. Electrical excitability of skeletal muscle postmortem in casework. *Forensic Sci. Int.* 1990; **47**: 207–27.

23 Raule P, Forster B, Joachim H, Ropohl D. Tierexperi-mentelle Untersuchungen zur Erregbarkeit des absterbenden Herzmuskels. *Z. Rechtsmed.* 1974; **74**: 99–110.

24 Partmann W. Zur Frage der postmortalen Reaktions-fähigkeit des kontraktilen Mechanismus der Muskulatur. *Naturwissenschaften* 1955; **42**: 161–2.

25 Nokes LD, Barasi S, Knight BH. Case report: co-ordinated motor movement of a lower limb after death. *Med. Sci. Law* 1989; **29**: 265.

26 Blasius W, Zimmermann H. *Pflügers Arch. Physiol.* 1962; **264**: 618.

27 Krause D, Klein A, Zett L. Todeszeitbestimmung mittels indirekter Muskelreizung über den N. ischiadicus und N. radialis. *Kriminal. Forens. Wiss.* 1976; **26**: 66–7.

28 Popwassilew J, Palm W. Über die Todeszeitbestimmung in den ersten 10 Stunden. *Z. Ärztl. Fortbildg.* 1960; **54**: 734–7.

29 Schourup K. Determination of the time since death (Danish, English summary). Diss. Med., Copenhagen, 1950.

30 Dotzauer G, Naeve W. Die aktuelle Wasserstoffionen-konzentration im Leichenblut. *Zentralbl. Pathol.* 1955; **93**: 360–70.

31 Dotzauer G, Naeve W. Wasserstoffionenkonzentration im Liquor post mortem. *Zentralbl. Allg. Path. Anat.* 1959; **100**: 516–24.

32 Silbernagel S, Despopoulos A. *Taschenatlas der Physiologie, 3.* Stuttgart: Thieme, 1988.

33 Joachim H. Mechanische und elektrische Erregbarkeit der Skelettmuskulatur. In: *Methoden zur Bestimmung der Todeszeit an Leichen.* (Henssge C, Madea B, eds.). Lübeck: Schmidt-Römhild, 1988: 32–82.

34 Dotzauer G. Idiomuskulärer Wulst und postmortale Blutung bei plötzlichen Todesfällen. *Dtsch. Z Gerichtl. Med.* 1958; **46**: 761–71.

35 Näcke P. Die Dauer der postmortalen mechanischen Muskelerregbarkeit bei chronisch Geisteskranken, speziell Paralytikern. *Z. d. ges. Neurol. u. Psychiatr.* 1911; **7**: 424–46.

36 Krause D, Klein A, Mattig W, Walz H. Praktische Erfahrungen mit dem Reizgerät "D 76" zur Todeszeitbestimmung. *Kriminal. Forens. Wiss.* 1980; **40**: 83–6.

Rigor mortis: estimation of the time since death by evaluation of cadaveric rigidity

THOMAS KROMPECHER

Rigor mortis is certainly the most fascinating cadaveric sign. Because it gives a petrified appearance to the deceased person, rigor mortis is noticed by everybody that encounters a corpse. It is therefore often used to estimate the time since death, even (and especially) by the non-initiated. It is generally accepted that a watch must be tested, perhaps even under various circumstances, before it is used to measure time. In addition, one is expected to read the user's manual. Alas, I fear we lack such a user's manual in the case of rigor mortis – and, if this is so, it is certainly not for want of related literature; in fact publications about cadaveric rigidity abound. A brief summary of our present knowledge concerning this phenomenon is presented below.

EXPLANATIONS OF THE MECHANISM OF RIGOR MORTIS

According to our current understanding, rigor mortis is the result of postmortem muscle contraction. Therefore, to understand the development of rigidity, we must first study the mechanism of muscle contraction and hence the structure of the muscle.

Szent-Györgyi, whose laboratory gave us numerous basic data concerning the composition and the function of the muscle, described the muscle fibre as, 'the loveliest toy ever provided by nature for the biochemist ... like most children, the biochemist, when he finds a toy, usually pulls it to pieces ...'

Szent-Györgyi's attempts to pull the muscle fibre to pieces resulted in the discovery of two proteins, which he named actin and myosin.[1,2] These two proteins form interdigitating thick (myosin) and thin (actin) filaments, which build the sarcomere, the contractile unit of the muscle. The sarcomeres are organized head-to-tail in series (4000 per cm) that form the fibrils. The muscle cell is a fibre composed of 1000 to 2000 fibrils (Fig. 5.11).

The contraction of the muscle can be explained by the ATP theory of Erdös[3] and the sliding filament model of contraction proposed by Hanson and Huxley.[4] According to this model, contraction or tension in the muscle is achieved by the contrary motion of the interdigitating filaments. The myosin filament carries myosin heads on both ends. These heads attach to the actin filament and act as cross-bridges to form the actin–myosin (Ac–My) complex. During contraction, the heads swivel and the thin filament is pulled past the thick one. As the heads on each end of the myosin filament swivel in opposite directions, the Z-lines approach each other and the sarcomere shortens. The limit of contraction is reached when the thick myosin filaments butt against the Z-line (Fig. 5.11).

Both filaments slide without changing their length. Motion is achieved by cyclic formation and breaking of the cross-bridges. The fibrils may shorten by 30 to 50%, thus requiring that the swivel cycle be repeated many times.

The driving force for the sliding motion comes

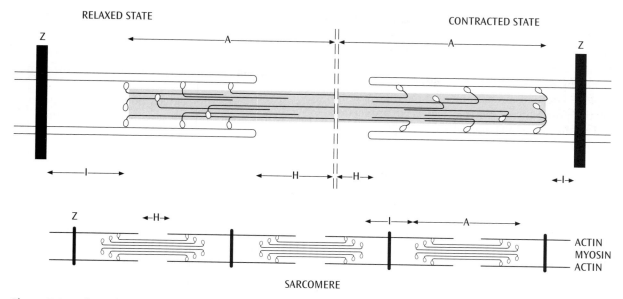

Figure 5.11 *Schematic representation of the contraction and relaxation of an isolated sacromere. The cross-bridges (myosin heads) pull the actin filaments and the attached Z-lines towards each other. The swivel cycle is repeated until the myosin filaments butt against the Z-line. The H zone and I band shorten, the A band remains constant.*

from the myosin heads. The kinetic energy is derived from chemical processes. The myosin heads bind ATP and form myosin–ATP, which in turn has a very high affinity for actin, resulting in the Ac–My complex. When the Ac–My complex is formed, the low ATPase activity displayed by free myosin heads is increased, and ATP is hydrolysed. The energy released through ATP hydrolysis is used for the dissociation of the Ac–My complex.

The ATP used is almost immediately regenerated. This may be achieved through three different processes:

1. The hydrolysis of creatine phosphate (CrP), which furnishes rapidly available energy within short time limits. As a consequence, brief but violent exercise may be accomplished (e.g. a 100-metre sprint). The CrP used in this process is restored by means of the energy generated by anaerobic glycolysis.
2. For continued exercise, the glycogen content of the muscle must be used. Glycogen can be transformed entirely to lactic acid by anaerobic hydrolysis. This process is limited by the accumulation of lactic acid.
3. Oxidative phosphorylation is the combustion of glucose in the presence of oxygen. It results in the production of CO_2 and H_2O and, although it

liberates great amounts of ATP, it is a relatively slow process.

If ATP is not regenerated, as is the case when ATP is consumed after death, the Ac–My complex is not split; rather, it persists and the muscle remains inextensible. This stable Ac–My complex is the basis for the development of rigor mortis in the postmortem state.

In summary, rigor mortis is a normal muscle contraction occurring after death and fixed by lack of ATP.

The *in vitro* experiments of Erdös,[3] and Krause and Zett[5] demonstrated that rigidity disappears after the addition of ATP or O_2. Consequently, the onset of rigor mortis can be considered as a supravital phenomenon: in fact, it is the last evident vital event in the muscle.

Given this explanation, it is easy to understand the mechanism of development of cadaveric rigidity, which unfolds in four different phases.

1st phase: delay period

After clinical death, the muscle survives in a normal state for a short time and stays relaxed as long as the ATP content remains sufficiently high to permit the splitting of the actin–myosin cross-bridges. This fact was first proven by Erdös,[3] who compared the hardness of the muscle with its ATP concentration. The two curves showed mirror images: the decrease in ATP levels was matched by an increase in hardness (confirmed by Bate-Smith and Bendall[6]). The rate of ATP depletion depends on its content at the time of death, on the possibility of postmortem ATP production, and on the rate of ATP hydrolysis.

2nd phase: onset period (reversible)

The ATP content of the muscle falls below a critical threshold. The cross-bridges remain intact and rigidity appears. However, this state is still reversible: the addition of ATP (Erdös,[3] confirmed by Bendall[7]) or O_2[5] results in relaxation, indicating that the muscle is still able to function.[8]

3rd phase: rigor (irreversible)

Rigidity is fully developed and becomes irreversible. Postmortem modifications of muscle fibres destroy their ability to relax.

4th phase: resolution

Rigidity disappears and the muscle becomes limp. The cause of resolution is not definitely established. Nevertheless, I believe that, according to our present knowledge, one can accept the suggestions of Erdös[3] and Szent-Györgyi[1] that resolution is a denaturation process. Morphological evaluations confirm this hypothesis.[9–12]

Bendall[7] proposed that the process is strongly pH-dependent and added, 'Thus there may be no further need to search about, apparently hopelessly, for a protease (cathepsin) which could break the rather specific linkages probably involved'.

The above phases are valid only for isolated fibres. In everyday practice, one is confronted with muscles which are built up of a multitude of fibres. The timing of the onset of rigor mortis cannot be determined precisely because rigor mortis is a progressive event, evolving from less to more pronounced. The progression can be explained by the coexistence of fibres at different stages of developing rigidity.

While the timing of the onset of rigor mortis in a fibre may depend on its ATP content, there are other reasons for heterogeneity.

The human skeletal muscles contain two types of fibre:

- Type I (red): rich in mitochondria, with a predominantly oxidative metabolism and slow myosin.
- Type II (white): relatively poor in mitochondria with a predominantly glycolytic metabolism[3–15] and fast myosin.[16]

The onset of rigor mortis in these two types of fibres is expected to occur at different times.

During a given period of time after the onset of rigor mortis, rigidity that is broken (by forcing the movement of a joint) is restored. This re-establishment of rigor mortis can be explained as follows: those fibres that are still slack, and perhaps those that are not fully contracted, retain their capacity for reversible binding of the myosin heads to the actin filaments. The contraction of such fibres causes the re-establishment of rigor mortis.

The progressive nature of the resolution of rigor mortis may be caused by a similar phenomenon. The different fibres will relax at different times, as the number of fibres destroyed by postmortem reactions increases.

DESCRIPTION OF CADAVERIC RIGIDITY IN THE LITERATURE

Description based on subjective examinations

NYSTEN'S LAW

In 1811, the French physician and chemist P. H. Nysten published the first scientific description of rigor mortis. The law named after him states: 'Cadaveric rigidity affects successively the masticatory muscles, those of the face and the neck, those of the trunk and arms and finally those of the lower limbs'. It is often added that resolution occurs in the same order. The development of rigor mortis is thus descending, a finding thought to be related to the varying distances between the different muscles and the central nervous system (CNS). However, Nysten himself noticed that the destruction of the CNS did not affect the order of the development of rigidity.

While Naumann[17] confirmed the descending development of rigor mortis, he added that in some special cases (e.g. in weak individuals, or those diminished by illness), rigidity may show an ascending pattern.

Based on 271 protocols carried out by the same forensic pathologist, Mittmeyer[18] concluded that: 'With increasing time interval from death, the joints were seen absolutely rigid and completely released in the following order: nape, elbow, jaw, knee and leaping joints'. Shapiro[19,20] wrote:

> It is difficult to understand why a physico-chemical process which takes place in recently dead tissues should follow the sequence usually described. It appears more likely that, because we are dealing with a physico-chemical process in what is virtually a lump of clay, this will take place *simultaneously* in all the recently dead muscles. If that be the case, it would be reasonable to expect that small masses of muscle would be involved completely much more rapidly than large masses of muscle.
>
> The account of the invariable progression of death stiffening from the top to the bottom of the body as generally given in the textbooks must, therefore, be modified. The explanation may have to be sought along the lines indicated, viz., that rigor mortis does not progress from the upper end to the lower end of the body in a well-defined fashion, but occurs simultaneously in the recently dead muscles; and that the fixation of a joint depends, among other things, on the involvement by rigor mortis of the quantity of muscle which controls that joint. Variations in the sizes of different joints and in the muscle masses which control them determine the surface, from where further heat loss occurs to the atmosphere by radiation and convection.

We found a possible confirmation of this hypothesis in the paper of Tarrant and Mothersill.[21] These authors found that in beef carcasses the pH values decreased with distance from the surface and as muscle temperature increased. The time required for the pH to fall to 6.0 in six major hindquarter muscles ranged from 2.2 to 13.6 hours, and varied with the muscle and depth in the carcass. Moreover, they observed a good correlation between the rate of ATP turnover and muscle temperature.

It should be mentioned that a fair part of our knowledge concerning the chemical changes underlying the rigor process were discovered in the laboratories working for the meat industry because the tenderness, i.e. the quality of the meat, depends on this process.

Textbooks of forensic medicine often suggest exceptions to Nysten's law, implying that:

- Nysten's law is often valid.
- Considering the exceptions, we must not rely on it.

The chronology of the development of rigor mortis

In this respect, it is interesting to recall the observations of Niderkorn,[22] who determined the times necessary for the completion of rigor mortis in 113 bodies. In 76 corpses (67%), rigor mortis was fully established after 4 to 7 hours (in 31 cases, after 4 hours; in 14 cases, after 5 hours; in 20 cases, after 6 hours; and in 11 cases, after 7 hours). In two cases, rigidity was complete 2 hours postmortem, and in two others, only 13 hours after death.

Mallach's chronology of the development of rigor mortis,[18,23,24] which was based on a survey of literature from 1811 to 1960, is shown in Table 5.3.

Table 5.3 *Time course of cadaveric rigidity*

Rigor phase	Mean with standard deviation(s)	Hours postmortem				Number of publications evaluated
		Limits of 95.5% probability (2 s)		Variations		
		Lower limit	Upper limit	Lower limit	Upper limit	
Delay period	3 ± 2	–	7	<1/2	7	26
Re-establishment possible	up to 5	–	–	2	8	–
Complete rigidity	8 ± 1	6	10	2	20	28
Persistence	57 ± 14	29	85	24	96	27
Resolution	76 ± 32	12	140	24	192	27

Mean and standard deviation calculated from the literature data of 150 years (1811 to 1960) by Mallach 1964 (Schleyer,[44] slightly modified).

This summary has been criticized, however.[25] Indeed, it is hazardous to compare and evaluate 'feelings' statistically: the observations are highly subjective, and were gathered by examiners over 150 years (1811 to 1960). Moreover, these observations were not codified: various authors often used different classifications in their determination of the state of development of cadaveric rigidity. Nonetheless, we lack a better survey.

In spite of their subjective nature, I believe that every individual estimate is highly valuable. In fact, our predecessors, with observation as the sole method at their disposal, used this simple means expertly, and their conclusions are of great worth. In our own work on cadaveric rigidity, we often base our experiments on statements provided by ancient authors. If our measurements happen to contradict these statements, we regard the results with scepticism. Once an experiment is repeated, and if our results are confirmed, we always seek a valid explanation for the discrepancy.

If these observations are valid (and in my mind, they indeed are in the overwhelming majority of cases), what are the reasons for the great differences in the development of rigor mortis between one corpse and another? The answer stems from the realization that the process is biological or, more precisely, biochemical, and that it can be affected by a number of intrinsic and extrinsic factors.

First, we must consider the physical condition of the individual prior to death, i.e. the factors that influence the energetic reserves.

H. A. Husband, in his *Student's Hand-Book of Forensic Medicine*,[26] summarized such factors as follows:

- Effects of enfeebling disease prior to death: rapid in its invasion, passing off rapidly.
- Effects of a robust frame at period of death: the accession may be prolonged but, other things being equal, it is more strongly manifested, and continues longer.
- Effects of violent exercise prior to death: supervenes, and disappears rapidly.
- Effects of poison. Poisons which cause violent contractions for some time prior to death, e.g. strychnine, influence the rapid invasion of the rigor mortis, its short duration, and the subsequent putrefaction.
- Where death in poisoning by strychnine is almost instantaneous, with a short convulsive stage, the rigor mortis comes on rapidly, and remains for a long time.

Today, more than 100 years later, textbooks include very similar statements.

Vock et al.[27] published a case of tetany involving instantaneous rigor. Electrocution may also hasten the onset of cadaveric rigidity. In the three electrocution cases reported by Schneider,[28] stiffness was complete after 1 hour 40 minutes, 1 hour 45 minutes, and 2 hours 5 minutes after death. In one of our cases,[29] rigidity was fully established 1 hour postmortem in the upper limbs located in the path of the electrical current, but no rigidity was observed elsewhere. Another individual who was found in the bath tub with a hairdryer, was in a state of complete rigidity only 3 hours after being seen alive for the last time.

Several cases of accelerated rigidity after certain intoxications have been reported recently (organophosphate compounds,[30] and strychnine[31]).

The influence of temperature

Considering that the onset of rigor mortis depends on biochemical processes, and that its resolution results from the degradation of cellular structures, it is easy to understand that its overall development is affected by the temperature of the body and consequently by that of the surroundings.

Naturally, this fact was noticed long ago. Nysten[32] states that rigidity persists longer in cold, wet air than in fresh, dry air.

Kussmaul[33] writes: 'The corpses of strong persons can stay stiff till 8 to 10 and more days in air of 2.5 to 7.5°C, while at 18.8 to 30°C the last traces of rigidity disappear in 4 to 6 days'.

In his textbook, Husband[26] sums up the effect of low temperature as follows: '[Rigor mortis is] prolonged by dry cold air and cold water'.

Bierfreund[34] examined the influence of temperature on the development of cadaveric rigidity on the lower limbs of rabbits. His observations are shown in Table 5.4.

Morgenstern's experiments on rabbits and cats of various ages showed that temperature has spectacular effects on the development of rigor mortis. These experiments also revealed the differences due to the species studied and the different ages of the animals. The same author recorded an important acceleration in the onset of rigidity when human corpses were immersed in warm water (35 to 37°C).[35]

Forster et al.[36] observed the duration of cadaveric rigidity in the lower limbs of human corpses kept at

Table 5.4 *Effect of temperature on the development of rigor mortis on the lower limbs of rabbits*[34]

Number	Temperature of air (°C)	Beginning of the onset of rigidity postmortem		Complete development of rigidity postmortem		Beginning of resolution postmortem		Complete resolution postmortem	
		Hours	Min	Hours	Min	Hours	Min	Hours	Min
1	4.0	1	30	7	–	38	–	48	–
2	20.0	1	–	5	15	26	–	36	–
3	22.5	1	–	4	20	–	–	36	–
4	29.0	–	50	3	20	24	–	28	–
5	37.5	–	35	2	–	2	25	4	10
6	41.0	–	45	1	5	1	22	2	30
7	52.5	–	15	–	45	1	–	1	40
8	54.0	–	–	–	50	1	–	1	50
9	55.0	–	2–5	–	37	–	40	1	40
10	60.0	Almost instantly		–	10	–	35	1	10

low temperatures (4 to 11°C). Based on the observations made during the entire period when the corpses were available, the following conclusions were made:

> If we address the question raised in the beginning specifically the persistence of complete rigidity 130 hours after death, we must come to the conclusion that at low temperatures, rigidity can be demonstrated well after this period, even if we take into account slight fluctuations in temperature and a possible error (of a few hours) in the estimate of time of death.

In one of Forster's cases, a corpse kept at +4°C exhibited strong rigidity, even after 234 hours.

In our practice, the opposite situation was illustrated by the case of two corpses found on an exceptionally hot summer day (40°C) in a closed car exposed to the sun. At the examination, carried out less than 8 hours after death, the corpses appeared strongly affected, with parts that were blackened and, naturally, without the faintest sign of rigidity. At the other temperature extreme, an interesting observation was made by Bendall:[7] 'If a muscle is frozen in the pre-rigor state while ATP and PC [phosphocreatine] levels are high, after thawing out rigor sets in'. However, because this experiment was carried out on very thin strips of muscle which were rapidly frozen at −20°C, it is difficult to imagine the occurrence of this phenomenon in the forensic practice.

The influence of the CNS

As noted above, the descending pattern in the development of rigor mortis was thought to be caused by the varying distances from the CNS. Fuchs[37] described the brain as the initial site of death, followed by the proximal part of the spinal cord, and suggested that the process then progressed towards the caudal spinal cord: the presumed impulsions arose from catabolic changes in the nerve cells.

Busch[38] observed that the removal of the brain and spinal cord resulted in an early onset of rigidity; moreover, rigidity was more pronounced and lasted longer.

In experiments conducted on animals, Eiselberg[39] demonstrated that when the ischiadicus nerve was sectioned on one side, in over 70% of the cases rigidity developed later than on the other side.

Gendre[40] and Aust[41] confirmed this finding. Aust, in particular, obtained this result in 12 out of a total of 13 experiments. Having conducted *in vivo* sectioning of the left side of the spinal cord in rabbits (underneath the pyramidal crossing), Bierfreund[34] made the following statement: 'I was very surprised to find that after a few hours following death, the right half of the body became very rigid, while the left half remained almost normally mobilisable'. Bierfreund thought that the 'accelerating' effect of the CNS on the appearance of cadaveric rigidity was the result of a weak excitation of the muscular system, and if this excitation really did exist, it was too weak to cause a visible contraction. To prove this hypothesis, Bierfreund conducted animal experiments that involved weak irritation by the sciatic nerve. The results were the very opposite of what he had hoped for.

Berg[42] determined that, following death, cholinesterase retains its full or partial activity in the muscle until an advanced stage of muscular degradation. Moreover, during the delay period, the muscular system was found to release small amounts of acetylcholine. The onset of cadaveric rigidity was found to be hastened by the inhibition of acetylcholinesterase, by the addition of acetylcholine, or by a thermal irritation of the contralateral motor region. The inhibition of transmitters retarded the onset of rigidity.

Krause et al.[10] made the following interesting observation: 'The irritation of sciatic and radial nerves in amputated arms and legs caused violent muscular reactions for up to two hours, but action potentials in the nerves were detectable even after this period of time'.

The experimental results described above are partially contradictory. Therefore, it remains unclear what role the nervous system may play in the development of cadaveric rigidity.

Instantaneous rigor or cadaveric spasm

Instantaneous rigor is defined as a complete rigor mortis occurring at the moment of death, and involving a hand, limb, or even the entire body. Baumann[43] surveyed the literature on this subject and concluded that the majority of instantaneous rigor mortis cases described involving lesions in the head, brain, brainstem and thorax were caused by death from internal lesions and also probably gas embolism. Laves[44] and Prokop[45,46] proposed that the cause could be a decerebrate rigidity.[47]

Polson and Gee[48] cited many such instances in the literature, but during their 20-year practice in Leeds they reported only two cases. In our own practice, I have never encountered an example of truly instantaneous rigor mortis, nor have I been able to gather acceptable examples in my colleagues' cases.

Some of the cases published in the literature, especially the more spectacular ones, were based on observations made during war time.[48,49] Interestingly, Mueller,[50] a German forensic pathologist, searched but failed to observe a case of instantaneous rigor during the war, in spite of his surveys of military medics.

We have encountered numerous cases of electrocution in which the body apparently remained in the position of the spasm caused by the electric shock.[28] In these cases, the facies was also found to be contracted. However, the term instantaneous rigidity does not apply here. Indeed, in all of our observed cases, the body remained in direct or indirect contact with the electrical current up to the moment of discovery of the cadaver. Because of the accelerated onset of rigor mortis (see above), it is reasonable to assume that rigor mortis fixed the body in a given position while the spasm was still occurring.

Ultimately, we believe that even if instantaneous rigor mortis does exist, it is a very rare event. Consequently, before accepting such an explanation, it is important to study all the other possibilities (changes in the position of the body and/or of the surrounding objects, electrocution, etc.).

Objective measurements of rigor mortis

Rigor mortis, the stiffening of the muscles after death, immobilizes the joints. The resistance in the joints can be used to make a qualitative or even a quantitative estimate of the degree of rigor.

In the situations described so far, the conclusions were drawn on the basis of estimates of the force necessary to bend a knee or an elbow immobilized by cadaveric rigidity. Such manual estimates are necessarily subjective and cannot be compared between different observers. Moreover, this method is not applicable when the degree of rigidity rises above a certain level. For example, one feels the same when asked to lift 200 or 500 kg – the weight makes no difference, as one cannot move either. The same situation can be found in the case of rigidity. When rigidity in a knee or jaw joint cannot be broken, it is not clear whether rigidity increases or decreases until its intensity falls down to the levels commensurate with human strength.

It is, of course, desirable to determine the exact degree of rigidity, to obtain reproducible numerical values that can be compared, and to extend the measurements in situations where human strength is insufficient.

As far as we know, the first objective measurements of rigidity were reported by Oppenheim and Wacker,[51] who gave a detailed description of their method to measure the force necessary to bend a leg with a knee joint immobilized by rigidity; this is referred to as 'breaking' the rigidity of a joint. Oppenheim and Wacker expressed their results relative to the mass of the relevant muscles. They discussed the influence of the cause of death on the development of rigor mortis, so their results could not be used to estimate the time of death.

Subsequently, two German research teams further developed methods to measure the force necessary to break the cadaveric rigidity of a knee joint. One team was headed by Forster in Freiburg, and the other by Beier in Munich. However, before reviewing their findings, a few general comments about the development of cadaveric rigidity may be useful.

In forensic practice, one examines the degree to which muscular rigidity fixes or immobilizes a joint. Hence, the measure of cadaveric rigidity is a measure of the force necessary to move a joint. The development of rigidity is the process of change in the intensity of rigidity over time. This intensity is weak at first, but it then increases, reaches a maximum, decreases, and finally practically disappears after a variable period of time. This process can be represented by a curve, although such a curve is valid only for one given corpse under clearly defined conditions.

Although only two points are necessary (and sufficient) to define a straight line, multiple points are needed to define a curve, which cannot be determined by a single point. This is the basis of the difficulty in attempting to characterize the development of cadaveric rigidity using a single measurement (it is not even possible to make two measurements, as the development of cadaveric rigidity is different in the two lower limbs of the same corpse; this will be discussed below). Forster et al.[52] proposed standardizing the measurements using the following formula:

FRR (Freiburger Rigor Index) = $p \cdot I_1 / U^2 \cdot I_2 \times 100$

where p is the traction force (kp); I_1 is the length of the leg (cm); I_2 is the distance from the rotation axis of the knee joint to the anterior surface of the knee cap (cm); and U is the circumference of the thigh (cm) (Table 5.5).

Table 5.5 *Proposed standardized measurements of cadavaric rigidity*

Rigor index	Degree of rigidity	Subjective observation
>5.5	1	Complete rigidity
<5.5–4.0	2	Very difficult to break
<4.0–2.5	3	Relatively easy to break
<2.5–1.3	4	Soft
<1.3–0.2	5	Weak
<0.2	6	Complete resolution

This formula may be used to correct (at least partially) for the differences between individual cases. However, it does not take into account individual factors, such as the difference in muscle mass between two thighs with the same circumference.

The actual worth of this formula remains unknown. While Forster et al. have published the formula on several occasions,[52–55] they have not communicated any numerical data to justify the entries made in their table. They have also published a schematic curve of the development of rigor mortis, [52–54] which was apparently based on the results calculated using their formula, but without explaining how they obtained it. Lacking conclusive reports, these conclusions should be treated with great caution.

Beier et al.[56] relied on a similar approach to measure the intensity of cadaveric rigidity. The experiments consisted of determining the torque necessary to break the rigor mortis of arms and legs. The measurements were made on 17 female and 35 male cadavers stored at a temperature of 4°C. The authors concluded that:

'The values show differences between male and female cadavers to an extent that both groups have to be treated separately. Relating the torque to the diameter of the cross-section of the limb does not eliminate the difference. Frequently, considerable differences between left and right limbs were obtained, however, without preference for one side over the other. There is no direct functional relationship between postmortem time and the intensity of rigor mortis, but the values occasionally allow estimates on the maximum time postmortem.'

In a second series of reports,[57,58] the following observations were made:

'The torque to overcome rigor mortis was determined for each leg by bending the lower leg of the prone cadaver toward the fixed thigh. The device ensures that the force is kept perpendicular to the tibia. The force is read from a spring balance with an accuracy of 5 Nm. For the lever arm, the distance from the knee joint, or the epicondylus lateralis, to the site of attachment of the spring balance was taken. Torque values ranging from 10 to 500 Nm were measured to an accuracy of 3 Nm and, above 100 Nm, to 3%. Before measurement the cadavers were kept in storage rooms at 4–6°C.

The rigor mortis of the legs of 101 male human cadavers were investigated. These were selected from the cadavers brought to the Institute by the following criteria: age at least 14 years, no pathological findings at the investigated extremities, time of death known exactly to within one hour.

There seems to exist an upper limit for the torque of rigor mortis, depending on the lay-time, above which no value was found. Below this limit, however, every value could be found. By calculating the 90% tolerance limits of lay-times grouped at 12-hourly intervals, this upper limit was found to decrease exponentially with lay-time. This plot may be used for the estimation of maximum lay-times from rigor mortis measurements.'

Beier's investigations and results have probably reached the limits of the possibilities offered by this method. Considering that only a single measurement can be made per joint (or limb), and that the obtained value represents a random time point in the development of rigor mortis, one can appreciate the large degree of freedom in constructing a curve depicting the development of rigidity. Given these limitations, we have developed a different method for the objective measurement of the intensity of cadaveric rigidity in rats.[59–62] The apparatus used is shown in Fig. 5.12. The principle of the method is to determine the force necessary to cause a movement of small amplitude (4 mm) in the limb under examination.

As this movement does not break rigor mortis, serial measurements can be taken. Our apparatus

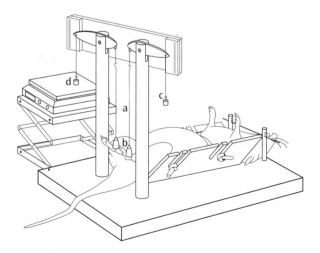

Figure 5.12 *Apparatus for the measurement of rigor mortis intensity.* (a) *Cord attached to hind limb.* (b) *Steel hooks permitting attachment of cord to limbs.* (c) *Hook supporting weights (previous technique).* (d) *Hook attached to a digital balance.*

measured the resistance caused by rigor both in the knee and in the hip joints.

Initially, the force was measured by hooking successively heavier weights to obtain the standardized movement of the limb.[59,60] Subsequently, a slight modification was introduced: the hook was attached to the plate of a digital balance which was placed on a jack (Fig. 5.12(d)). When the balance was lowered to produce the standardized small amplitude movement of the limb, the resistance caused by rigidity could be read directly from the balance (a negative value, as traction was exerted).

All the experiments were conducted on male albino rats, with each study involving animals of the same age and body weight.

We reproduce here the curve of the development of the rigor mortis as first obtained on a rat at a temperature of 24.5°C (Fig. 5.13).

In the following experiment,[59] we demonstrated that there is essentially no difference in the time course of the development of rigor mortis in the hind and front limbs, in spite of the fact that the muscular mass of the hind limbs is 2.89 times greater than that of the front limbs. At the same time, it should be noted that, in the initial phase, rigor mortis was more pronounced in the front limbs. Moreover, resolution was initially faster in the front limbs, although both hind and front limbs reached complete resolution at the same time.

The development of rigor mortis was also studied in rats of varying ages and weights.[62] While the time course of the development was always the same, the intensity of rigor was found to be directly proportional to the increase in the animal's body weight.

Because the method appeared to be suitable for studying the development of rigor mortis in rats, we decided to determine the effects of physical exercise prior to death.[60] The animals were subjected to a treadmill exercise lasting 1 hour, with the distance covered being approximately 1020 metres. For rats raised in small cages, a 1000-metre run must represent a considerable effort, but the experimental animals tolerated it quite well. The results of this experiment are presented in Fig. 5.14.

The development of rigor mortis in rats that had exercised prior to death differed from that of the control. The following features were noted for the exercised animals:

- There was a higher intensity in the initial phase.
- Maximum development was reached at the same time as in the controls.

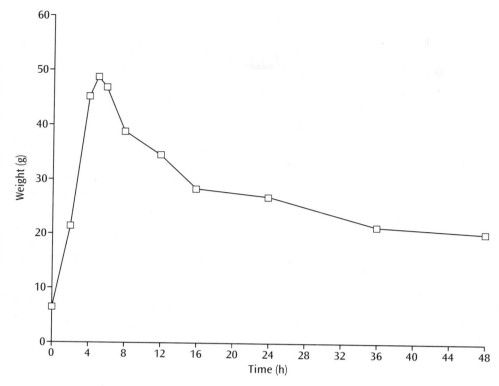

Figure 5.13 *Evolution of the intensity of rigor mortis in the hind limb of a rat of body weight 350 g.*

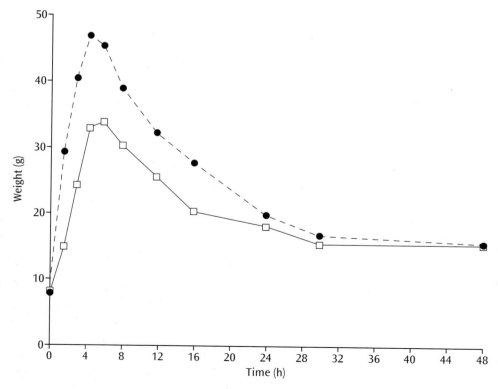

Figure 5.14 *The evolution of rigor mortis in the hind limbs of rats in control* —□— *and exercised* —— ● —— *groups. Values given are always an average for ten animals (20 hind limbs).*

Table 5.6 *The evolution of rigor mortis in the two groups relative to the maximum value of the control group (33.8 g) taken as 100%*

	Time postmortem (h)						
	1.66	**3**	**4.5**	**6**	**8**	**12**	**16**
Treadmill exercise (%)	86.5	119.5	139.2	134.6	115.8	95.6	82.3
Control (%)	44.4	72.3	97.8	100.0	89.8	76.0	60.3

- Higher maximum values were reached (in our experiments, 1.39 times the maximum values in the controls).
- The higher values were maintained from 100 minutes to 16 hours, with statistically significant differences.
- Resolution occurred at the same time.

Table 5.6 summarizes the development of rigor mortis in the exercised and in the control groups, relative to the maximum value of the control group (33.8 g) normalized to 100%. The results illustrate the types of errors that can occur when a single, manual estimate of rigor made on a cadaver with an unknown history is used to establish the time of death. For example, the values obtained at 100 minutes and 16 hours in the exercised group are both very close to 100%, which could be interpreted, erroneously, as fully developed rigidity (compared with the control group).

The development of rigor mortis at different temperatures is shown in Fig. 5.15; Fig. 5.16 illustrates the development of rigor at 6°C. By transferring the cadavers to 24°C for 24 hours between 216 and 240 hours postmortem, we wished to accelerate decomposition, thus causing the possible remnants of rigor mortis to disappear. The consecutive transfer to 6°C for 24 hours was made to determine whether the decrease in temperature alone could cause rigidity.

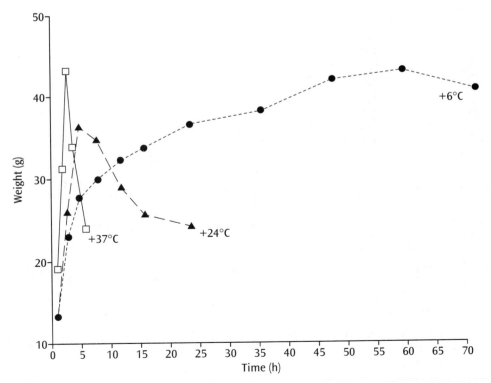

Figure 5.15 *The evolution of the intensity of rigor mortis in the hind limbs of rats at different temperatures. Values given are always an average for ten animals (20 hind limbs).*

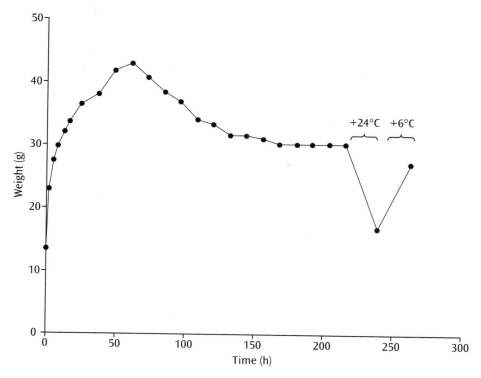

Figure 5.16 *The evolution of the intensity of rigor mortis in the hind limbs of rats at +6°C. Values given are always an average for ten animals (20 hind limbs).*

Indeed, a marked increase in resistance could be seen between the measurements taken at 240 hours post-mortem at 24°C and those taken 24 hours later at 6°C. The only difference between the specimens at these two time points was the decrease in rectal temperature from 24 to 6°C (note that the muscles were not frozen). The increase in resistance (from 17.3 to 27.6 g) led us to conclude that a decrease in temperature alone enhances the stiffness of the muscles, and perhaps the resistance in the joints as well, leading to what can be called 'cold rigidity'. The increase in our case was 59.53%, which was highly significant.[63]

Figure 5.17 illustrates the effects of fatal intoxication by strychnine, carbon monoxide and curare on the development of intensity of rigor mortis.[31] Our findings can be summarized as follows:

- Strychnine intoxication hastens the onset and the passing of rigor mortis.
- Carbon monoxide intoxication delays the resolution of rigor mortis.
- The intensity of rigor may vary depending on the cause of death.

In the electrocution case (see page 150), our first investigation at the scene of death revealed that the arms of the victim, which were in direct contact with the electrical current, displayed severe rigor. The victim's husband, suspected of the murder of his wife, asserted that he had left her alive 1 hour earlier.

Our experiments on electrocution[29] were conducted on animals as follows:

- Group 1, a control set killed in the usual manner by nitrogen asphyxia.
- Group 2, electrocution with 140 V, 50 Hz alternating current applied for 50 seconds, with the electrodes clamped on the left front and the right hind limb of the animal.
- Group 3, same as group 2, but electrocution for 90 seconds.
- Group 4, animals killed by nitrogen asphyxia, followed by electrocution (same as group 3), 10 minutes later.

The results of this experiment, shown in Fig. 5.18, led to the following conclusions:

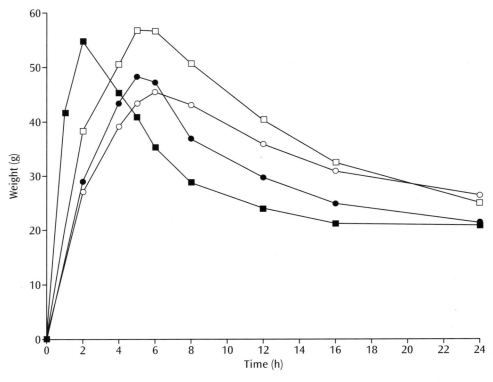

Figure 5.17 *Evolution of the intensity of rigor mortis in the hind limbs of rats in the case of nitrogen asphyxia —□—; fatal intoxication by strychnine —■—; carbon monoxide —○—; and curare —●—. Mean values are for ten animals (20 hind limbs).*

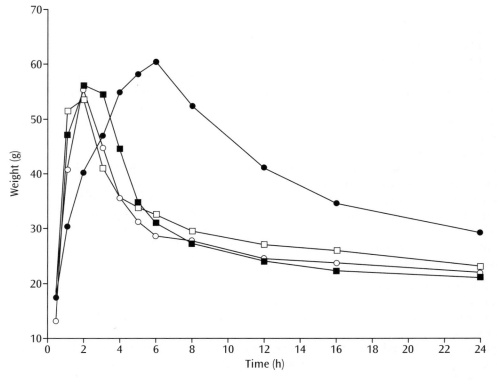

Figure 5.18 *Evolution of the intensity of rigor mortis in the hind limbs of rats in the case of nitrogen asphyxia —●—; 'direct' electrocution 50 s —○—; 'direct' electrocution 90 s —□—; 'direct' postmortem electrocution 90 s —■—; Mean values are for ten animals (20 hind limbs) in the control group and for ten animals (10 hind limbs) in the 'electrocution' groups.*

1. Electrocution hastens the onset of rigor mortis. After a 90-second electrocution, rigor mortis developed as rapidly as 1 hour postmortem, compared with 5 hours for the controls.
2. Electrocution hastens the disappearance of rigor mortis.
3. In the case of postmortem electrocution, the observed changes were slightly less pronounced.

The changes in the development of rigor mortis were less pronounced in the limbs that were not directly affected by the electrical current (left hind limbs in our experiments).

Although it is clear that the results of our experiments are not directly applicable to humans, our method is the only means to evaluate the effects of different intrinsic and extrinsic factors on the development of rigor mortis, under a set of well-defined conditions. Moreover, these experiments do provide us with an overall idea on the time course of the various changes.

In terms of practical applications based on our experiments, if the stage of rigidity is used to estimate the time of death, it is necessary to: (i) perform a succession of objective measurements of the intensity of rigor mortis; and (ii) verify the possible presence of factors that can play a role in the modification of the development of rigor mortis.

We applied these two principles and tested our method by deriving an estimate of time elapsed since death.[64] The experiment consisted of monitoring the development of the intensity of rigor mortis in nine groups of six rats each. The animals were killed by nitrogen asphyxia at an ambient temperature of 24°C. Measurements were initiated after 2, 4, 5, 6, 8, 12, 15, 24 and 48 hours postmortem, and lasted 5 to 9 hours, which would be the usual procedure when a corpse is discovered.

The results of these experiments are shown in Fig. 5.19 and Table 5.7. The measurements, which were initiated 2 hours postmortem and covered a period of 9 hours, resulted in a curve composed of a rising portion, a plateau, and a descending slope. When the measurements were started 4 hours postmortem, the rising portion was small, and this was followed by a long descending slope. At the later time points, the rising part was absent: after 8 hours postmortem, for example, the curve showed a plateau and a descent.

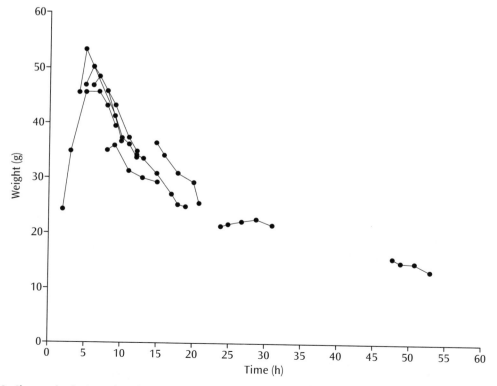

Figure 5.19 *Changes in the intensity of rigor mortis in rats in different postmortem periods.*

Table 5.7 *Experimental evaluation of rigor mortis*

Time postmortem (h)	Intensity changes 1/2/3/4/5/6/7/8/9/10/11/12/13/14/15/16/17/18/19/20/21/	/24/25/26/27/28/29/30/31/	/48/49/50/51/52/53
2–9	2↑3↑5−7↓8↓9		
4–10	4↑5−7↓9↓10		
5–12	5↑6−8↓10−11↓12		
6–12	6−7↓9↓11↓12		
8–15	8−9↓11−13−14−15		
12–19	12−13↓15↓17↓18−19		
15–21	15−16↓18−20↓21		
24–31		24−25−27−29−31	
48–53			48−49−51↓53

↑ Increase; ↓ decrease : significant changes; : no significant changes.

Thus, three different phases were observed that can help estimate the time since death:

1. If an increase in intensity is observed, measurements are made no later than 5 hours postmortem.
2. If a decrease in intensity is observed, measurements are made no earlier than 7 hours postmortem.
3. At 24 hours postmortem, the resolution is complete; there are no more changes in intensity.

It should also be noted that the totality of the curves assembled in Fig. 5.19 gives a form very similar to that of a normal curve (compare this with Fig. 5.13).

The results presented above demonstrate that, in comparison with the single measurement method used earlier, repeated measurements of the intensity of rigor mortis in rats allow the derivation of a more accurate estimate of the time since death.

The question remains as to whether this method is applicable to human corpses. In theory, it should be, and while we can attest that its practical realization is not simple, we are nevertheless attempting to build a measuring device.

Recommendations for practice

First, I would like to quote a remark made by Keith Simpson:[65] 'Rigor mortis is the best known, though the most uncertain and unreliable postmortem event'.

I hope that this section has convinced readers of the validity of this statement, and that they should exercise great caution if they use cadaveric rigidity to estimate the time since death.

Having studied cadaveric rigidity for a long time, I have come to believe that it is not the 'good method', or not '*the* method' to estimate the time since death. Indeed, it requires experience, i.e. regular examinations of corpses made over a long period of time. Moreover, one must remember that there are no tables with values necessarily applicable to a given case.

Nevertheless, I am sure that rigor mortis could be a useful complement for the estimation of the time since death. Under such circumstances, I can only make the following recommendations:

1. We must base estimates on our own personal experience.
2. It is important to consult the data in the literature, in particular the descriptions of individual experiences made by a number of persons.
3. In Mallach's table (Table 5.3), the extreme values, and not the averages, must be considered.
4. We must always seek and appreciate factors that may affect the development of rigor mortis.

Finally, I hope that the method of repeated measurements of the intensity of rigor mortis, once adapted to the human corpse, will permit a better use of this phenomenon for the estimation of time since death.

REFERENCES

1 Szent-Györgyi A. Studies on muscle. *Acta Physiol. Scand.* 1945; **9** (Suppl. XXV).
2 Szent-Györgyi A. *Chemistry of Muscular Contraction*. New York: Academic Press, 1947.
3 Erdös T. Rigor, contracture and ATP. *Stud. Inst Med. Chem. Univ. Szeged.* 1943; **3**: 51–6.

4 Hanson J, Huxley HE. The structural basis of contraction in striated muscle. *Symp. Soc. Exp. Biol.* 1955; **9**: 228–64.

5 Krause D, Zett L. Experimentelle Untersuchungen über den Einfluss von Sauerstoff auf Mechanogramm und Membranpotential bei der Ausbildung der Totenstarre. *Beitr. Gerichtl. Med.* 1973; **30**: 252–7.

6 Bate-Smith EC, Bendall JR. Rigor mortis and adenosine triphosphate. *J. Physiol.* 1947; **106**: 177–85.

7 Bendall JR. Postmortem changes in muscle. In: *The Structure and Function of Muscle, Vol. II, Structure, part 2* (Bourne GH, ed.). London: Academic Press, 1973: 244–309.

8 Krause D, Zett L. Physiologische und morphologische Untersuchungen zu Mechanismus und Verlauf der Totenstarre. *Z. Rechtsmed.* 1973; **72**: 245–54.

9 David H, David S. Submikroskopische Veränderungen der Skelettmuskulatur während der postmortalen Autolyse. *Acta Biol. Med. Germ.* 1965; **14**: 423–35.

10 Krause D, Klein A, Zett L. Todeszeitbestimmung mittels indirekter Muskelreizung über den N. ischiadicus und N. radialis. *Kriminalistik und Forens. Wiss.* 1976; **26**: 66–7.

11 Eisenmenger W, Peschel O, Bratzke H, Welsch U, Herzog V. Elektronenoptische Untersuchungen zur Totenstarre. In: *Gerichtsrnedizin; Festschrift fur W. Holczabek* (Bauer G, ed.). Wien: F. Deuticke Verlag, 1988: 251–66.

12 Peschel O, Bratzke H, Eisenmenger W, Welsch U. Zur Mikromorphologie der Totenstarre im menschlichen Skelettmuskel. *Beitr. Gerichtl. Med.* 1989; **47**: 31–42.

13 Brooke MH, Kaiser KK. The use and abuse of muscle histochemistry. *Ann. N. Y. Acad. Sci.* 1974; **228**: 121–44.

14 Essen B, Jansson E, Henriksson J, Taylor AW, Saltin B. Metabolic characteristics of fibre types in human skeletal muscle. *Acta Physiol. Scand.* 1975; **95**: 153–65.

15 Meijer AEFH, Elias EA. The value of enzyme histochemical techniques in classifying fibre types of human skeletal muscle. 1. Adult skeletal muscles with no apparent disease of the neuromuscular system. *Histochemistry* 1976; **48**: 257–67.

16 Billeter R, Weber H, Lutz H, Howald H, Eppenberger HM, Jenny E. Myosin types in human skeletal muscle fibres. *Histochemistry* 1980; **65**: 249–59.

17 Naumann E. Untersuchungen über den Gang der Totenstarre. *Pflügers Arch.* 1917; **169**: 517–36.

18 Mittmeyer HJ. Abhängigkeit der Totenstarre und Totenflecke vom Leichenalter. *Beitr. Gerichtl. Med.* 1971; **28**: 101–7.

19 Shapiro HA. Rigor mortis. *Br. Med. J.* 1950; **2**: 304.

20 Shapiro HA. Medico-legal mythology – some popular forensic fallacies. *J. Forensic Med.* 1953/54; **1**: 144–69.

21 Tarrant PV, Mothersill C. Glycolysis and associated changes in beef carcasses. *J. Sci. Fd. Agric.* 1977; **28**: 739–49.

22 Niderkorn PF. Cited by Polson CJ. *The Essentials of Forensic Medicine.* Oxford: Pergamon Press, 1962.

23 Mallach HJ. Zur Frage der Todeszeitbestimmung. *Berl. Med.* 1964; **18**: 577–82.

24 Mallach HJ, Mittmeyer HJ. Totenstarre und Totenflecke. *Z. Rechtsmed.* 1971; **69**: 70–8.

25 Henssge CI, Madea B. *Methoden zur Bestimmung der Todeszeit an Leichen.* Lübeck: Schmidt-Römhild, 1988.

26 Husband HA. *The Student's Hand-Book of Forensic Medicine and Medical Police.* Edinburgh: E. and S. Livingstone, 1877.

27 Vock R, Hein PM, Metter D. Tod im tetanischen Anfall. *Z. Rechtsmed.* 1984; **92**: 231–7.

28 Schneider V. Zum Elektrotod in der Badewanne. *Arch. Kriminal.* 1985; **176**: 89–95.

29 Krompecher T, Bergerioux C. Experimental evaluation of rigor mortis. VII. Effect of ante and postmortem electrocution on the evolution of rigor mortis. *Forensic Sci. Int.* 1988; **38**: 27–35.

30 Maresch W. Die Vergiftung durch Phosphorsäureester. *Arch. Toxikologie* 1957; **16**: 285–319.

31 Krompecher T, Bergerioux C, Brandt-Casadevall C, Guler H-R. Experimental evaluation of rigor mortis. VI. Effect of various causes of death on the evolution of rigor mortis. *Forensic Sci. Int.* 1983; **22**: 1–9.

32 Nysten PH. *Recherches de physiologie et chimie pathologiques pour faire suite a celles de Bichat sur la vie et la mort.* Paris, 1811.

33 Kussmaul A. Ueber die Todtenstarre und die ihr nahe verwandten Zustände von Muskelstarre, mit besonderer Berücksichtigung auf die Staatsarzneikunde. *Vierteljahrsschr. prakt. Heilk. (Prag)* 1856; **13**: 67–115.

34 Bierfreund M. Untersuchungen über die Totenstarre. *Pflügers Arch.* 1888; **43**: 195–216.

35 Morgenstern S. Experimentelle Ergebnisse zur Frage des Temperatureinflusses auf die Leichenstarre. *Dtsch. Z. ges. Gerichtl. Med.* 1927; **9**: 718–22.

36 Forster B, Ropohl D, Prokop O, Riemer K. Tierexperimentelle und an menschlichen Leichen gewonnene Daten zur Frage der Dauer der Totenstarre. *Kriminal. Forens. Wiss.* 1974; **13**: 35–45.

37 Fuchs. *Z. allg. Physiol.* 1904; **4**: 359. Cited by Berg S, Nervensystem und Totenstarre. *Dtsch. Z. ges. Gerichtl. Med.* 1948/49; **39**: 429–34.

38 Bush. Experimenta quaedam de morte. Halae, 1819. Cited by Bierfreund M, Untersuchungen über die Totenstarre. *Pflügers Arch.* 1888; **43**: 195–216.

39 Eiselberg AV. Zur Lehre von der Todtenstarre. *Pflügers Arch.* 1881; **24**: 229–31.

40 Gendre AV. Ueber den Einfluss des Nervensystems auf die Todtenstarre. *Pflügers Arch.* 1885; **35**: 45–8.

41 Aust G. Zur Frage über den Einfluss des Nervensystems auf die Todtenstarre. *Pflügers Arch.* 1886; **39**: 241–4.

42 Berg S. Nervensystem und Totenstarre. *Dtsch. Z. ges. Gerichtl. Med.* 1948/49; **39**: 429–34.

43 Baumann J. Ueber kataleptische Totenstarre. *Dtsch. Z. ges. Gerichtl. Med.* 1923; **2**: 647–70.

44 Laves W. Ueber die Totenstarre. *Dtsch. Z. ges. Gerichtl. Med.* 1948/49; **39**: 186–98.

45 Prokop O. Die Totenstarre (Rigor Mortis). In: *Forensische Medizin* (Prokop O, Gohler W, eds.). Stuttgart: G. Fischer Verlag, 1976.

46 Schleyer F. Leichenveränderungen. Todeszeitbestimmung im früh-postmortalen Intervall. In: *Gerichtliche Medizin, Bd. 1.* (Müller B, ed.). Berlin: Springer Verlag, 1975.

47 Sherrington CS. *The Integrative Action of the Nervous System.* London: A. Constable and Co., 1908.

48 Polson CJ, Gee DJ. *The Essentials of Forensic Medicine.* Oxford: Pergamon Press, 1973.

49 Prokop O. Supravitale Erscheinungen. In: *Forensische Medizin* (Prokop O, Gohla W, eds.). Berlin: Volk und Gesundheit Verlag, 1975: 16–27.

50 Mueller B. *Gerichtliche Medizin.* Berlin: Springer, 1953.

51 Oppenheim F, Wacker L. Das Ausbleiben der postmortalen Säurebildung im Muskel als Ursache der verschiedenen Intensität der Totenstarre menschlicher Leichen. *Berl. Klin. Wschr. II.* 1919; **42**: 990–4.

52 Forster B, Ropohl D, Raule P. Eine neue Formel zur Beurteilung der Totenstarre: Die Feststellung des FRR-Index. *Z. Rechtsmed.* 1977; **80**: 51–4.

53 Forster B. Der Arzt am Tatort. Todeszeitbestimmung. *Hippokrates* 1978; **49**: 22–40.

54 Forster B, Ropohl D. *Rechtsmedizin 2.* Stuttgart: Ferdinand Enke Verlag, 1979.

55 Forster B, Ropohl D. *Medizinische Kriminalistik am Tatort.* Stuttgart: Ferdinand Enke Verlag, 1983.

56 Beier G, Liebhardt E, Schuck M, Spann W. Totenstarremessungen an menschlichen Skelettmuskeln in situ. *Z. Rechtsmed.* 1977; **79**: 277–83.

57 Schuck M, Beier G, Liebhardt E, Spann W. Zur Schätzung der Liegezeit durch Messungen der Totenstarre. *Beitr. Gerichtl. Med.* 1978; **36**: 339–43.

58 Schuck M, Beier G, Liebhardt E, Spann W. On the estimation of lay-time by measurement of rigor mortis. *Forensic Sci. Int.* 1979; **14**: 171–6.

59 Krompecher T, Fryc O. Experimentelle Untersuchungen an der Leichenstarre. II. Das Entstehen der Leichenstarre unter Einfluss von körperlicher Anstrengung. *Beitr. Gerichtl. Med.* 1978; **36**: 345–9.

60 Krompecher T, Fryc O. Experimental evaluation of rigor mortis. III. Comparative study of the evolution of rigor mortis in different sized muscle groups in rats. *Forensic Sci. Int.* 1978; **12**: 97–102.

61 Krompecher T, Fryc O. Experimental evaluation of rigor mortis. IV. Change in strength and evolution of rigor mortis in the case of physical exercise preceding death. *Forensic Sci. Int.* 1978; **12**: 103–7.

62 Krompecher T, Fryc O. Zur Frage der Todeszeitbestimmung auf Grund der Leichenstarre. *Beitr. Gerichtl. Med.* 1979; **37**: 285–9.

63 Krompecher T, Fryc O. Experimental evaluation of rigor mortis. V. Effects of temperature on the evolution of rigor mortis. *Forensic Sci. Int.* 1981; **17**: 19–26.

64 Krompecher T. Experimental evaluation of rigor mortis. VIII. Estimation of the time since death by repeated measurements of the intensity of rigor mortis on rats. *Forensic Sci. Int.* 1994; **68**: 149–59.

65 Simpson K. *Forensic Medicine.* London: Edward Arnold, 1974.

Postmortem mechanical excitation of skeletal muscle

BURKHARD MADEA

Zsako's phenomenon and idiomuscular contraction are different phases of postmortem mechanical excitability of skeletal muscle. While Zsako's phenomenon seems to be a propagated excitation of muscle fibres, the idiomuscular contraction or idiomuscular pad is a local contraction of the muscle.

Investigations on postmortem mechanical excitability of skeletal muscle were mainly carried out

Table 5.8 *Investigations on idiomuscular pad with random samples, muscles investigated and results obtained*

Reference	Random sample	Results	Muscles investigated
Näcke[8]	20 mentally ill men	Mechanical excitability of skeletal muscle expired after 3–4 hours	Mimic muscles, neck muscles muscles on the limb
Dotzauer[1]	595 examinations on 176 bodies	Idiomuscular pad can be induced up to 12 hpm; $\bar{x}$ = 6.9 hpm	M. pectoralis M. deltoideus M. biceps brachii
Popwassilew and Palm[5]	60 examinations	Idiomuscular pad can be induced in the interval 1.5–8 hpm; $\bar{x}$ = 4.25 hpm	M. biceps brachii
Semmler[7]	102 bodies	2 hpm idiomuscular pad positive in 90.3%, 8 hpm negative in all cases; $\bar{x}$ = 4.21 hpm	Right thigh

during the nineteenth century and the first half of the twentieth century[1,2] (the more recent investigations are listed in Table 5.8).

In these older investigations, different muscles were investigated and different modes of excitation were used (including pinching, hitting with the hand, the back of the hand, the back of a knife or a chisel). The heavier the blow, the stronger the reaction. Different names were used for the same phenomenon, for instance 'Zsako's muscle phenomenon', which is just a propagated contraction of the muscle after mechanical excitation in the very early postmortem interval. Some authors confined their experiments to the very early postmortem period,[3,4] and recommended as many as eight different places to examine this phenomenon (Fig. 5.20); however, clear values for the duration of postmortem excitability of these different muscles are lacking. Therefore, the literature on mechanical excitation of skeletal muscle is somewhat confused and different studies are hardly comparable. For practical use, the last two extensive studies on idiomuscular contraction should be considered[1,5] because they present relatively detailed information on the mode of excitation and the results obtained (Table 5.9; Figs 5.21 and 5.22).

According to Dotzauer[1] and the detailed review of Joachim[2] on postmortem mechanical excitability of skeletal muscle, three phases or degrees of mechanical

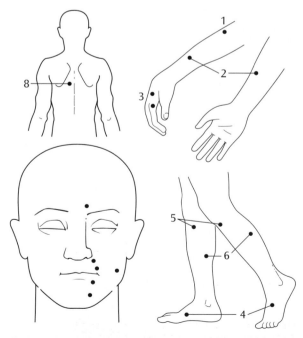

Figure 5.20 *Examining Zsako's phenomenon (mechanical excitability of skeletal muscle in the very early postmortem interval). The points give the places where optimal reactions can be obtained.*[2]

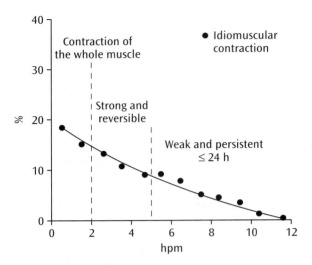

Table 5.9 *Postmortem mechanical excitability*[28]

Zsako's phenomenon/idiomuscular pad		
	++	+
Idiomuscular pad	0–5.5	1.5–8
(M. biceps brachii)	$\bar{x} = 2.25$	$\bar{x} = 4.25$
	$n = 77$	$n = 60$
Zsako's phenomenon		0–2.5
(hitting on the Mm. interossei		$\bar{x} = 1.5$
at the back of the hand;		$n = 41$
hitting on the M. quadriceps femoris)		

+ = only weak reaction, IMP just to touch; ++ = stronger reaction, IMP is good, visible. IMP, idiomuscular pad.

Figure 5.21 *Percentage frequency of positive results in mechanical excitability of skeletal muscles. The mechanical excitability is graded in three phases (see also* Table 5.10*).*[1]

methods of examining mechanical excitability of skeletal muscle at different regions of the body (Fig. 5.20); Although quoted in the literature, very few authors seem to have experience with Zsako's methods, as stated by Dotzauer.[1] Prokop[6] recommends from Zsako's methods the following: hitting the lower third of the thigh four to five cross-fingers above the patella. This first degree of idiomuscular contraction (propagated excitation) can be seen up to 1.5–2.5 hours postmortem.[1,2] Figure 5.23 shows the frequency of idiomuscular contraction postmortem in three temperature classes.

excitability of skeletal muscle can be distinguished (Fig. 5.21; Table 5.10):

1. In the first phase, mechanical excitation of the muscle reveals a contraction of the whole muscle (propagated excitation). This first phase of idiomuscular contraction is identical to Zsako's muscle phenomenon.[3,4] Zsako himself gave eight

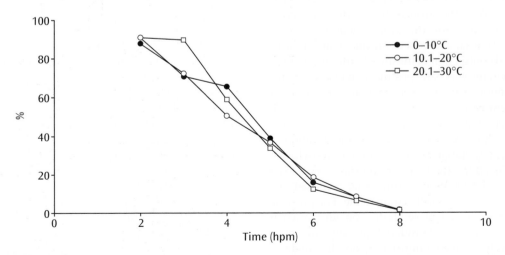

Figure 5.22 *Percentage frequency of positive results in mechanical excitability of skeletal muscle (idiomuscular pad and Zsako's phenomenon). There is no obvious temperature dependence for the duration of mechanical excitability. The shorter postmortem period in which idiomuscular pad could be induced, compared with* Fig. 5.21*, is probably due to the fact that Semmler used hospital cases, whereas Dotzauer (*Fig. 5.21*) used coroner cases for investigation. The figure was drawn using original data from Semmler.*[7]

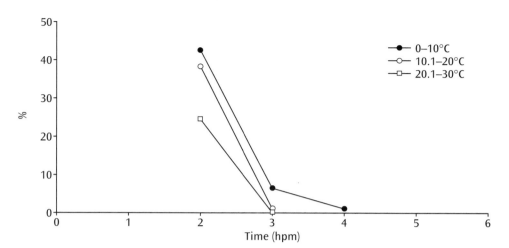

Figure 5.23 *Percentage frequency of Zsako's phenomenon in three temperature classes. Mode of excitation: hitting onto the Mm. interossei between metacarpal 3 and 4 with a reflex hammer. Drawn using original data from Semmler.*[7]

2. In the second phase, a strong and typically reversible idiomuscular pad develops. This phase may be seen as long as 4 to 5 hours postmortem. The mechanical excitation of the muscle causes a membrane depolarization. The shortening of the muscle spreads very slowly, at only 0.2 cm/second, over the whole muscle length, the duration of shortening being 0.7 second. Shortening is initiated by action potentials. The local excitation and contraction is a relatively stable process, mechanical excitability lasting longer than electrical excitability, according to older literature referenced by Dotzauer.[1]

3. In the last phase, a weak idiomuscular pad develops which may persist over a long period (up to 24 hours). The weak idiomuscular pad can be seen in the time interval up to 8–12 hours postmortem.)

Semmler,[7] working on the influence of ambient temperature on the duration of electrical excitability, also examined idiomuscular contraction and Zsako's phenomenon. The idiomuscular pad was examined by hitting with a reflex hammer on the right thigh. At 2 hours postmortem, an idiomuscular pad was present in 90.3% of the bodies investigated; at 8 hours postmortem it was absent in all 102 bodies (median value 4.21 hours postmortem). No temperature-dependence of the idiomuscular pad could be demonstrated (see Fig. 5.22). The shorter time period in which the idiomuscular pad could be demonstrated in Semmler's study compared with Dotzauer's study[1] may be due to the composition of the sample. Dotzauer worked on forensic pathology material, and Semmler on clinical pathology material.

Zsako's phenomenon was also investigated by hitting the interosseous muscles between metacarpals 3 and 4 with a reflex hammer. At 2 hours postmortem, Zsako's phenomenon was seen in 35.5% of all bodies, but at 3 hours postmortem only two bodies were positive, and at 4 hours postmortem, none was positive. (Figure 5.23 shows the frequency of Zsako's phenomenon.) For practical use in death-time estimation in casework, we recommend that the data in Table 5.10 be used (see Chapter 7).

Table 5.10 *Mode of excitation and grading of the three phases of postmortem mechanical excitability of skeletal muscle*

Mode of excitation: hit vigorously with the back of a knife or chisel on the M. biceps brachii at right angles to the arm axis	
Phase one	Contraction of the whole muscle; 1.5–2.5 hpm
Phase two	Strong and typical reversible idiomuscular pad; 4–5 hpm
Phase three	Weak idiomuscular pad which may persist for a longer period (up to 24 hours); 8–12 hpm

REFERENCES

1 Dotzauer G. Idiomuskuläter Wulst und postmortale Blutung (German). *Z. gericht. Med.* 1958; **46**: 761–71.
2 Joachim H. Mechanische und elektrische Erregbarkeit der Skelettmuskulatur. In: *Methoden zur Bestimmung der Todeszeit an Leichen.* (Henssge C, Madea B, eds.). Lübeck: Schmidt-Römhild, 1988: 32–82.
3 Zsako St. Die Bestimmung des Todeszeitpunktes. *Psychiatr. Neurolog. Wschr.* 1941; 66–9.
4 Zsako St. Die Bestimmung der Todeszeit durch die muskelmechanischen Erscheinungen. *Münch. Med. Wschr.* 1916; **3**: 82.

5 Popwassilew J, Palm W. Über die Todeszeitbestimmung in den ersten zehn Stunden. *Z. ärztl. Fortbildung* 1960; **54**: 734–7.
6 Prokop O. *Forensische Medizin.* Berlin: Verlag Volk und Gesundheit, 1975.
7 Semmler J. *Einfluss der Umgebungstemperatur auf die Todeszeitbestimmung durch elektrische Reizung der Oberlidmuskulatur menschlicher Leichen.* Magdeburg University: MD Thesis, 1979.
8 Näcke P. Die Dauer der postmortalen mechanischen Muskulaturerregbarkeit bei chronisch Geisteskranken, speziell Paralytikern. *Z. gesamte Neurol. Psychiatr.* 1991; **7**: 424–46.

Postmortem electrical excitability of skeletal muscle in casework

BURKHARD MADEA

INTRODUCTION: HISTORICAL REVIEW

Studies on the electrical excitability of skeletal muscle postmortem began with Luigi Galvani's discovery of 'animal electricity'.[1]

The great period of electrophysiology during the nineteenth century was accompanied by many studies on the postmortem electrical excitability of skeletal muscle, which were performed mainly by physiologists, but also by French and German pathologists. At the beginning of the nineteenth century the aim of these studies was mainly to exclude apparent death (Table 5.11), and only those bodies in which electrical excitability had ceased completely were buried.

As late as 1872, Rosenthal[2] wrote that the loss of electrical excitability was the most reliable sign of death. However, as early as 1811, Nysten[3] described (in analogy to the onset of rigor mortis – Nysten's rule) the regular loss of electrical excitability in different regions of the body, '*In musculis trunci citius periit irritabilitas, quam in musculis membrorum; musculi extremitatum inferiorum eam citius perdunt quam musculi extremitatum superiorum*'. This rule proved to be quite exact in succeeding investigations.[4]

Several papers on anatomical and physiological investigations on executed bodies have provided information on the duration of electrical excitability.[5,6] According to these authors, indirect electrical excitability of skeletal muscle ceases some minutes after death. However, Du Bois Reymond (in Kölliker and Virchow[6]) and Kölliker and Virchow[6] have seen intensive muscle contractions after exciting the nerve at 1.5 hours postmortem. This was confirmed 100 years later by Krause *et al.*[7] on amputated limbs.

Table 5.11 *Development of electrical excitability of skeletal muscle postmortem in the nineteenth century*

Galvani	1780	⎫	Animal electricity
Klein	1794		
Creve	1796	⎬	
Hüpsch	1800		Studies on electrical excitabilty
Heidmann	1804		of skeletal muscle postmortem to
Struwe	1805		detect and prevent apparent death
Sommer	1833		
Rosenthal	1872	⎭	
Bichat	1800	⎫	
Nysten	1811		Studies on electrical excitability
Devergie	1841		of skeletal muscle postmortem
Harless	1851	⎬	which provide some knowledge
Kölliker	1851		for determining the time since
Rosenthal	1871		death
Onimus	1880	⎭	

Figure 5.24 shows experiments by Aldini on human bodies after decapitation.[8] Aldini examined electrical excitability of the muscles of the trunk, limbs and facial muscles of two criminals decapitated in Bologna in 1804.

On direct excitation, excitability remained preserved for several hours, according to Nysten[3] up to 26 hours postmortem. On several executed bodies (decapitation) he was able to detect the following intervals of electrical excitability:

1. Left chamber of the heart: 'short'.
2. Bowel and stomach: 45 minutes.
3. Right chamber of the heart: 3 hours.
4. Oesophagus: 1.5 hours.
5. Iris: 1.75 hours
6. Muscles of the trunk shorter than muscles of the lower limbs shorter than muscles of the upper limbs.

Nysten investigated the influence of the cause of death on electrical excitability in 40 hospital cases, and found a loss of electrical excitability after:

- 2.75 hours in peritonitis.
- 3 to 6 hours in cases with phthisis, scirrhus, carcinoma.
- 9 hours in cases of fatal haemorrhage or injuries of the heart.
- 12 hours in cases with apoplexy with paralysis.
- 10 to 15 hours in cases with 'adynamic fever'.
- 13 to 15 hours in cases with pneumonia.
- 5 to 27 hours in cases with aneurysm of the heart.

In 1872, Rosenthal[2] stated that the sphincter palpebrarum remains the longest excitable; this was confirmed 100 years later by Klein and Klein.[9]

The fact that Rosenthal was working in the 1870s indicates that it was recognized quite early that electrical excitability of skeletal muscle may be a suitable method for determining the time since death in the early postmortem interval. This conclusion was also reached by Onimus[10] and Tidy.[11] However, Lochte[12] and Puppe[13] rejected electrical excitability as a method of death-time estimation – Lochte having no experimental experience and Puppe working with already outdated time intervals.

The renaissance of postmortem electrical excitability of skeletal muscle began with investigations stimulated by Prokop.[14,15] Several papers on the construction of square-wave generators[16–22] and a large series on human bodies followed.[9,17,23–28]

CURRENT STATE

Most investigations on the postmortem electrical excitability of skeletal muscle have worked with a verbal description and subjective grading of the muscular response to excitation – the muscular contraction – according to:

1. The strength of contraction.
2. The spread of movement to areas distant from the electrodes.

For example, the results of the first large study on electrical excitability of orbicularis oculi, orbicularis oris muscle and muscles of the hand and forearm on 102 bodies are shown in Fig. 5.25 and Table 5.12. The muscle contraction is graded into three degrees.

During the early postmortem interval there is a

Table 5.12 *Grading by Popwassilew and Palm*[15]

	Grading		
	+++	++	+
Orbicularis oculi	Contraction of of the whole mimic muscles	Contraction of the eyelids	Fibrillar twitching
Orbicularis oris	Contraction of orbicularis oris, neck muscles and eyelids	Contraction of orbicularis oris	Fibrillar twitching
Hand	Contraction of the whole arm	Contraction of the hand and the forearm	Fibrillar twitching

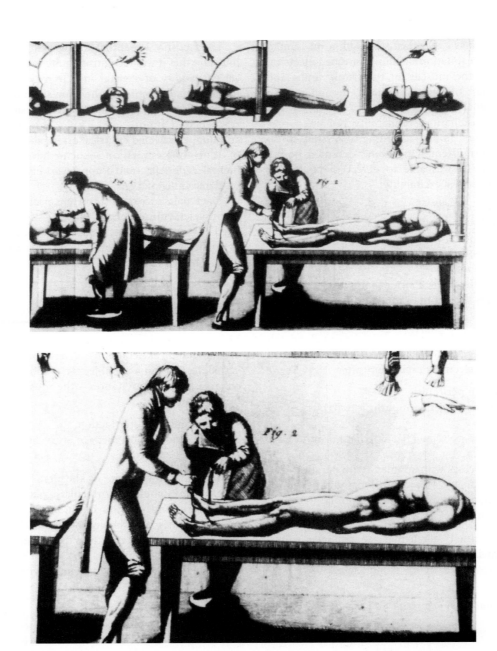

Figure 5.24 *Experiments on electrical excitability of skeletal muscle postmortem conducted after decapitation, by J. Aldini in 1804. Aldini (1762–1834) was a nephew of Galvani. After having performed animal experiments he wanted to study further questions regarding 'animal electricity' on human bodies. He thought that the bodies of persons dying from chronic diseases were not suitable for his experiments because the diseases would destroy the 'fiber structure of muscles'. Therefore he used bodies whose vital force would be preserved after death. 'Therefore I stood so to speak near the scaffold to receive from the hangman's hand the exsanguinated bodies ... It was for advantage to me that two criminals in Bologna were decapitated and the government understood my physical curiosity.' The copperplate print shows the experiments being carried out.*

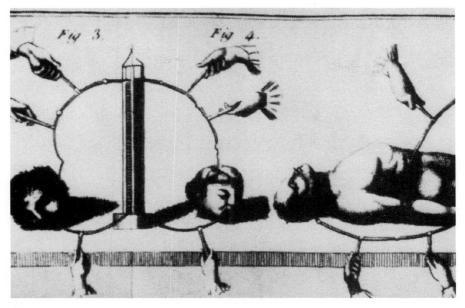

Figure 5.24 continued

strong contraction of the muscles and the excitation will spread to muscles distant from the electrodes (+++; Fig. 5.26), while with increasing postmortem interval, the contraction will become weaker and the muscular response will be confined to the place of excitation (+). Table 5.13 gives the results of this first major investigation (mean value for the special degree, range of scatter and number of cases).

Succeeding investigations modified the subjective grading of electrical excitability for electrode position in the orbicularis oculi muscle: the three degrees by Popwassilew and Palm[15] were changed into six degrees

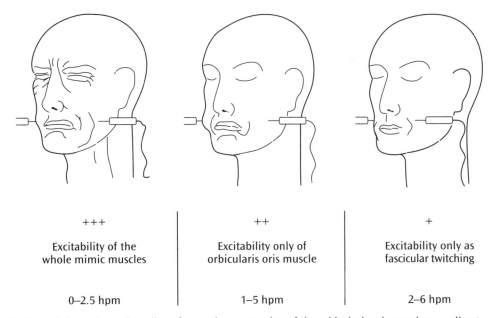

+++	++	+
Excitability of the whole mimic muscles	Excitability only of orbicularis oris muscle	Excitability only as fascicular twitching
0–2.5 hpm	1–5 hpm	2–6 hpm

Figure 5.25 *Position of electrodes and grading of muscular contraction of the orbicularis oris muscle according to Popwassilew and Palm[15] with the postmortem duration of electrical excitability for the special degree. + This degree is in any case found up to 2 hours postmortem, in some up to 6 hours postmortem.*[80]

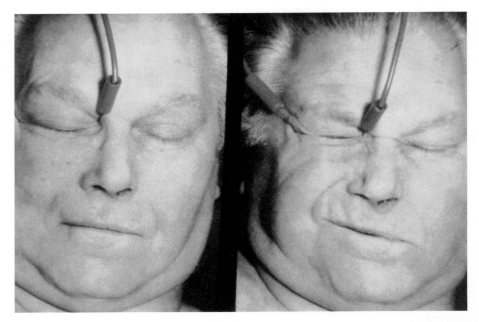

Figure 5.26 *Contraction of the whole mimic muscles on excitation. Degree +++ according to Popwassilew and Palm[15] or degree VI according to Klein and Klein[9] (Table 5.12).*

by Klein and Klein[9] and four degrees by Krause *et al.*[24] (Table 5.14.)

Not only the subjective grading was changed but also the position of electrodes, even for the same investigated muscle (Table 5.15). Most investigators use puncture electrodes; only Zink and Reinhardt[19] recommend surface electrodes.

The depth of insertion of the puncture electrodes varies between 3 mm and 2 cm.

Table 5.13 *Random sample of Popwassilew and Palm[15] 102 cases; for grading see Table 5.12*

	Grading		
	1 +++	**2** ++	**3** +
Orbicularis oculi			
range	0–2.5 h	1–5 h	2–8 h
mean	1.25 h	2.25 h	4.25 h
n	64	79	75
Orbicularis oris			
range	0–2.5 h	1–5 h	2–6 h
mean	1 h	1.75 h	3.75 h
n	56	67	56
Hand			
range	0–2.5 h	1–4 h	1–5.5 h
mean	0.75 h	1.25 h	3.25 h
n	53	55	51

Lastly, the physical parameters of excitation also differ (Table 5.16). Some authors work with differing repetition rate–voltage combinations,[9,24] for example rectangular-like impulses of some millisecond duration, a repetition rate of 10, 30, 70 and 120 per second, and a voltage of 10, 30 or 50 V, which means 12 repetition rate–voltage combinations.[9] Together with the six (seven) degrees of muscular reaction, 75 combinations between mode of excitation and degree of reaction result. In this way, examining electrical excitability becomes very complicated, without any rise in the precision of the death-time estimation.[29]

These few tabular summaries show that all elements of methods (position of electrodes, parameters of excitation, grading of muscular contraction) have been modified. Therefore, it is not surprising that the results of different authors are hardly comparable (Table 5.17). For instance, the Popwassilew and Palm[15] three degrees are comparable with the six degrees of Klein and Klein[9]; however, according to the parameters of excitation and the position of electrodes, the mean values and range of scatter for the degrees differ widely. The same is true for the results on the orbicularis oris muscle.

In practice, there is the question of which investigation (mode of excitation and results) to refer to. If experts wish to use different studies as references, they must employ different square-wave generators.

Table 5.14 *Subjective grading of muscular response to excitation for the orbicularis oculi muscle*

Popwassilew and Palm[15]	Klein and Klein[9]	Krause *et al.*[24]
+++ Whole mimic muscles	VI upper and lower eyelid + forehead + cheek V upper and lower eyelid + forehead	IV heavy contraction spreading to the surrounding muscles III contraction in whole length of the excited muscle
++ Upper and lower eyelid	IV upper and lower eyelid III whole upper eyelid	II incomplete contraction of the excited muscle
+ Fibrillar twitching	II ⅓–⅔ upper eyelid I local upper eyelid	I fibrillar twitching

Table 5.15 *Position of electrodes in the orbicularis oculi muscle according to different authors*

Position of electrodes	Reference
Puncture electrodes in a horizontal distance of 10 mm in the medial part of the left upper eyelid 3 mm deep *or* Puncture electrodes in a vertical distance of 10 mm into the right upper eyelid, inner angle, 3 mm deep	Krause *et al.*[24]
Surface electrodes beside the eye angles of the same eye	Zink and Reinhardt[19]
Puncture electrodes from lateral into the upper eyelid (musculus orbicularis oculi, pars palpebralis)	Popwassilew and Palm[15]
Needle electrodes in a distance of 15 to 20 mm into the nasal part of the upper eyelid 5 to 7 mm deep	Klein and Klein[9]
Like Popwassilew and Palm – 2 cm deep	Walz and Mattig[20]

RECOMMENDATIONS FOR PRACTICAL USE

One of the most extensive investigations was presented by Klein and Klein[9] on case material of 447 bodies. The position of electrodes and the grading of muscular contraction is seen in Tables 5.14 and 5.15 and Figs 5.27 and 5.28. From this extensive case material, Henssge[29] calculated the 95% confidence limits for the six degrees of muscular contraction.

The data originally refer to stimulation by rectangular-like impulses of some milliseconds duration, with a repetition rate of 30 to 70 per second, a voltage of 50 V, and resistance of 1 kOhm. They are completely transferable to excitation with constant-current rectangular impulses of 30 mA, 10 ms duration, and repetition rate 50 per second. At the scene of crime, we use a small self-constructed generator (Fig. 5.29), with the above-mentioned physical parameters of excitation.

The 95% confidence limits for the six degrees of electrical excitability of the orbicularis oculi muscle were calculated on forensic pathology case material. In cases with a longer terminal episode (clinical pathology), the duration of electrical excitability is shorter (Table 5.18).

In cases with haematoma or emphysema of the

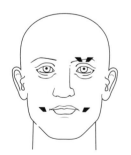

Electrical excitability of mimic muscles

Eye: puncture electrodes in a distance of 15 to 20 mm in the nasal part of the upper eyelid 5 to 7 mm deep

Mouth: puncture electrodes on both sides 10 mm besides angle of the mouth

Figure 5.27 *Position of electrodes for stimulation of mimic muscles (musculus orbicularis oculi, musculus orbicularis oris) according to Klein and Klein.*[9]

Table 5.16 *Differing parameters of excitation according to different authors*

Parameters of excitation	Investigated muscles	Reference
Probably rectangular impulses of 6 ms duration, 9 V, repetition rate 100/s; voltage peaks >4000 V	M. orbicularis oculi M. orbicularis oris Flexors of the forearm	Popwassilew and Palm[15]
Rectangular impulses of some ms duration, repetition rate 10 to 120/s; 10, 30, 50 V; resistance 1 kOhm	M. orbicularis oculi M. orbicularis oris	Klein and Klein[9] Klein et al.[23]
Triangular impulses; repetition rate probably 50/s; 10 voltage steps between 9 and 70 V		Mattig and Waltz[93]
Rectangular impulses of 'a few ms duration', 10 to 50 V, repetition rate between 10 and 100/s	M. orbicularis oculi M. orbicularis oris M. biceps brachii M. brachioradialis	Krause et al.[24]
Constant-current rectangular impulses of 10 ms duration, 30 mA, repetition rate 50/s	M. orbicularis oculi M. orbicularis oris	Henssge and Madea[97,98]
Rectangular impulses of 1 s duration; 200 V; current intensities according to the muscular threshold	Different muscles	Joachim and Feldmann[78] Madea[4] Madea and Henssge[94,95] Ravache-Quiriny[28,83]
Rectangular impulses of 30 V; repetition rate 50/s		Waltz and Mattig[20]
Non sinus-like voltage with voltage peaks up to 1000 V	M. orbicularis oculi	Zink and Reinhardt[19]
Constant-current rectangular impulses of 1 s duration, current intensity between 0.1 and 80 mA according to muscular threshold or definite supraliminal strength	Thenar, hypothenar, M. biceps brachii, M. quadriceps femoris, M. orbicularis oculi	Madea[4]

eyelid, electrical excitability may last much longer than that corresponding to the upper 95% confidence limits for the special degree of the forensic pathology case material (Table 5.19; Fig. 5.30). This may be due to aerobic glycolysis in these cases, with a 19-fold greater energy profit[30–33] and a postmortem Feng effect.[34]

Re-examination of the data of Klein and Klein[9]

We performed investigations on 30 bodies (traumatic or sudden natural death without long-lasting terminal episodes) with about 300 excitations, in order to re-examine whether or not the calculated 95% confidence limits for the different degrees are valid.

The time period investigated was 2 to 13 hours postmortem. The mode of excitation was constant-current rectangular impulses of 1 second duration and 30 mA. The boxes (Fig. 5.31) represent the upper and lower 95% confidence limits for the special degree.

In spite of the slightly differing mode of excitation, the 95% confidence limits proved to be valid (Fig. 5.31). Each point represents one single excitation and all points are within the boxes, except some

Table 5.17 *Mean values and 95% limits of confidence (Klein and Klein[9]) or range of scatter (Popwassilew and Palm[15]) of differing degrees of electrical excitability (in hours). The three degrees of Popwassilew and Palm are comparable to the six degrees of Klein and Klein. Different time values according to position of electrodes and mode of excitation*

		Klein and Klein[9]		Popwassilew and Palm[15]	
		x	95% limits	x	Range of scatter
M. orbicularis oculi					
I	upper eyelid, nasal part	13.5	5–22 ⎫+++	4.25	2–8
II	⅓–⅔ upper eyelid	10.5	5.16 ⎭		
III	whole upper eyelid	8.25	3.5–13 ⎫+++	2.25	1–5
IV	plus lower eyelid	5.5	3–8 ⎭		
V	plus cheek	4.5	2–7 ⎫+	1.25	0–2.5
VI	plus forehead	3.5	1–6 ⎭		
M. orbicularis oris		7	3–11	3.25	2–6

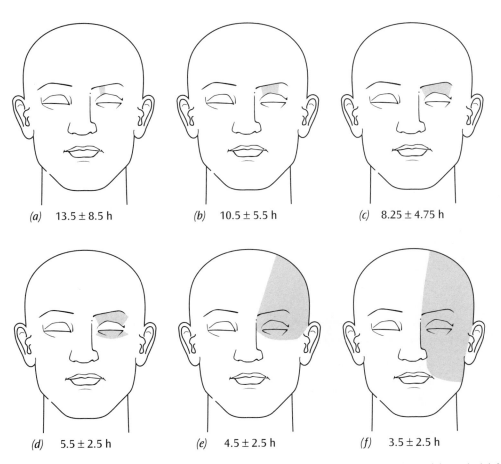

(a) 13.5 ± 8.5 h   (b) 10.5 ± 5.5 h   (c) 8.25 ± 4.75 h

(d) 5.5 ± 2.5 h   (e) 4.5 ± 2.5 h   (f) 3.5 ± 2.5 h

Figure 5.28 *Degrees of a positive reaction for stimulating the orbicularis oculi muscle according to Klein and Klein[9] with mean values and 95% limits of confidence (in hours) for the special degree (calculated by Henssge on the material of Klein and Klein[9]).*

Table 5.18 *Upper and lower 95% limits of confidence for the six degrees of electrical excitability in two different random samples: forensic pathology and clinical pathology. In clinical pathological cases (longer lasting terminal episode) the duration of electrical excitability is shorter*

Degree		Forensic pathology	Clinical pathology (longer lasting terminal episode)
I	local upper eyelid	5–22	3–16
II	⅓–⅔ upper eyelid	5–16	0–16
III	whole upper eyelid	3.5–13	1.5–9
IV	upper and lower eyelid	3–8	1–7
V	upper and lower eyelid + forehead	2–7	1–7
VI	upper and lower eyelid + forehead + cheek	1–6	1–6

points for the degrees IV to VI, which represent several excitations in two cases of fatal hypothermia. In hypothermia, electrical excitability may last much longer.

CONCLUSIONS

Examining the electrical excitability of skeletal muscle postmortem is a very easy procedure, which can be performed at the scene of crime. It takes less than 1 minute to perform, and information on the time since death is available immediately.

Since, in almost all previous papers, either the mode of excitation or the grading of muscular contraction has changed, the investigator must adhere to one method. We recommend examining electrical excitability using a square-wave generator with rectangular impulses of 10 ms duration, 30 mA and a repetition rate of 50 per second. The position of electrodes and grading of muscular contraction is according to Klein and Klein,[9] with the 95% confidence limits calculated by the method of Henssge.[29] These times are valid for forensic cases (exceptions: fatal hypothermia; haematoma or emphysema of the eyelid, where longer times are possible).

Combining electrical excitability with the nomogram method of Henssge *et al.*[35] in the early postmortem interval, the precision and accuracy of the death-time estimation may be raised considerably (see Chapter 7). Using two independent methods to obtain a common result increases the investigator's confidence in the calculation on the time since death. When the temperature method cannot be used, examining electrical excitability alone may provide valuable information on the time of death. In our opinion, the examination of electrical excitability should be included in the minimal standard of methods used in the early postmortem interval for determining the

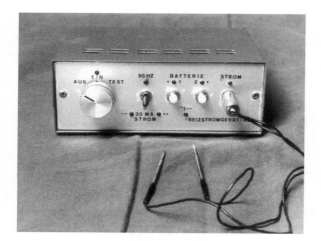

Figure 5.29 *Self-constructed generator for examining electrical excitability at the scene of crime. The output is constant-current rectangular impulses of 30 mA, 10 ms duration at a repetition rate of 50/s.*

Table 5.19 *Duration of electrical excitability in cases of traumatic emphysema, postmortem artificial emphysema and traumatic haematoma of the eyelid*

Circumstances	Duration of electrical excitability (hpm)
Traumatic emphysema (vital)	up to 29
Postmortem emphysema (air insufflation into the eyelid)	27.3–52
Traumatic haematoma of the eyelid	up to 32

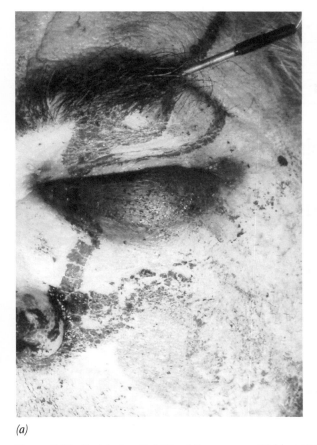

(a)

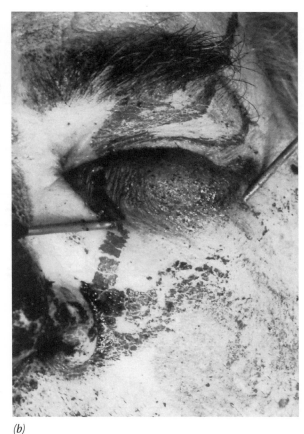

(b)

Figure 5.30 *Electrical excitability of the upper eyelid (a) at 16 hours postmortem while the whole bloodshot lower eyelid is still contracting.*

time since death. In those countries where, for legal reasons, the insertion of needle electrodes before autopsy is not permitted, the use of surface electrodes may be an alternative. However, this would require further investigations if the 95% confidence limits for the six degrees are to be valid for this modified mode of excitation.

LONGITUDINAL STUDIES ON ELECTRICAL EXCITABILITY

Introduction

One of the main reasons for the unsatisfactory comparability of different studies on electrical excitability of skeletal muscle is that the subjective grading of muscular contraction was made only by visual

perception of the muscular reaction or its intensity (spread). The first improvement must therefore be the introduction of a method for objectifying muscular contraction. Another reason for the lack of comparability of different studies is that different authors worked with:

- different modes of excitation; and
- insufficiently defined physiological parameters of excitation.

This second point for improvement must therefore be the introduction of well-defined electrical stimuli.

An electrical stimulus is defined, according to its biological efficiency, by:

1. Strength or intensity.
2. Rise.
3. Duration in one direction.
4. Repetition rate.

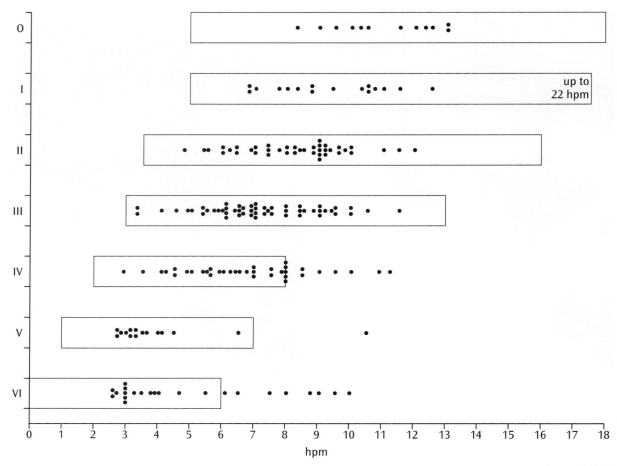

Figure 5.31 *Re-examination of the calculated 95% limits of confidence for the forensic pathology case material. I–VI: degree of electrical excitability according to the grading by Klein and Klein.[9] The boxes represent the upper and lower 95% limits of confidence. Each point corresponds to one excitation (about 300 excitations on 30 bodies). The points outside the boxes (the upper 95% limits of confidence) for the degrees IV–VI were observed in two cases of fatal hypothermia.*

The preceding studies had variation in all elements of excitation. The aim of the present study was to analyse the objectified muscular contraction in relation to electrical stimuli. Therefore, according to the practice in clinical neurophysiology, we used only constant-current rectangular impulses of 1 second duration as single impulses. These are characterized by an infinitely high rise, sufficient duration in one direction, and a defined strength. Our experimental studies with a much shorter duration of stimulus – for instance 0.2 ms, as is usual in physiology – revealed that even by 2 hours postmortem the muscle failed to give any response on excitation (see page 200).

The third defect in preceding investigations was that longitudinal studies on the electrical excitability of the same muscle, until excitability expired, were virtually non-existent (with the exception of the post-mortem rise of galvanic threshold; see page 194).

After an encouraging pilot study in 1984 which avoided these three defects in the preceding investigation,[36] an accurate, standardized and reproducible method was developed for assessing the contraction of skeletal muscle after death by means of electrical stimulation, assessing this phenomenon serially and then relating it to the time elapsed since death.[4,37–39]

Material and methods

For objectifying muscular contraction we used a sensitive force transducer (originally constructed for investigations in experimental cardiac surgery[40,41]) inserted

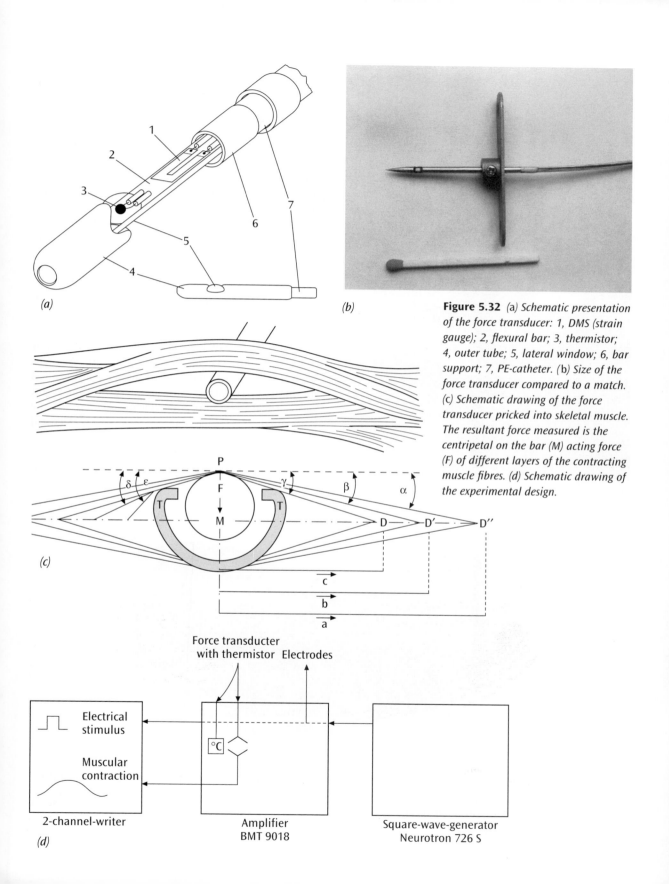

Figure 5.32 (a) *Schematic presentation of the force transducer: 1, DMS (strain gauge); 2, flexural bar; 3, thermistor; 4, outer tube; 5, lateral window; 6, bar support; 7, PE-catheter. (b) Size of the force transducer compared to a match. (c) Schematic drawing of the force transducer pricked into skeletal muscle. The resultant force measured is the centripetal on the bar (M) acting force (F) of different layers of the contracting muscle fibres. (d) Schematic drawing of the experimental design.*

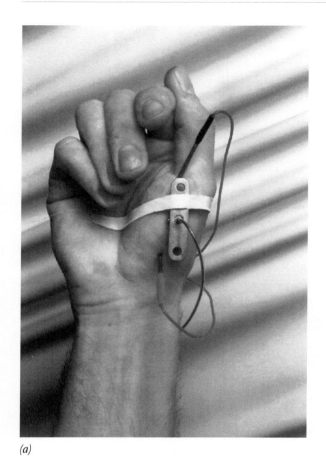

(a)

in a hypodermic needle. Below the top of the force transducer is a lateral window, in which a flexural bar can be seen (Fig. 5.32(a)).

When the force transducer is inserted into the muscle, the contracting muscle fibres will press on the flexural bar, causing it to lose its axial position in the force transducer; this signal will be quantified by the strain gauge. The signal measured the centripetal force acting on the bar due to the contracting muscle fibres (Fig. 5.32(c)).

The measured force of the muscle fibres compressing the bar, as well as the electrical stimulus, were registered by a two-channel writer (Fig. 5.32(d)).

The force transducer was pricked into the muscle, and puncture electrodes were inserted on either side (Fig. 5.33). Investigations were performed mainly on the thenar and hypothenar muscles. The muscle was stimulated half-hourly, using rectangular impulses of 1 second duration of 2, 4, 8, 16, 32, 64 and/or 80 mA, by use of a commercial square-wave generator (Siemens Neurotron 726 S) until the electrical excitability expired for the applied or highest current intensity (Table 5.20).

Electrical excitation and registration were usually performed at contralateral positions. When electrical excitability expired at one position, the electrodes and the force transducer were inserted into another muscle. The random sample consisted of 50 cases of

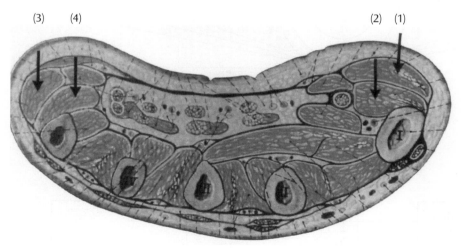

(b)

Figure 5.33 *(a) In corpore insertion of force transducer and puncture electrodes on the right thenar. (b) Cross-section of the hand with muscles investigated: thenar (M. abductor pollicis brevis (1)); M. opponens pollicis (2); hypothenar (M. abductor digiti minimi (3)); M. opponens digiti minimi (4).*

Table 5.20 *Experimental procedure and equipment*

Measurement mostly at contralateral positions (thenar, hypothenar, biceps of the right and left side)

Mode of excitation: rectangular impulses of 1 s duration of supraliminal strength (2, 4, 8, 16, 32, 64, 80 mA) each half-hour until electrical excitability expired for the applied or highest current intensity. Then change to another place (of the same muscle) or to another muscle

Puncture electrodes (steel, 2 mm diameter, 10 mm long) were pricked into the muscle at a distance of 3 to 4 cm, 5 to 7 cm deep

Generator: Neurotron 726 S (Siemens)

Objectifying muscular contraction by a force transducer pricked into the muscle (see text)

Table 5.21 *Composition of the reference and control samples*

Random sample	Control sample
50 cases of sudden natural or traumatic death with a short terminal episode	21 cases of sudden natural or traumatic death with a short terminal episode
male: 26; x̄ 54.2 years (21–80 years)	10; x̄ 38.3 years (19–69 years)
female: 24; x̄ 53.5 years (16–76 years)	11; x̄ 66.3 years (40–79 years)
Beginning of the experiments: 2 to 11 hpm (x̄ 3.9 hpm)	2 to 8 hpm (x̄ 4.3 hpm)
Duration of the experiments: 1 to 9 h (x̄ 4.9 h)	1 to 9 h (x̄ 4.3 h)

sudden natural or traumatic death. Afterwards, a control group of 21 cases was also investigated. The experiments took place in a constant ambient temperature of 20°C (Table 5.21). Continuous measurement of the deep rectal temperature was made, as well as the local temperature at the location of measurement.

Graphical form of muscular contraction

Two graphical forms of muscular contraction must be distinguished:

1. A two-peak shape during the first hours after death.
2. A one-peak shape in the later postmortem interval (Fig. 5.34)

The continuous change of the shape of muscular contraction could be studied in some cases where the start

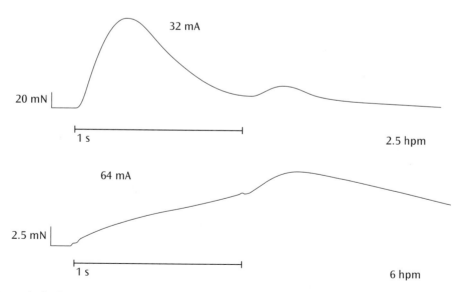

Figure 5.34 *Two principal graphical forms of muscular contraction after stimulation with rectangular impulses of 1 second duration and supraliminal strength. Top, two-peak-shaped contraction corresponding to a closing and opening contraction at the beginning and end of the stimulus. Fast relaxation of the closing as well as the opening contraction. Bottom, one-peak-shaped muscular contraction. The maximum force is achieved after the end of the stimulus; an opening contraction is missing. Return of the contracted muscle fibres to the starting tension is retarded.*

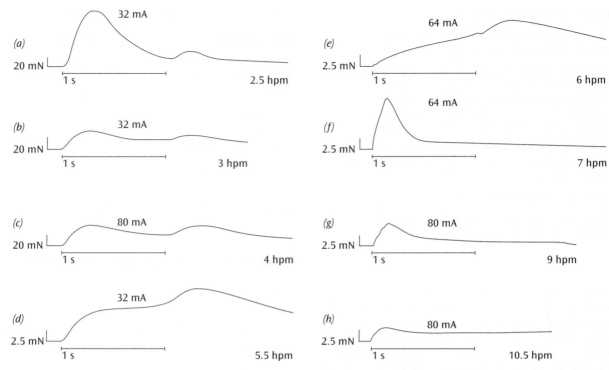

Figure 5.35 *Postmortem change in the shape of muscular contraction. Left, force in mN; bottom, duration of the 1 s electrical stimulus in relation to the time course of muscular contraction; current intensities; time since death in hours. The curves (a) to (e) were registered at 100 mm/s, the curves (f) to (h) at 10 mm/s paper speed.*

of investigation could be made very soon after death, with a long duration of electrical excitability (Fig. 5.35(a)).

In the early postmortem interval, the muscular contraction is characterized by a two-peak shape: a closing and opening contraction at the beginning and the end of the 1-second electrical stimulus (Fig. 5.35). The closing, as well as the opening, contractions have their own contraction and relaxation period.

In the early postmortem interval the closing contraction has a higher maximum force than the opening contraction (Fig. 5.35(a)). When the relaxation period of the closing contraction becomes weaker, the opening contraction begins at a higher force level and shows a higher force maximum (Fig. 5.35(d)). This results in a superimposition of the closing contraction on the opening contraction.

As the contraction velocity of the closing contraction decreases, the contraction period of the closing contraction is continued through the contraction period of the opening contraction. Consequently, a one-peak shape of muscular contraction results. At 80 mA current intensities, the one-peak shape appeared, on average, at 5 hours postmortem (Table 5.22).

This one-peak shape of muscular contraction becomes increasingly weaker with the increasing postmortem interval (Fig. 5.35(f–h)). That this pattern of muscular contraction has not yet been described in the literature may be due to the fact that long-lasting stimuli as used here are not normally used in physiology investigations.

Another example of the continuous change of the graphical form of muscular contraction is shown in Fig. 5.36.

The first appearance of a one-peak shape of muscular contraction depends not only on the current intensity used for stimulation (see Table 5.20) but also on the temperature history of the body. The deeper the rectal temperature at the beginning of the investigations, the later the one-peak shape of muscular contraction will appear (Fig. 5.37).

Decrease of muscular force

Figure 5.38 shows that, with stable current intensity, the maximum force developed on excitation decreases

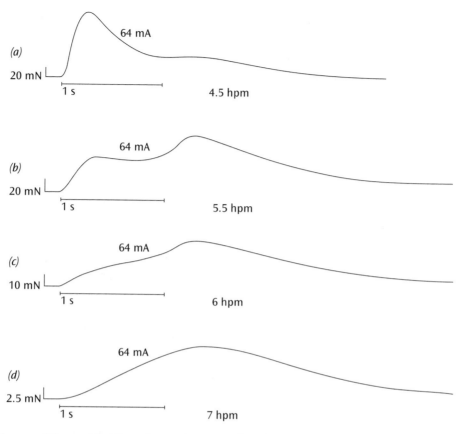

Figure 5.36 *Changes of the graphical form of muscular contraction after excitation with a current intensity of 64 mA. Left, calibration of force; bottom, duration of the electrical stimulus in relation to the graphical form of muscular contraction.*

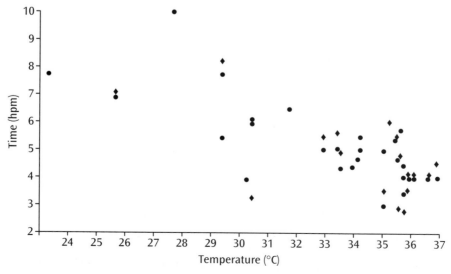

Figure 5.37 *Moment of the first appearance of a one-peak shape of muscular contraction on the right (●) and left (◆) thenar after excitation with 80 mA current intensity over the rectal temperature of the body (temperature at the beginning of the experiments).*

Table 5.22 *Postmortem time for the change in the shape of muscular contraction. First appearance of a single-shaped curve for the right and left thenar and different current intensities. Mean value and range of scatter in minutes postmortem*

J (mA)	Right thenar			Left thenar		
	n	x̄ (min)	Range of scatter (min)	n	x̄ (min)	Range of scatter (min)
2	9	214	135–405	12	203	110–330
4	16	227	150–405	13	230	110–420
8	19	255	160–520	18	252	140–420
16	22	275	180–545	20	254	140–420
32	23	295	180–575	21	282	140–495
64	26	316	180–605	20	290	140–495
80	26	322	180–605	18	289	165–495

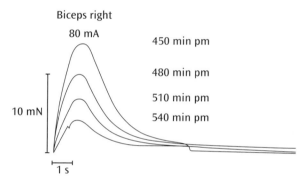

Figure 5.38 *Decrease in the maximum force on the right M. biceps brachii over the postmortem interval. Current intensity 80 mA; time since death in minutes postmortem; left, gauge for 10 mN.*

with increasing postmortem interval. There is virtually a linear relationship between the natural logarithm of the maximum force and the time since death (Fig. 5.39). Figure 5.39(a) shows the decrease of the maximum force of the same muscle after excitation with current intensities between 4 and 80 mA. The higher the current intensity, the longer the muscular contractions may be demonstrated. In a few cases the force maximum of the second registration was higher than that of the first (Fig. 5.39(b)).

This 'paradoxical' rise of force can be explained both by muscular fatigue and by the breaking of the stiffening of some fibres during the first muscle contraction. By this breaking such stiffening, the inner resistance of muscle during developing rigor mortis, is overcome and the later contractions can develop a higher force maximum.

In contralateral muscles the decrease in the maximum force is almost identical (Fig. 5.40). In different muscles of the same body, the decrease in the maximum force differs widely (Fig. 5.41(a, b)). For example, the decline in the biceps muscle is nearly always faster than in the thenar or hypothenar muscle (Fig. 5.41(a)). While the biceps has lost electrical excitability at 6.5 hours postmortem, excitability of the hand muscles is preserved for 4 hours more, most likely for the following reasons:

• Variations in the glycogen content of different muscles of the body at the moment of death. We should note that, in healthy individuals, the glycogen content of the rectus femoris muscle varies by a factor of 2.5.
• A different cooling velocity, depending on the diameter of the muscle and its topographical localization.
• Probably the extension of the muscle: the greater the extension, the sooner the electrical excitability expires.

There is great interindividual variability in the decrease of the maximum force after stimulation with stable current intensity (Fig. 5.42(a–c)). Even in cases that had the same postmortem period and were kept under similar experimental conditions, the duration of electrical excitability varied between 6 and 12 hours postmortem (Fig. 5.42(c)).

Extrapolation of the time since death

As there is an almost linear relationship between the natural logarithm of the decrease of the maximum

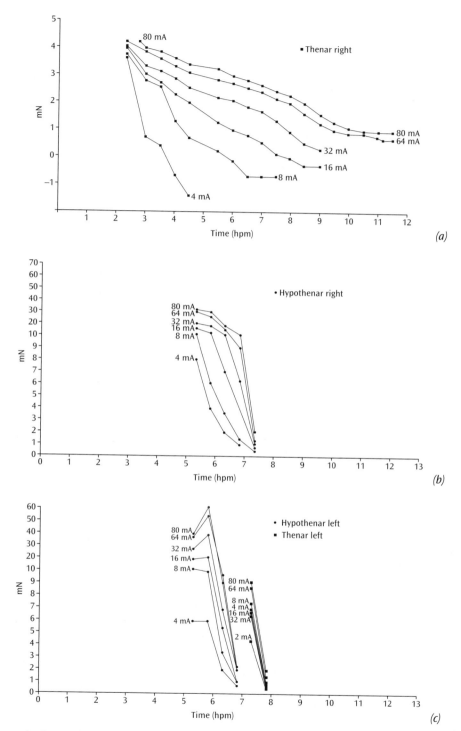

Figure 5.39 *Decrease in the maximum force of the same muscle after excitation with current intensities between 4 and 80 mA. x axis = time since death in hours; y axis = natural logarithm of the maximum force (mN). Almost linear relationship between decrease of the force (ln mN) and time since death. Decrease of maximum force on the right (b) and left (c) hypothenar, on the left hypothenar with a 'paradoxical' rise of force for current intensities between 16 and 80 mA between first and second series of stimulation.*

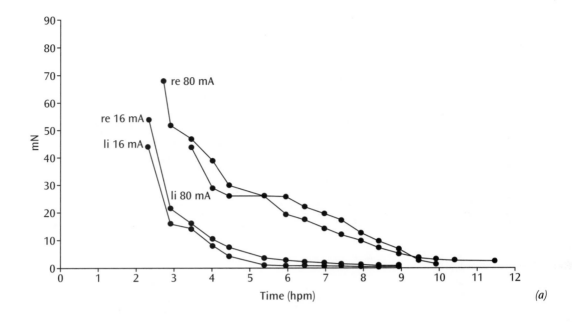

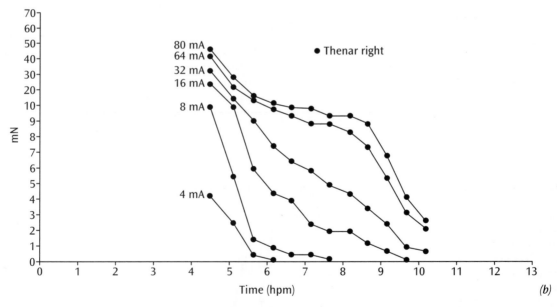

Figure 5.40 *(a) Decrease in maximum force (mN) over the time since death (hpm) at contralateral muscles (right and left thenar) for two current intensities (16 and 80 mA). (b) Decrease in the maximum force at contralateral positions over the time since death. At the left thenar (c) two measuring positions. Although the force developed on excitation and the decrease in force differs, there is nearly the same PMI of preserved excitability.*

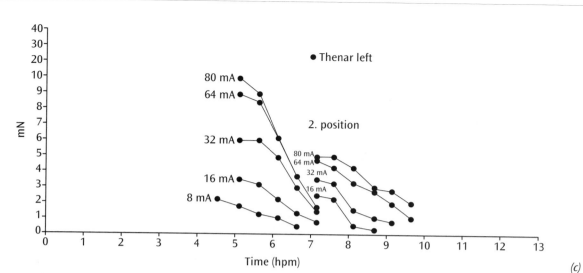

Figure 5.40 continued

force and time since death, linear regression analysis was performed for all cases using current intensities of 8, 32 and 80 mA for all forces measured at the right and left thenar. From this regression analysis, mean values for the slope and intercept were calculated (Table 5.23). With these collective mean values the time since death was calculated as follows:

$$t = a_i - \frac{\bar{a}}{\bar{b}}$$

where t = time since death in minutes; a_i = registered maximum force; and $\bar{a}/\bar{b}$ = collective mean values for slope and intercept.

The 95% confidence limits of estimated time of death are shown in Table 5.23. With increasing current intensity, i.e. with increasing postmortem interval of demonstrable reagibility, the 95% confidence limits vary between ± 2.31 hours (8 mA) and ± 4.27 hours (80 mA current intensity). These calculated 95% confidence limits were checked on an

Table 5.23 *Statistical parameters of precision in estimating the time since death (thenar)*

	Decrease of maximum force			Force-related relaxation
Experimental group				
Current intensity	8 mA	32 mA	80 mA	
Mean values for:				
intercept *a*	7.7	8.4	8.2	−3.18
slope *b*	−0.024	−0.019	−0.016	4.9
No. of measurements	248	426	445	346
Mean (h)	−0.222	0.059	−0.136	0.049
Standard deviation (h)	1.176	1.41	2.18	1.371
95% limits of confidence (h)	2.31	2.76	4.27	2.69
Control group				
Current intensity	8 mA	32 mA	80 mA	
No. of measurements	50	106	113	90
Mean (h)	−0.43	−0.21	−0.17	0.25
Standard deviation (h)	1.08	1.31	1.45	1.27
95% limits of confidence (h)	2.23	2.62	2.91	2.54

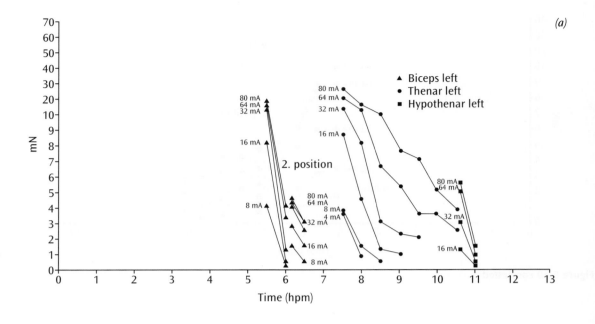

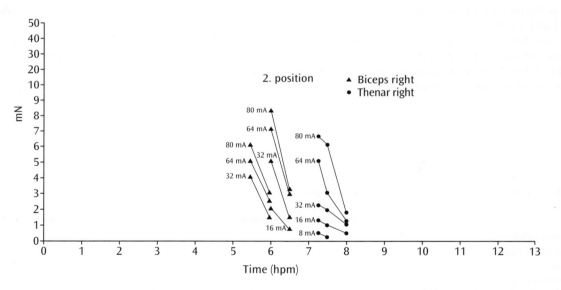

Figure 5.41 (a) Decrease in maximum force of different muscles of the same body (intraindividual variability) over the PMI. While the excitability of the left biceps brachii examined at two different positions expired 6.5 hours postmortem, the thenar and hypothenar muscles remained excitable up to 11 hours postmortem. (b) Decrease of maximum force at contralateral positions, right and left thenar and hypothenar. In only a few cases could such marked differences in the duration of electrical excitability between thenar and hypothenar be observed. While the excitability of the contralateral thenar muscle has already expired 7 hours postmortem, excitability at the hypothenar was preserved for 4 more hours.

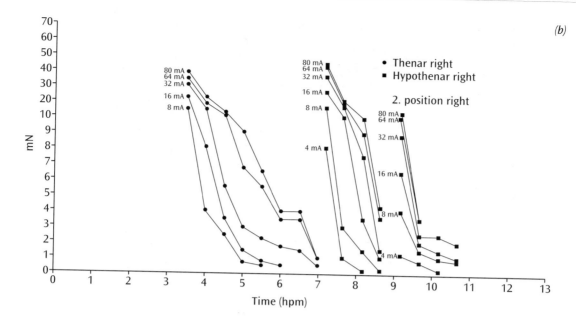

(b)

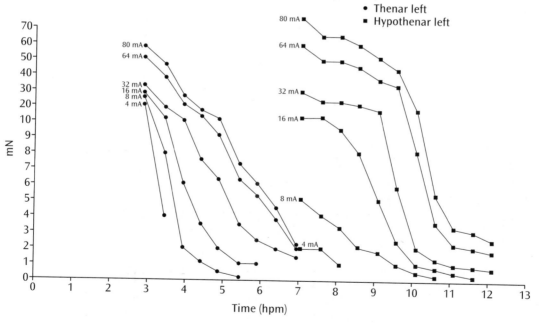

Figure 5.41 continued

independent group of 21 bodies, and proved to be reliable (Table 5.23; Fig. 5.43).

The time of death estimated from the force values measured on the hypothenar is reliable within the same limits; for the biceps brachii the ranges are much wider (Table 5.24).

Relaxation time

The graphic record of muscular contraction consists of a latency period, a contraction period and a relaxation period (Fig. 5.44).

These periods can be quantified as follows:

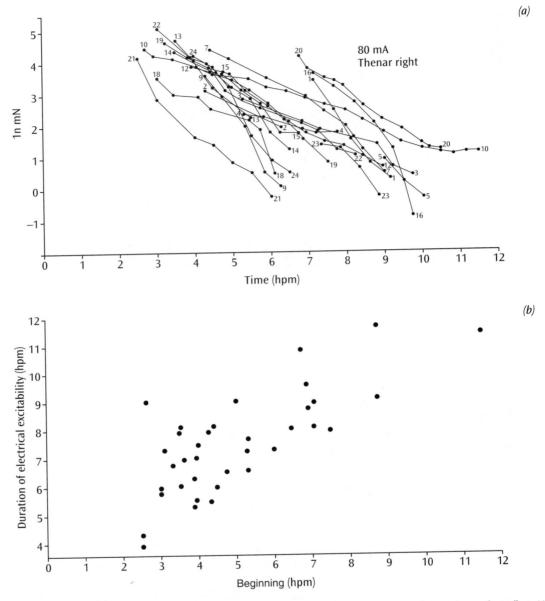

Figure 5.42 (a) Interindividual variability of the duration of electrical excitability. Decrease in the maximum force (ln mN) over the postmortem interval (hpm) on the right thenar, current intensity 80 mA; 20 bodies with known time since death. The small numbers at the curves are case numbers. Cases 10 and 21, with almost identical beginnings of the excitations and identical experimental conditions, show an interindividual variability in the duration of electrical excitability of 6 hours. (b) Duration of electrical excitability over the postmortem beginning of experiments. Duration of electrical excitability (decrease in maximum force until a force value of 5 mN has been reached; stimulation with 80 mA current intensity) for 36 cases with known time since death over the postmortem beginning of experiments. Even in cases with the same postmortem beginning the duration of electrical excitability differs widely. (c) Differing duration of electrical excitability in two cases with the same postmortem beginning. Decrease in maximum force for two cases with beginning of the experiments 3 hours postmortem. The duration of electrical excitability differs by about 6 hours.

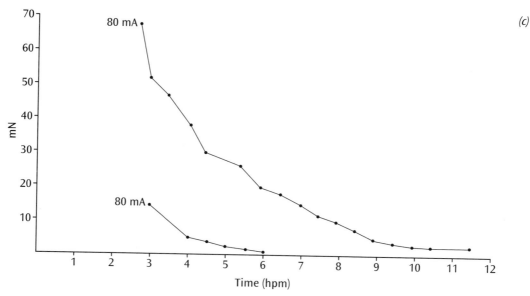

(c)

Figure 5.42 continued

contraction time until 25, 50 or 100% of the maximum force is achieved during contraction; or relaxation time until 50 or 25% of the maximum force is reached again in the relaxation period. The shape of muscular contraction, which becomes weaker with increasing postmortem interval, is characterized by a maximum force reached after the 1-second stimulus (increasing contraction time) and an increasingly

retarded return of the contracted fibres to the starting tension (increasing relaxation time) (see Fig. 5.34).

Compared to the contraction time, the relaxation time (time until the maximum force has decreased to 25%) shows the most notable change over the time period since death (Fig. 5.45). The relaxation time also shows an exponential correlation with the maximum force (Fig. 5.46). Therefore, we devised a quotient* of

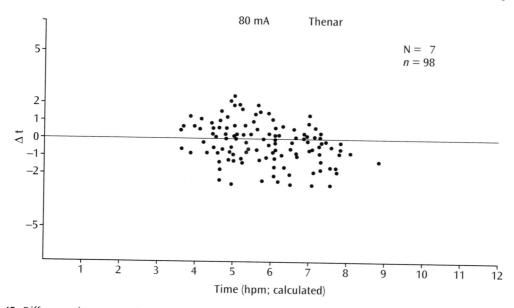

Figure 5.43 *Differences between real and extrapolated time since death of the control sample over the extrapolated time since death. Seven cases, thenar, 80 mA current intensity. All values within the calculated 95% limits of confidence.*

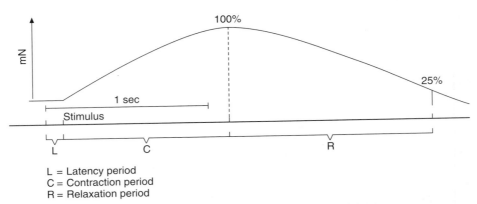

L = Latency period
C = Contraction period
R = Relaxation period

Figure 5.44 *Schematic presentation of a muscular contraction in relation to the electrical stimulus. With the beginning of the stimulus as starting point the record of a contraction is composed of a latency period, a contraction period and a relaxation period.*

Table 5.24 *Precision of death-time estimation using the criterion 'decrease of maximum force'*

	Decrease of maximum force					
	Hypothenar			**Biceps brachii**		
Current intensity	8 mA	32 mA	80 mA	8 mA	32 mA	80 mA
Mean values for:						
slope a	9.76	9.93	11.3	10	7.8	9.41
intercept b	−0.024	−0.019	−0.020	−0.029	−0.020	−0.025
No. of bodies	18	18	18	4	6	6
No. of measurements	107	162	181	25	57	63
Mean (h)	−0.33	0.05	0.23	0.39	0.19	−0.43
Standard deviation (h)	1.01	1.16	1.29	1.45	1.47	1.44
95% limits of confidence (h)	2.02	2.29	2.56	3.06	2.95	2.89
PMI (h)	3–10	3–12	3–12	2–7	2–9	2–9

the relaxation time and the maximum force. In the form of its natural logarithm, a very strong linear relationship with the natural logarithm of the time since death exists (Fig. 5.47). This quotient, called 'force-related relaxation time', contains two criteria of objectified muscular contraction, changing throughout the postmortem period:

1. A vertical component (the decrease of the maximum force); and

2. A horizontal component (the increase of relaxation time).

Extrapolation of the time since death

Again, regression analysis was performed with these values, and collective mean values for slope and intercept were calculated. By using these collective mean

---

*Each half-hour the muscle was stimulated with different current intensities, the relaxation time of three curves was measured, a mean value was formed, and a fixed value for the contraction time was subtracted ($t25\% - 1.100$ ms). The increase of the contraction time can be neglected as compared with the increase in relaxation time. This value ($t25\% - 1.100$ ms) was divided through the mean maximum force of the curves evaluated:

$$\frac{t25\% - 1.100 \text{ ms}}{A \text{ mN}}$$

This value is called 'force-related relaxation time'. An example for calculating this is given in Table 5.25.)

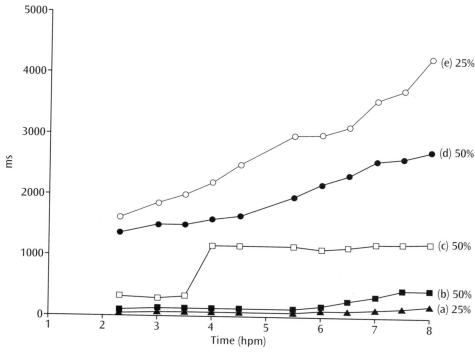

Figure 5.45 *Contraction and relaxation time over the PMI. Contraction time up to 25% (a), 50% (b), 100% (c) of the maximum force during muscular contraction. Relaxation time up to 50% (d) and 25% (e) during the relaxation period. The relaxation time up to 25% of maximum force shows the steepest slope over PMI. Presentation is for one case. Each point is a mean value for at least three 'contraction or relaxation times' of different muscular contractions registered at the same time postmortem after excitation with different current intensities. The increase of the contraction time (curve (c) at 3.5 hours postmortem) has its reason in the change of the shape of muscular contraction: the opening contraction now has a higher force than the closing contraction.*

values (see Table 5.23) for all relaxation times, the time since death could be estimated

The calculated 95% confidence limits of estimated time of death are ± 2.7 hours up to 13 hours postmortem (see Table 5.23). These limits were re-checked on an independent sample of 21 bodies, and proved to be reliable (Table 5.23; Fig. 5.48).

Discussion

For the first time, longitudinal studies on electrical excitability of skeletal muscle (with simultaneous registration of stimuli and the objectified muscular contraction) were carried out on a large case series. Altogether, about 20,000 muscular contractions were recorded from 71 bodies. By objectifying the muscular contraction, the muscular response to excitation is demonstrably much longer, as contractions are

visible.[36] The long duration of stimuli was also of great advantage since, compared with shorter durations, muscular contractions can be induced over a longer postmortem period and the threshold intensities are much lower.

Using long-lasting stimuli of 1000 ms, the beginning and the end of the stimulus are biologically effective.[42] Correspondingly, in the early postmortem interval, a closing and an opening contraction could be objectified (being visible as two twitches). The irritation at the beginning of the stimulus is always greater than at the end,[42] which becomes evident on comparing the amplitude of the closing and opening contraction.[43]

The change in the shape of muscular contraction is due mainly to an increase of the relaxation time, then of the contraction time of the closing contraction, and later also of the opening contraction. With the increasing relaxation time of the closing contraction, the

Table 5.25 *Example for calculating the force-related relaxation time: case no. 10; right thenar. At the same PMI time after excitation with different current intensities (I_1–I_3) different maximum forces (A_1–A_3) and relaxation times ($t_1 25$–$t_3 25$) were registered. From these values the force related relaxation time is calculated*

hpm	I_1	A_1	$t_1,25$	I_2	$_2$	$S_2,25$	I_3	A_3	$t_3,25$	$\bar{A}$	$\bar{t}_{25}$	$\bar{t}_{25}$-1100	$\dfrac{\bar{t}_{25}-1100}{\bar{A}}$	$\ln\dfrac{\bar{t}_{25}-1100}{\bar{A}}$	ln hpm
2^{20}	32	54	1600	16	48	1500				51	1550	450	8.82	2.17	0.83
3	32	30	1800	64	46	1850				38	1725	625	16.45	2.80	1.1
3^{30}	32	24	1950	64	40	2000				32	1975	875	27.3	3.31	1.25
4	32	16	2400	64	28	2350	80	36	2200	26.6	2316	1216	45.7	3.82	1.38
4^{30}	32	12.25	2350	64	22	2700	80	30	2500	21.4	2516	1416	66.2	4.19	1.5
5^{30}	32	11	2550	64	17	3050	80	22	3000	16.6	2866	1766	106.2	4.67	1.71
6	32	8.5	2550	64	15	2750	80	18.5	3000	14	2766	1666	119.1	4.78	1.79
6^{30}	32	7	2850	64	13.25	3150	80	16.5	3150	12.25	3050	1950	159.2	5.1	1.87
7	32	5.75	3600	64	11.25	3600	80	14,25	3600	10.4	3600	2500	240.4	5.48	1.95
7^{30}	32	4	3500	64	8.75	3800	80	11.5	3760	8.1	3683	2583	318.9	5.77	2.02
8	64	7.25	3700	80	10	4300				8.63	4000	2900	337.2	5.82	2.1

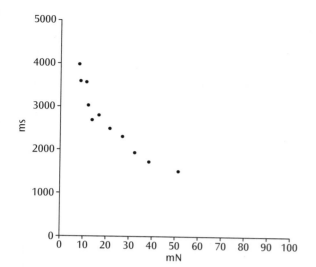

Figure 5.46 *Relation between relaxation time (up to 25% of maximum force) and maximum force. Although the maximum force decreases over the PMI, the relaxation time increases. Each point represents mean values of 'relaxation times' over the mean values of the maximum force registered at the same time postmortem after excitation with different current intensities.*

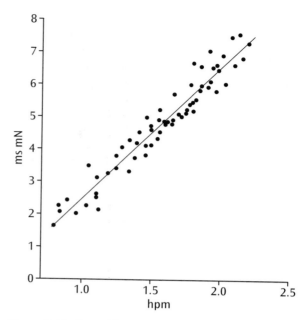

Figure 5.47 *Natural logarithm of the force-related relaxation time and the natural logarithm of the time since death. Strong linear relationship.*

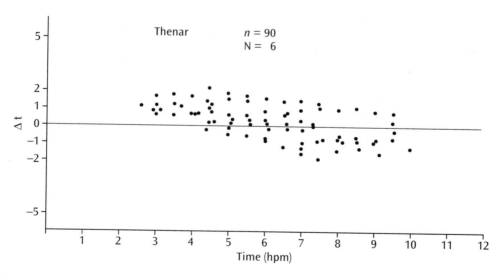

Figure 5.48 *Force-related relaxation time. Differences between extrapolated and real time since death for ten cases of the control sample. Differences within the calculated 95% limits of confidence.*

opening contraction starts on a higher force level and the amplitudes of the closing and opening contractions are equal. When the contraction velocity of the closing contraction decreases, a one-peak shape of muscular contraction results because the closing contraction has not achieved its maximum force at the end of the 1-second stimulus and is continued by the contraction period of the opening contraction.

Both the retarded relaxation and the decreasing contraction velocity of the closing contraction (later also of the opening contraction) have long been known from muscle physiology as a sign of muscular fatigue.[44-48] Signs of muscular fatigue are not only consequences of frequent stimulation, but also of muscle anoxia.

When the investigations started at a later postmortem interval, there was primarily a single-shaped muscular contraction. Discontinuous biphasic curves of muscular contractions after electrical stimulation have already been reported in the older physiological literature.[49-55] As the recording was usually made using a kymograph, direct comparison of muscular contractions with the duration of stimulation was not possible. These biphasic curves were related to:

- The innervation of muscles.[52,54,56]
- The differing modes of contraction of white and red muscles.[53-55]
- Muscular fatigue.[50-54]
- Temperature.[54,60,61]
- Intensity of stimulation.[49,61]

However, there is no relationship between the curves reported in the literature and the shape of muscular contraction reported here.

The 'paradoxical' increase of force (amplitude) of muscular contraction after repeated stimulation of the muscle with the same current intensity is also known to be a sign of muscular fatigue – the 'phenomenon of the treppe (stairs)'.[44,45,47,62,67] This rise of force (amplitude) was seen in our own investigations not only after stimulating the muscle with the same current intensity at 30-minute intervals, but also when, at the same time, the muscle was stimulated with different current intensity (at first 80 mA, then a higher force when stimulating with 64 mA). An additional reason for this paradoxical rise of amplitude may be that the stiffening of single muscle fibres during the asynchronous rigor process within one muscle is 'broken' by the first muscular contraction. The shortening of muscle during muscular fatigue[45] was recorded in our own investigations as a rise in the tension of muscle in the interval between two series of stimulations. This rise in muscular tension can be explained by experimental findings on whole isolated muscles or single muscle fibres during the development of rigor mortis (stiffening is increasing, plasticity decreasing, shortening of muscle fibres).[68-76]

As a third sign of muscular fatigue, the duration of muscular contraction increases in living persons. This increase is mainly due to the retarded relaxation.[47,66,67,77] Correspondingly, increase of relaxation time and decrease of maximum force are the two quantifiable criteria of supravital muscular contraction. All findings on postmortem electrical excitability of human muscle 'in corpore' (change of shape of muscular contraction, increase of duration of contraction, decrease of amplitude) can be explained by the results of classical physiology on muscular fatigue. The longitudinal studies make possible a continuous recording of the death time-dependent criteria of muscular contraction and form the basis for intra- and interindividual comparisons.

In agreement with Joachim and Feldmann,[78] the thenar and hypothenar muscles (M. abductor pollicis brevis, M. opponens pollicis, M. abductor digiti minimi, M. opponens digiti minimi) show the longest duration of postmortem excitability (excluding the M. orbicularis oculi, which could not be used for implantation of the force transducer). Contractions of the thenar and hypothenar muscles could not only be recorded during a longer postmortem interval than other muscles (for instance M. biceps brachii), but the death-time estimation is also more precise. Both objectified and quantified criteria of supravital muscular contraction are suitable for extrapolating the time since death (decrease of maximum force, force-related relaxation time). The force-related relaxation time provides the most precise death-time estimation in the interval up to 13 hours postmortem (Table 5.26) with a 95% confidence limit of ± 2.7 hours. Compared with the most practical methods of examining electrical excitability in casework, according to Klein and Klein,[9] in the same postmortem interval the 95% confidence limits could be reduced from ± 4.75 hours (degree III of electrical excitability of M. orbicularis oculi) to ± 2.7 hours.

Compared with the first extensive study on electrical excitability on the thenar muscles,[15] the postmortem interval, where contractions can be registered, could be augmented from 5.5 to 13 hours by objective measurement of electrical reagibility. Compared with the precision of estimating the time since death on the basis of the postmortem rise of galvanic threshold,[78] a death-time estimation on the basis of the force-related relaxation time is also more precise (± 2.7 hours compared with ± 3.3 hours). For the hypothenar muscles, the precision of death-time estimation using the criterion 'decrease of maximum force' is even greater than for the thenar (see Tables 5.23 and 5.24). However, the random sample on the hypothenar was much smaller than with the thenar. Whether this tendency for the hypothenar to be more

Table 5.26 *Precision of death-time estimation using different criteria of electrical excitability*

Criterion/source	95% limits of confidence (h)	Investigated postmortem period (h)
Decrese of maximum force	2.85*	< 13
Force-related relaxation (Joachim and Feldmann[26])	2.7	< 13
Rise of galvanic threshold (Madea and Henssge[95])	3.3	< 10
Degree of electrical excitability of mimic muscles (Klein and Klein[9])	4.75	3.5–13, $\bar{x} = 8.25$
Weakest reaction after stimulating the thenar (Popwassilew and Palm[15])	2.25	1–5.5, $\bar{x} = 3.25$

* Calculated on the basis of all deviations between real and extrapolated time since death for the current intensities 8, 32 and 80 mA.

reliable can be proved on an augmented random sample is still unclear. Joachim and Feldmann,[78] in performing their investigations on postmortem rise of galvanic threshold on 11 different muscles, found the M. flexor digiti quinti to be the most reliable muscle. The biceps brachii muscle, like the other muscles of the trunk or limbs, loses its electrical excitability much earlier than the thenar or hypothenar muscles. Nevertheless, the precision of death-time estimation on the biceps is (in a shorter postmortem interval than the hypothenar) lower than with the muscles of the hand. It was considered that, for statistical analysis, only those cases where electrical reagibility was preserved at the beginning of the experiments should be used, not those where it had already expired, because it remains unclear at what time reagibility expires. In many cases the biceps had already lost electrical excitability at the beginning of the experiment, whilst the hand muscles were still excitable. It is uncertain whether this is due to the slower postmortem cooling of the biceps compared with the muscles of the hand and/or different modes of contraction (isometric–isotonic).

Technically, the measurement of muscular contractions in the biceps muscle was difficult, due to its high tension.

Conclusion

The main aim of the present study was to evaluate criteria that describe muscular excitability quantitatively and that change with time. The decrease of the maximum force on excitation with stable current intensity and the increase of the relaxation time are quantifiable criteria. A considerable increase in the precision of death-time estimation using both these criteria has been achieved. However, a greater interindividual variability of the duration of electrical excitability remains.

According to Bate-Smith and Bendall,[69] one of the main factors determining the time course of the delay period, i.e. the period of unchanged elasticity of muscle before onset of rigor mortis, is the glycogen content of the muscle at the moment of death. Therefore investigations with simultaneous measurement of electrical excitability and parameters of anaerobic glycolysis – probably lactate – are necessary in order to reduce the 95% confidence limits of estimation of the time since death even further.

The second factor determining the time course of electrical excitability is the environmental temperature. Our results obtained on the experimental material presented here suggest that the electrical excitability lasts longer in the presence of a low local muscular temperature (Fig. 5.49).

The possibilities of the technique described regarding the theoretically derived and expected precision of death-time estimation have not yet been exhausted. At the present moment, the technique can be applied only within our department, but not at the scene of death. First results in practical cases are encouraging and confirm the precision of death-time estimation within the limits given here.[4,37,38] The technique seems to be useful for evaluating the importance of the influence of temperature and glycogen content at the moment of death in relation to the duration of electrical excitability.

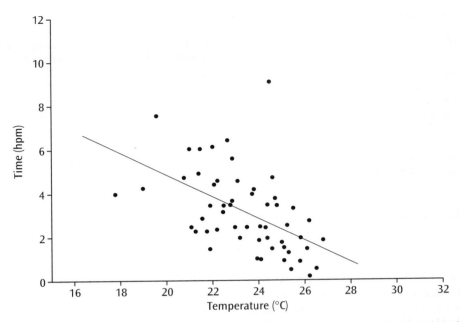

Figure 5.49 *Postmortem duration of electrical excitability over the median local muscular temperature since death. The median local muscular temperature was calculated from the measured values assuming a starting temperature at the thenar of 33°C and a linear fall in temperature. Although with a great range of scatter, there is a statistically significant correlation between the duration of electrical excitability and the median local muscular temperature since death.*

POSTMORTEM RISE IN GALVANIC THRESHOLD

Introduction

Rheobase is the current intensity with extremely long duration (1000 ms) that just causes a muscular contraction. Joachim[79] was the first to describe a strong correlation between postmortem interval and the postmortem increase of the muscular threshold to galvanic stimuli (rectangular impulses of 1 second duration, strength ranging between 0.2 and 80 mA). In 1980, Joachim and Feldmann[78] were able to confirm the original animal experiments on 11 human bodies (Fig. 5.50(a)).

A criterion of death-time is the postmortem increase of galvanic threshold after excitation with rectangular impulses of 1 second duration. A positive reaction of the muscle excited is defined as a good visible contraction of the muscle. Good results can be obtained on the finger muscles (M. flexor digiti V and M. flexor digitorum communis brevis) because movements are easily visible. Surface-ball electrodes for excitation were used.

The muscular threshold is determined four times in 3 hours at the times t_0 to t_3 (with about a 30-minute interval between two measurements) (Fig. 5.50(b)). There is a strong linear relationship between the logarithm of galvanic threshold and time of investigation.

From the values of t (in minutes) and ln of galvanic threshold:

$$Yt \text{ (ln mA)}$$

a linear regression is calculated:

$$Yt = a_0 + b \times t \qquad (5.1)$$

Time since death is obtained by extrapolation on a 'primary galvanic threshold' (a^*) of the muscle in its logarithmic form (ln) according to:

$$t^* = \frac{a_0 - a^*}{b} \qquad (5.2)$$

where t^* = time of death; a_0 = ln of galvanic threshold at the beginning of the investigation; b = slope of the regression; and a^* = ln of the primary postmortem threshold.

The 'primary postmortem threshold' of different muscles was calculated on cases with known time since death using eqn 5.2 and assuming a linear relationship up to death.

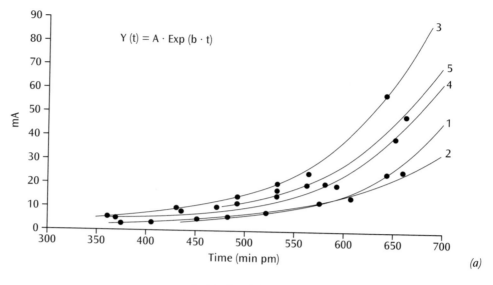

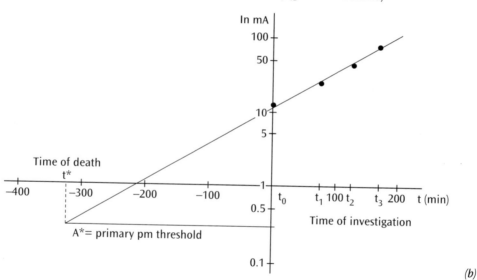

Figure 5.50 (a) Exponential rise in galvanic threshold of various skeletal muscles of a 75-year-old man (cause of death: cardiac failure; excitation with rectangular impulses of 1 s duration). 1, postmortem galvanic threshold (mA) of M. flexor digitorum superficialis brevis; 2, left M. flexor digiti V(5); 3, left M. flexor pollicis longus; 4, left M. fibularis longus; 5, M. flexor digitorum communis brevis. (b) Linear rise in logarithm of galvanic threshold over the time of investigation. Extrapolation on a primary postmortem threshold of the muscle reveals the time since death.

The basis for these calculations was measurement on two to eight bodies (different cause of death, different ambient temperature, different postmortem period of investigation). For practical use, measurements on several muscles are recommended and the resulting death-times should be averaged.

According to Joachim,[80] the great advantage of the method is that by measuring the galvanic threshold four times in 2 to 3 hours, the individual rise is determined; the factors determining the time course of electrical excitability (temperature, glycogen content of muscle) are not to be taken into consideration. Using this procedure, reference samples would not be necessary.

However, the primary postmortem threshold itself is influenced by many factors, for instance cause of death and environmental temperature.[81]

Joachim and Feldmann[78,80] published their investigations in detail (including the complete statistics) in 1980 and in 1988. The following muscles are recommended for measurements:

- M. flexor digiti V.
- M. flexor digitorum communis brevis.
- M. sternocleidomastoideus.
- M. levator palpebrae.

The calculated 95% confidence limits are ± 2.5 hours in the postmortem interval, up to 8 hours postmortem.[82]

The advantage of Joachim's method, compared with other means of examining electrical excitability, is that for the first time a physiological parameter (galvanic threshold) was investigated and formed the basis for the extrapolation of the time since death, and also that longitudinal studies were carried out.

Ravache-Quiriny[28,83] found (in a few cases only) a linear relationship between ln of galvanic threshold and time since death. She carried out her experiments (19 bodies, two cases with electrolyte imbalances, one multiple sclerosis victim, one cachexia of malignancy) in part on the muscles exposed after incision into the skin and subcutaneous tissue (Table 5.27). However, her final statement that 'the use of the fairly simple technique seems rather limited'[83] cannot be evaluated on her published material because the raw data and statistics are missing.

The paper of Ramme and Staak[84] contributes little to the topic because the necessary information (which muscles were investigated, postmortem period of investigation, which mathematical relationship between threshold and time of investigation, precision of death-time estimation) is entirely missing, and the conclusions drawn by the authors are incorrect.

Joachim[80] stated that objectification and quantification of muscular threshold should be attempted, to ensure that, with increasing threshold, there was always an equally strong contraction.

Table 5.27 *Tabular summary of published investigations on postmortem rise of galvanic threshold*

Reference	Cases investigated	Muscles investigated	PMI	Precision of death-time estimation (95% limits of confidence)
Joachim and Feldmann[26]	n = 11; statistical analysis for only 8 cases; in 3 cases too few measurements	Orbicularis oculi and oris, levator palpebrae, sternocleidomastoideus, biceps brachii, flexor pollicis longus, flexor + opponens pollicis brevis, flexor digiti V, quadriceps femoris, gastrocnemius, fibularis longus, flexor digitorum communis	2–15 hpm	± 2.5 h
Ravache-Quiriny[28,83]	n = 19; 2 cases with disturbance of electrolyte homoeostasis, 1 multiple sclerosis, 1 cachexia of malignancy; no statistical analysis	Orbicularis oculi and oris, sternocleidomastoideus, flexor digitorum communis, flexor digiti V	Up to 12.25 hpm. No data on pm beginning of investigation	No data
Ramme and Staak[84]	25 cases with only partial known time since death. No further data on random sample, no statistical analysis, not even for the cases with known time since death	No data	Up to 16 hpm. No data on the beginning of experiments	No data
Madea[4]	20 cases with known time since death (statistical analysis for these cases), 8 cases with not exactly known time since death	Abductor pollicis brevis, opponens pollicis, abductor digiti minimi, opponens digiti minimi, biceps brachii	2–13 hpm	± 3.27 h

Materials and methods

The correlation between galvanic threshold and time since death was investigated for a random sample of 20 cases (sudden, natural or traumatic death). Muscular contraction was objectified using a sensitive force transducer pricked into the muscle (right and left thenar). The muscle was stimulated each half-hour with rectangular impulses of 1 second duration and intensities between 0.1 and 80 mA using needle electrodes; these were pricked into the muscle beside the force transducer. A current intensity, which causes a muscular contraction of 2.5 mN, was defined as threshold intensity (rheobase).

Results

There was a strong linear relationship ($r = 0.965$; Fig. 5.51) for ln of muscular threshold and time since death. The time since death was extrapolated for all threshold values for all 20 cases with mean values for slope and intercept (calculated from the random sample) according to:

$$t^* = \frac{a_0 - \bar{a}}{\bar{b}} \qquad (5.3)$$

where t^* = time of death; a_0 = ln of galvanic threshold at the beginning of investigation; $\bar{a} = -1.748$; and $\bar{b} = 0.0129$; $\bar{a}$ and $\bar{b}$ are mean regression parameters calculated from the random sample.

The resultant differences between real and extrapolated time since death are shown in Fig. 5.52. The 95% confidence limits of death-time estimation was ± 3.3 hours.

In a second step, the time of death was calculated according to Joachim[78,80] for the first of four consecutively (in 30-minute intervals) measured thresholds using the individual slope according to:

$$t\times = \frac{a_0 - \bar{a}}{b_{ind}} \qquad (5.4)$$

where t^* = time of death; $\bar{a} = -1.748$; a_0 = ln of galvanic threshold at the beginning of the investigation; and b_{ind} = slope of the regression between ln of threshold values and time of investigation.

For the same values ($n = 67$) the time since death was also extrapolated according to eqn 5.3 with the collective mean value for the slope.

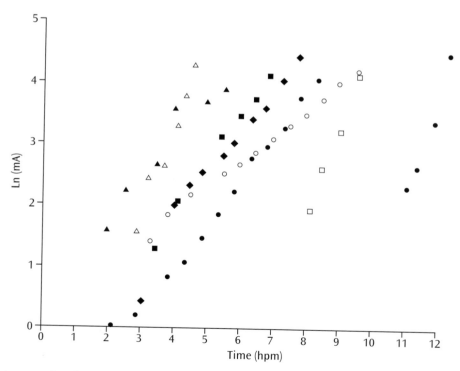

Figure 5.51 *Postmortem rise of galvanic threshold (ln I) for eight cases marked with different symbols. Linear relationship between logarithm of rheobase and time since death.*

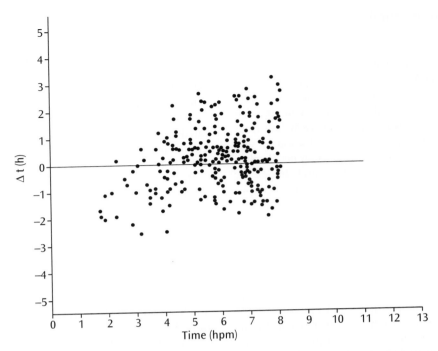

Figure 5.52 *Differences between real and extrapolated time since death (Δ t) over the extrapolated time since death for 267 threshold values. For extrapolation of the time since death a collective mean value for the slope was used.*

Surprisingly, extrapolation of the time since death with mean values for the slope revealed a much more precise death-time estimation than using an individual slope. Figure 5.53 shows the differences between real and extrapolated time since death using mean values (•) and individual values (o) for the slope (Table 5.28).

The intercept (primary postmortem threshold) is a calculated value which is determined by the time since death and the individual slope. Extrapolation of the time since death with an individual slope can provide a more precise death-time estimation only when the individual intercept is also known. However, in cases of unknown time since death, the intercept also remains unknown and obviously there is a great interindividual variability of the intercept.

A second point is that different cases investigated at different postmortem intervals have almost the same intercept and slope of galvanic threshold (Fig. 5.54).

Checking of the proposed procedure (extrapolation of the time since death with mean values for the slope) on eight independent cases revealed that the calculated 95% confidence limits of ± 3.3 hours are reliable (Fig. 5.55).

Conclusions

1. The strong linear relationship between ln of galvanic threshold and time since death that has been reported by Joachim and Feldmann[78] can be confirmed using a modified technique with objectification of muscular response to electrical stimulation.
2. Extrapolation of the time since death with mean values for the slope reveals a much more precise death-time estimation than extrapolation with an individual slope – which requires repeated measurements of the threshold at intervals of 30 minutes.

Table 5.28 *Postmortem rise of galvanic threshold; accuracy of death-time estimation in hours*

	b_{ind}	$\bar{b}$	$\bar{b}$
n	67	67	267
$\bar{x}$	2	−0.12	−0.11
s	8.13	1.69	1.67

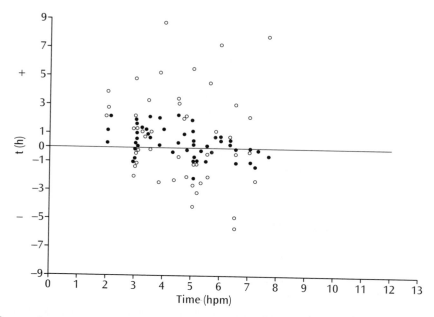

Figure 5.53 *Differences between real and extrapolated time since (± t (h)) for several threshold values using a collective mean value for the slope (●) or an individual slope (○) calculated on the basis of four threshold values. There are much wider differences between real and extrapolated time since death using an individual slope.*

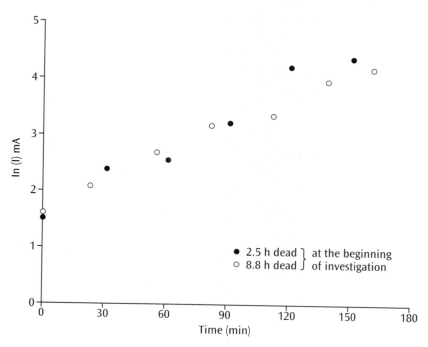

Figure 5.54 *Postmortem rise in galvanic threshold over time of investigation for two cases. Although at the beginning of the experiments time since death differs by about 6 hours, both cases have the same intercept and rise in galvanic threshold.*

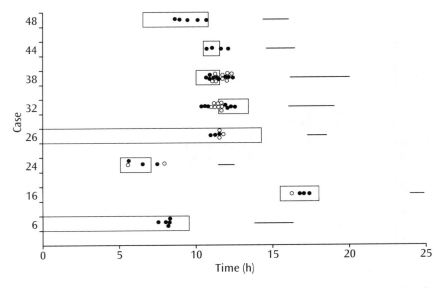

Figure 5.55 *Application of the method in casework. y axis, case numbers; x axis, time; boxes, time since death as a result of investigation of the police (last time seen alive – found dead); lines, time of investigation. Extrapolated time since death for the right (●) and left (○) thenar (mean value).*

3. The calculated 95% confidence limits of death-time estimation of ± 3.3 hours were confirmed as being reliable.
4. With 95% confidence limits of ± 3.3 hours up to 10 hours postmortem, Joachim's method in its modified form is only a little more precise than methods of examining electrical excitability with a subjective grading (see page 169) and less precise than other criteria of objectified muscular contraction (see page 193).

The heuristic value of Joachim's work on postmortem rise in galvanic threshold is without question, but the method must be tested thoroughly before it can be recommended for practical use.

POSTMORTEM STRENGTH–DURATION CURVES

Strength–duration curves (*i/t* curves) describe the dependence of the threshold intensity of rectangular impulses from their duration: the shorter the duration of the stimulus, the higher the threshold intensity; *i/t* curves have the approximate form of a hyperbola (Fig. 5.56). In clinical neurophysiology, they help to clarify whether or not a muscle is denervated.[85–89]

The postmortem changes of strength–duration curves in the postmortem interval from 2 to 9 hours postmortem were investigated on 17 bodies.[90] Muscular contraction was objectified using a sensitive force transducer pricked into the muscle. The muscle was stimulated with constant-current rectangular impulses of 5 to 1000-ms duration and current intensities that produced a force of muscular contraction of 2.5 mN every 30 minutes.

The strength–duration curves of human bodies taken in the earliest postmortem period (2 hours postmortem) show the pattern of partial or total denervation (steep rise of threshold values for stimuli shorter than 100 ms; Fig. 5.57), whilst in animal experiments the *i/t* curves obtained at 60, 90 and 120 minutes postmortem show the normal hyperbola-like pattern (Fig. 5.58).

As for the rheobase, there is a strong linear rela-

Table 5.29 *Collective mean values for slope and intercept and correlation coefficient for different duration of stimuli (T)*

T (ms)	ā	b̄	r̄
500	−0.8064	0.0118	0.9702
300	−0.9209	0.0129	0.973
200	−1.1977	0.0140	0.9723
100	−1.4269	0.0163	0.9695
50	−1.3423	0.0176	0.9527
20	0.4978	0.013	0.935

ā = intercept; b̄ = slope of regression line.

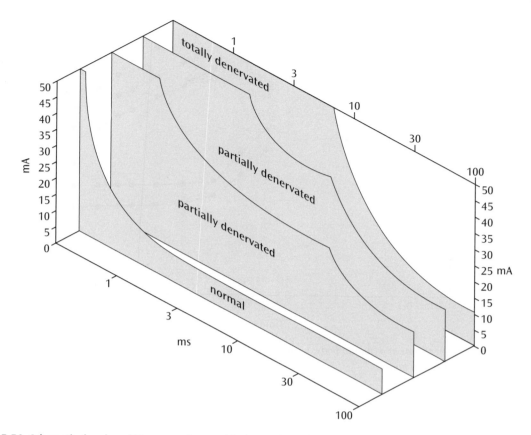

Figure 5.56 *Schematic drawing of i/t curves of normal innervated, partially and totally denervated muscle. y axis, current intensity in mA; x axis, duration of stimulus in ms.*

tionship between ln of threshold and time since death for the durations of stimuli below 1000 ms (Fig. 5.59; Table 5.29).

Extrapolation of the time since death on the basis of threshold values of different duration of stimuli of an *i/t* curve reveals only a small increase in precision of death-time estimation compared with the extrapola-

tion of the time since death using only the rheobase (Table 5.30). This means that strength–duration curves are of no additional value in estimating the time since death, since the information can be obtained by easier means.

The following conclusions can be drawn from the experiments on strength–duration curves:

Table 5.30 *Precision of estimating the time since death (95% limits of confidence/h). Extrapolation of the time since death using threshold values for different duration of stimuli*

| | | | | | **T (ms)** | | | |
	1000	500	300	200	100	50	20	Σ
n	59	58	52	49	38	26	20	302
$\bar{x}$	0.2	−0.2	−0.3	−0.2	−0.003	−0.003	−0.9	−0.1
s	±1.2	±1.2	±1.1	±1.1	±1	±1	±1.6	±1.1
95%	±2.42	±2.42	±2.23	±2.23	±2.05	±2.31	±2.43	±2.16

n, number; $\bar{x}$, mean; s, standard deviation; 95%, 95% confidence limits.

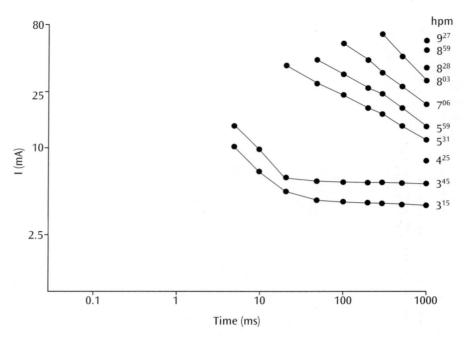

Figure 5.57 *i/t curve; right thenar of a human body; y axis, current intensity in mA; x axis, duration of stimulus in ms; on the right margin, time since death in hours.*

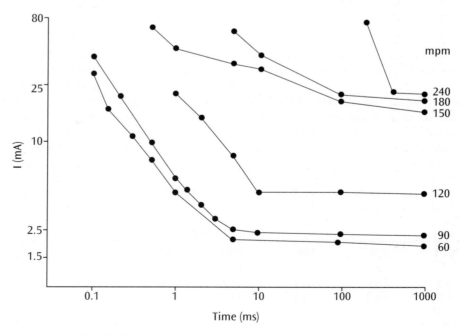

Figure 5.58 *i/t curve taken at the left thigh of a dog.*

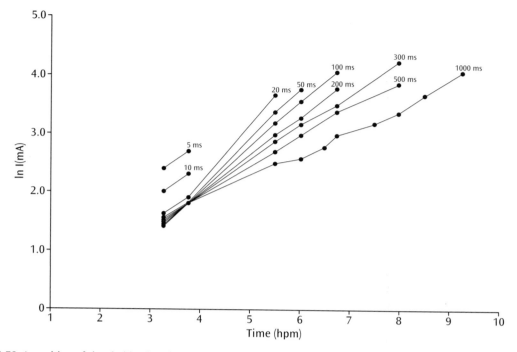

Figure 5.59 *Logarithm of threshold values (1n I(mA)) for different durations of stimuli (5–1000 ms) of one case over the PMI. Linear relationship between threshold values and time since death.*

The *i/t* curves in animal experiments taken 60, 90 and 120 minutes postmortem show the pattern of normal innervation of muscle. This confirms the literature regarding the survival period of mammalian nerve after global ischaemia.[7,91,92]

The *i/t* curves taken on human bodies at the earliest time possible (2 hours postmortem) correspond to the pattern of partial or total denervation, with a steep rise of threshold values using durations of stimuli below 100 ms.

For postmortem investigations on skeletal muscle, long-lasting stimuli are to be preferred.[4,36–39,78] No muscular contraction could be obtained when using shorter durations of stimuli – for instance 0.2 ms, as is usual in physiology – at only 2 hours postmortem.

REFERENCES

1 Galvani L. Cited by Rothschuh KE. In: *Physiologie. Der Wandel ihrer Konzepte, Probleme und Methoden vom 16. bis 20. Jahrhundert.* Freiburg-München: Karl Alber, 1968.

2 Rosenthal M. Untersuchungen und Beobachtungen über das Absterben der Muskeln und den Scheintod. *Wiener Medizinisches Jahrbuch* 1872: 389–413.

3 Nysten PH. Von der Erstarrung, welche die Körper der Menschen und Tiere nach dem Tode befällt. Recherches de physiologie et chemie pathologique, Paris 1811. Übersetzt und mit Zusätzen begleitet von A. C. Mayer, Bern. *Huieland-Journal* 1816; **43**.

4 Madea B. *Supravitale elektrische Erregbarkeit der Skelettmuskulatur: Längsschnittuntersuchungen zur Objektivierung der muskulären Reaktion an 70 Leichen.* Habil. Schrift, Köln, 1989.

5 Harless E. Untersuchungen an einem Hingerichteten. *Jenaer Analen II* 2, 1850; Zit. nach *Schmids Jahrbuch* 1851; **72**: 10–11.

6 Kölliker A, Virchow R. Über einige an der Leiche eines Hingerichteten angestellte Versuche und Beobachtungen. *Wiss. Zool.* 1851; **III**: 37–52.

7 Krause D, Klein A, Zett L. Todeszeitbestimmung mittels indirekter Muskelreizung über den N. ischiadicus und N. radialis. *Kriminal. Forens. Wiss.* 1976; **26**: 66–7.

8 Vogt H. *Das Bild des Kranken.* Munich: JF Bergman, 1980.

9 Klein A, Klein S. *Die Todeszeitbestirnmung am menschlichen Auge.* Med Diss., B., Med. Akad., Dresden, 1978.

10 Onimus M. Modification de l'excitabilitie des nerfs et des muscles apres la mort. *J. l'anat. Physiol. normale pathol.* 1880: 629.

11 Tidy CM. *Changes in the muscle and in the general condition of the body after death. Legal Medicine. Part 1.* London: Smith-Elder, 1882.

12 Lochte Th. Über die Absterbeerscheinungen der Skelettmuskulatur, insbesondere über die Totenstarre in gerichtlich-medizinischer Beziehung (Dtsch). *Z. Ges. Gerichtl. Med.* 1923; **2**: 169–90.

13 Puppe G. Der Scheintod und seine Diagnose. (Dtsch). *Med. Wochenschr.* 1920; **14/15**: 383–5.

14 Prokop O. *Lehrbuch der gerichtlichen Medizin.* Berlin: Verlag Volk und Gesundheit, 1960.

15 Popwassilew J, Palm W. Über die Todeszeitbestimmung in den ersten 10 Stunden. *Z. ärztl. Fortbild.* 1960; **54**: 734–7.

16 Radam G. Ein elektronisches Reizgerät zur Todeszeitbestimmung (German). *Gesundheitswes.* 1963; **18**: 1400–1.

17 Nagy J. The postmortem excitability of the skeletal muscles. *Acta Med. Leg. Soc. (Liege)* 1968: 177–8.

18 Raszeja S, Bardzik St. Studies on the "intralethal" excitability of muscles following stimuli obtained from an electronic stimulator. *Bull. Poll. Med. Sci. Hist.* 1971; **14**: 93.

19 Zink P, Reinhardt G. Die Todeszeitbestimmung bei der ärztlichen Leichenschau. *Bayer. Ärztebl.* 1972; **27**: 109–15.

20 Waltz H, Mattig W. Elektrische Messungen an Leichen für die Konstruktion eines elektronischen Reizgerätes zur Todeszeitbestimmung. *Kriminal. Forens. Wiss.* 1974; **16**: 159–78.

21 Kliese U, Henssge C, Madea B. *Reizgenerator zur Prüfung der elektrischen Erregbarkeit der Skelettmuskulatur.* Unveröffentlichtes Manuskript, 1985.

22 Böhm E. Anmerkungen zu Reizbarkeit und Starreeintritt der Skelettmuskulatur. *Beitr. Gerichtl. Med.* 1986; **44**: 439–50.

23 Klein A, Krause D, Hamann B. Praktische Erfahrungen mit einem neuen elektronischen Reizgerät zur Todeszeitbestimmung. *Kriminal. Forens. Wiss.* 1975; **19**: 126.

24 Krause D, Klein A, Mattig W, Waltz H. Praktische Erfahrungen mit dem Reizgerät D 76 zur Todeszeitbestimmung. *Kriminal. Forens. Wiss.* 1980; **40**: 83–6.

25 Krause D, Schöning R, Kuchheuser W. Stimulator M 85 – Ein kommerzielles Reizgerät zur Todeszeitbestimmung. In: *Medizin und Recht. Festschrift fur Wolfgang Spann.* (Liebhardt E, Schuck M, Eisenmenger W, eds.). Berlin: Springer, 1986: 639–44.

26 Joachim H, Feldmann U. Eine quantitative Methode der Todeszeitbestimmung durch Untersuchung der galvanischen Reizschwelle. *Z. Rechtsmed.* 1980; **85**: 5–22.

27 Ravache-Quiriny J. The time of death: some thoughts on the trustworthiness of our response. *Int. Acad. Leg. Med. Soc. Med.* 1982; **1** (Newsletter): 9–11.

28 Ravache-Quiriny J. *Les moments de la mort. Cahiers de Médiane légale, Droits medicales no.* 3: Association Lyonnaise Médicine regale. Lyon: Editions Alesandre Lacasagne, 1986.

29 Henssge C. Methoden zur Bestimmung der Todeszeit-Leichenabkühlung und Todeszeitbestimmung. Diss B, Humboldt-Universität Berlin, 1982.

30 Bendall JR. Postmortem changes in muscle. In: *The Structure and Function of Muscle, Vol. II, Structure, part 2* (Bourne DH, ed.). London: Academic Press, 1973: 244–309.

31 Döring G, Falsafi A. Der Einfluss von Dehnung und Sauerstoff auf den postmortalen ATP-Stoffwechsel des Skelettmuskels (Dtsch). *Z. Gerichtl. Med.* 1967; **59**: 88–98.

32 Döring G, Patzer A, Forster B. Untersuchungen über den postmortalen ATP-Stoffwechsel der Magenmuskulatur der Ratte. *Pflügers Arch.* 1965; **285**: 229–40.

33 Forster B, Hummelsheim G, Döring G. Tierexperimentelle Untersuchungen über die postmortale Magenperistaltik bei Leuchtgas- und Parathionvergiftung. (Dtsch). *Z. Gerichtl. Med.* 1965; **56**: 148–59.

34 Feng TP. The effect of length on the resting metabolism of muscle. *J. Physiol.* 1932; **74**: 441–54.

35 Henssge C, Madea B, Gallenkemper E. Death time estimation in case work II. Integration of different methods. *Forensic Sci. Int.* 1988; **39**: 77–87.

36 Henssge C, Lunkenheimer PP, Salmon O, Madea B. Zur supravitalen elektrischen Erregbarkeit der Muskulatur. *Z. Rechtsmed.* 1984; **93**: 165–74.

37 Madea B. Längsschnittuntersuchungen zur supravitalen elektrischen Erregbarkeit der Skelettmuskulatur. I. Objektivierung der supravitalen Muskelkontraktion. *Z. Rechtsmed.* 1992; **2**: 107–21.

38 Madea B. Längsschnittuntersuchungen zur supravitalen elektrischen Erregbarkeit der Skelettmuskulatur. II. Quantifizierung der supravitalen Muskelkontraktion. *Z. Rechtsmed.* 1993; **3**: 44–50.

39 Madea B. Estimating time of death from measurement of the electrical excitability of skeletal muscle. *J. Forensic Sci. Soc.* 1992; **32**: 117–29.

40 Lunkenheimer PP, Lunkenheimer A, Stroh N, Köhler F, Welham K, Graham G, Kirk E, Sonnenblick E, Kröller J. Vergleich klassischer und neuer Zugänge zum intramyokardialen Kraftverteilungsmuster. *Zentralbl. Vet. Med. A.* 1982; **29**: 557–601.

41 Lunkenheimer PP, Lunkenheimer A, Torrent-Guasp F. *Kardiodynamik: Wege zur strukturgerechten Analyse der Myokardfunktion.* Beiträge zur Kardiologie Bd. 33. Erlangen: Perimed-Fachbuch-Verlagsges, 1985.

42 Pflüger E. *Untersuchungen über die Physiologie des Electrotonus.* Berlin: August Hirschwald, 1859.

43 Basler A. Über den Einfluss der Reizstärke und der Belastung auf die Muskelkurve. *Arch. f. d. ges. Physiol.* 1904; **102**: 254–68.

44 Landois L. *Lehrbuch der Physiologie des Menschen. I I. Aufl., Bearb. v. Rosemann R.* Berlin: Urban und Schwarzenberg, 1905.

45 Landois L, Rosemann R. *Lehrbuch der Physiologie.* Berlin: Urban und Schwarzenberg, 1935.

46 Von Frey M. Allgemeine Physiologie der quergestreiften Muskeln. In: *Handbuch der Physiologie des Menschen* Bd. 4, 2. Hälfte, 1. Teil. (Nagel W, ed.). Vieweg Verlag, Braunschweig, S427–S543.

47 Fenn WO. Der zeitliche Verlauf der Muskelkontraktion. In: *Handbuch der Normalen und Pathologischen Physiologie 811.* (Bethe A, v Bergmann G, Emwen G, Ellinger A, eds.). Berlin: Springer Verlag, 1925: 166–91.

48 Ciba Foundation Symposium. *Human Muscle Fatigue: Physiological Mechanisms.* London: Pitman Medical, 1981.

49 Fick A. *Studien über elektrische Nervenreizung.* Arbeiten aus dem physiologischen Labor der Würzburger Hochschule, 1872.

50 Funke O. Über den Einfluss der Ermüdung auf den zeitlichen Verlauf der Muskelthätigkeit. *Pflügers Arch.* 1874; **8**: 213–52.

51 Joteyko J. *La Fonction Musculaire.* Paris, 1909.

52 De Boer CC. Die Bedeutung der tonischen Innervation für die Funktion der quergestreiften Muskeln. *Z. f. Biol.* 1915; **65**: 239–354.

53 Hartree W, Hill AV. The nature of the isometric twitch. *J. Physiol.* 1921; **55**: 389–411.

54 Harmon PM. Influence of temperature and other factors upon the two-summited contraction curve of the gastrocnemius of the frog. *Am. J. Physiol.* 1922; **62**: 261–281.

55 Ebbecke U. Der idiomuskuläre Wulst. *Skand. Arch. f. Physiol.* 1923; **43**: 138–64.

56 Brown GT. Der Einfluss des Nervensystems auf die Form der Zuckungskurve des Frosch-Gastrocnemius. *Pflügers Arch.* 1908; **125**: 491–505.

57 Roesner A. Über die Erregbarkeit verschiedenartiger quergestreifter Muskeln. *Arch. ges. Physiol.* 1900; **81**: 105–30.

58 Fischer H. Zur Physiologie der quergestreiften Muskeln der Säugetiere. *Arch. f. d. ges. Physiol.* 1908; **125**: 541–83.

59 Riesser O. Untersuchungen an überlebenden roten und weissen Kaninchenmuskeln. *Arch. ges. Physiol.* 1921; **190**: 137–57.

60 Brunton LT, Cash JT. Influence of heat and cold upon muscles poisoned by veratrea. *Am. J. Physiol.* 1883/84; **4**: 1–7.

61 Yeo GF, Cash T. On the relation between the active phases of contraction and the latent period of skeletal muscle. *Am. J. Physiol.* 1884; **4**: 198–221.

62 Biedertnann W. *Elektrophysiologie.* Jena: Gustav Fischer Verlag, 1895.

63 Fröhlich FW. Über die scheinbare Steigerung der Leistungsfähigkeit des quergestreiften Muskels im Beginn der Ermüdung. *Z. f. Physiol.* 1905; **5**: 288–316.

64 Frohlich FW. Das Prinzip der scheinbaren Erregbarkeitssteigerung. *Ergebnisse d. Physiol.* 1918; **16**: 40–86.

65 Lee FS. The cause of the treppe. *Am. J. Physiol.* 1907; **18**: 267–82.

66 Taskinen K. Beitrag zur Erkenntniss der Ermüdung des Muskels. *Skand. Arch. Physiol.* 1910; **23**: 1–54.

67 Uhlmann F. Über Ermüdung der willkürlich oder elektrisch gereizten Muskeln. *Pflügers Arch. ges. Physiol.* 1912; **146**: 517–42.

68 Bate-Smith EC, Bendall JR. Rigor mortis and adenosine-triphosphate. *J. Physiol.* 1947; **106**: 177–85.

69 Bate-Smith EC, Bendall JR. Factors determining the time course of rigor mortis. *J. Physiol.* 1949; **110**: 47–65.

70 Nakamura L. Untersuchungen über die elastischen Eigenschaften der Muskeln bei verschiedenen funktionellen Zuständen. III. Mitteilung: Die Änderungen der Zugresistenz des quergestreiften Kaltblutermuskels während der Toten- und Wärmestarre. *Pflügers Arch. ges. Physiol.* 1924; **205**: 92–197.

71 Forster B. *Über die plastische, elastische und kontraktile Verformung des totenstarren Skelett- und Herzmuskels.* Göttingen: Habil. Schr., 1962.

72 Forster B. The plastic and elastic deformation of skeletal muscle in rigor mortis. *J. Forensic Med.* 1963; **10**: 91–110.

73 Forster B. The contractile deformation of skeletal muscle in rigor mortis. *J. Forensic Med.* 1963; **10**: 133–47.

74 Zink P. *Über das Verhalten des menschlichen Skelettmuskels bei Dehnung während des Verlaufs der Totenstarre.* Erlangen: Habil. Schr., 1970.

75 Zink P. Mechanische Eigenschaften lebensfrischer und totenstarrer menschlicher Skelettmuskelfasern und ganzer Muskeln. *Z. Rechtsmed.* 1972; **70**: 163–77.

76 Zink P. Das mechanische Verhalten menschlicher Skelettmuskulatur während des Verlaufs der Totenstarre. *Z. Rechtsmed.* 1972; **71**: 47–63.

77 Reichel H. *Muskelphysiologie.* Berlin, Springer, 1960.

78 Joachim H, Feldmann U. Eine quantitative Methode der Todeszeitbestimmung durch Untersuchung der galvanischen Reizschwelle. *Z. Rechtsmed.* 1980; **85**: 5–22.

79 Joachim H. *Probleme der frühen Todeszeitbestimmung und die sogenannten supravitalen Reaktionen des Muskels im Tierversuch.* Freiburg: Habil.-Schrift, 1976.

80 Joachim H. Mechanische und elektrische Erregbarkeit der Skelettmuskulatur. In: *Methoden zur Bestimmung der Todeszeit an Leichen* (Henssge C, Madea B, eds.). Lübeck: Schmidt-Römhild, 1988: S32–S82.

81 Harris R. Chronaxy. In: *Electrodiagnosis and Electromyography* (Licht S, ed.). Baltimore, Maryland: Waverly Press, 1971.

82 Henssge C. *Methoden zur Bestimmung der Todeszeit-Leichenabkühlung und Todeszeitbestimmung.* Diss. B, Berlin Humboldt-Universität: MD Thesis, 1982.

83 Ravache-Quiriny J. The time of death: some thoughts on the trustworthiness of our response. *Int. Acad. Leg. Med. Soc. Med,* 1982; newsletter no. 1: 9–11.

84 Ramme H, Staak M. Vergleichende Untersuchungen zur Methodik der Todeszeitschätzung. *Beitr. Gerichtl. Med.* 1983; **41**: 365–9.

85 Scheidt W. *Lehrbuch der Neurologie.* Stuttgart: Thieme, 1982.

86 Bruggencate G. *Medizinische Neurophysiologie: Zellfunktionen und Sensomotorik unter klinischen Gesichtspunkten.* Stuttgart: Thieme, 1984.

87 Edel H. *Fibel der Elektrodiagnostik und Elektrotherapie.* Berlin: VEB-Verlag Volk und Gesundheit, 1983.

88 Lullies H. *Taschenbuch der Physiologie, Bd. II. Animalische Physiologie I. Allgemeine Nerven- und Muskelphysiologie.* Stuttgart, G. Fischer, 1973.

89 Senn E. *Elektrotherapie. Gebräuchliche Verfahren der physikalischen Therapie – Grundlagen, Wirkungsweisen, Stellenwert.* Stuttgart: Thieme, 1990.

90 Madea B. Zum postmortalen Verhalten von Reizzeit – Reizstromstärkekurven. *Beitr. Gerichtl. Med.* 1991; **49**: 233–46.

91 Gerard RW. The response of nerve to oxygen lack. *Am. J. Physiol.* 1930; **92**: 498–541.

92 Wright E. A comparative study of the effects of oxygen lack on peripheral nerve. *Am. J. Physiol.* 1946; **147**: 78–89.

93 Mattig W, Waltz H. Untersuchungen zur Todeszeitbestimmung mittels elektrischer Reizung. *Kriminal. Forens. Wiss.* 1976; **26**: 68–71.

94 Madea B, Henssge C. Zum postmortalen Verhalten der Rheobase. *Z. Rechtsmed.* 1990; **103**: 435–52.

95 Madea B, Henssge C. Electrical excitability of skeletal muscle postmortem in casework. *Forensic Sci. Int.* 1990; **47**: 207–27.

96 Kölliker A, Virchow R. Über einige an der Leiche eines Hingerichteten angestellte Versuche und Beobachtungen. *Wiss. Zool.* 1851; **III**: 37–52.

97 Henssge C, Madea B, Gallenkemper E. Todeszeitbestimmung – Integration verschiedener Teilmethoden. *Z. Rechtsmed.* 1985; **95**: 185–96.

98 Henssge C, Madea B, Gallenkemper E. Death time estimation in casework. – II. Integration of different methods. *Forensic Sci. Int.* 1988; **39**: 77–87.

Hypostasis and timing of death

BERNARD KNIGHT

Hypostasis is one of the most obvious postmortem changes; alternative names are 'postmortem lividity' and the older term, 'suggilation'.

Hypostasis is the staining of the skin surface – and internal organs – by the settling of blood under the influence of gravity after the circulation has ceased.

Red blood cells and plasma sink to the most dependent parts of the body under gravitational attraction, filling the now inert vascular channels, particularly the veins and capillaries. This leads to a red or blue discoloration of the skin at the lowest parts, usually the back of the trunk, neck and thighs in bodies that lie in the usual supine position after death.

Where the body presses on a firm supporting surface, these contact areas remain pale, as the vascular channels are closed by the pressure; this is commonly seen on the buttocks and shoulder blades.

Hypostasis also occurs in internal organs, and inexperienced pathologists have often been misled into mistaking hypostasis in the intestines and myocardium for true infarction, due to the dark, congested appearance.

The colour of hypostasis varies, being darker red or blue where the contained haemoglobin is less oxygenated. In hypothermia, or where the body has been in refrigeration or cold environmental surroundings, the colour may be bright pink. Other tints may be seen in various toxic states, such as those due to carbon monoxide, cyanide or nitro-compounds.

The value of hypostasis in estimating the time since death is slight, though recent research is now attempting to improve upon this situation. First, hypostasis may not appear at all, especially in old and anaemic persons. In those with heavy racial pigmentation, hypostasis may be partly or even totally masked by the skin colour.

It has been said that hypostasis can even appear before death, as in deep coma such as that due to barbiturate poisoning or a dense stroke. This must be very rare, but the skin blistering seen in dependent parts of victims of deep coma, formerly known as 'barbiturate blisters', is due to cutaneous oedema caused by cessation of venous return following muscle flaccidity – the same mechanism potentially allowing hypostatic pooling of blood in the subcutaneous veins.

True postmortem hypostasis develops at a very variable rate following cardiac arrest. The standard forensic medicine textbooks offer a wide range of the time of onset (Table 5.31).

Several authors have attempted to use subjective measurements of hypostasis, using stages such as 'beginning, confluence, maximum intensity, displacement by slight pressure, complete shifting and incomplete shifting'. Mallach[1] analysed such data, but the wide scatter of results and the doubtful specificity of such subjective descriptions make the results of little practical value in casework, other than to add a further general corroboration to better results obtained by other techniques.

Given these wide ranges, it is obvious that the use of hypostasis in estimating the time of death is of little evidential use. All that can be said is that it usually

appears between 30 minutes and 4 hours, reaches maximum intensity in up to about 12 hours, and persists in an undisturbed corpse until putrefactive changes set in, usually several days later. In tropical conditions, hypostasis may be destroyed by decomposition on the first day after death, if the body undergoes rapid dissolution.

Apart from the initial time of onset of hypostasis, it has long been claimed that its permanent fixation is time-related. Many textbooks have stated that, after a certain (but very variable) time, primary hypostasis becomes fixed and will not then move again under the influence of gravity if the body position is altered.

This claim was justified on the premise that, immediately after death, blood remains fluid, but that at a later time it clots within the vessels so that further movement cannot occur. This theory is patently untrue, or at least is extremely unreliable.

Postmortem blood coagulation and subsequent fibrinolysis has a very irregular timeframe, and clotting may not occur at all.

As every observant pathologist will know, hypostasis will sometimes flow completely from one part of the body to another, if the cadaver is moved to a new position. Sometimes it does not move at all, and often it partly moves and partly remains fixed. The inconstancy of secondary shifting thus makes this a virtually useless indicator of the length of the postmortem interval.

Crude methods of detecting fixation have been used, in which local pressure is applied to the hypostatic skin, to determine whether the colour can be blanched.

Suzutani et al.[2] examined 430 bodies by pressing the side of a forceps against the dependent skin. These authors discovered that hypostasis could not be squeezed out in about 30% of cases where death had occurred 6 to 12 hours previously. Over 50% of cases were fixed after a postmortem interval of 12 to 24 hours, and no fading took place in about 70% who had died 1 to 3 days earlier.

Suzutani et al.[2] also found that there was a significant number of cases where hypostasis was not fixed up to at least 3 days. In addition, there was some seasonal variation, with less movement in the summer months; in addition, asphyxial deaths and those with intracranial lesions had delayed fixation rates.

Fechner et al.[3] examined 28 cases of sudden death which were stored at different temperatures, and found a variation of hypostatic fixation with temperature, but no linear relationship and a very wide individual variation relative to the time of death.

Table 5.31 *Time of onset of hypostasis*

Reference	Onset	Maximum hours
Andelson	30 min–4 h	8–12
Polson and Gee	30 min–2 h	6–12
Spitz and Fisher	2 hr–4 h	8–12
Taylor (ed. Simpson)	0 h	12
Taylor (ed. Mant)	1 h	12
Gradwohl (ed. Camps)	20–30 min	6–12
Glaister	–	8–12
DiMaio	30 min–2 h	8–12
Sydney Smith	0 h	12
Mant	0 h	12
Gordon and Shapiro	'few' h	12

Although the foregoing commentary seems to indicate that hypostasis is almost valueless in the determination of time since death, recent research – and some which is still in progress – is attempting to improve this situation with the use of sophisticated optical equipment.

Schuller *et al.*[4] began to use colorimetry on hypostasis. When examining seven corpses over a period from 3 to 35 hours after death, they observed an increasing paleness of the hypostasis between 3 and 15 hours postmortem. These authors concluded that there was a colour change from a wavelength of 575 nm at 3 hours at an average rate of 2 nm per hour.

On-going research by Dr Peter Vanezis[5] uses a tri-stimulus colorimeter. A standard xenon light source and filter illuminates the bodies, conforming to standard illumination D 65, which resembles daylight. A constant, small area of hypostasis on each corpse is illuminated, and the reflected light is split into blue, green and red for measurement. The body, which had developed its primary hypostasis in the supine position, was turned into the prone position and an area of lumbar skin was examined at 30-minute intervals to determine changes in colour as secondary movement takes place over a period of 3 to 8 hours.

In a pilot study on 41 corpses, Vanezis claims that there is a linear relationship between the fading colour of the hypostasis and time during the first 24 hours, after which the relationship is unpredictable.

In 1995, Vanezis and Trillo[6] reported further on the use of colorimetry in measuring the hypostasis from 93 corpses. Measurements were taken over a 4-hour period, and the rate of change of colour intensity of the hypostasis plotted over a post-mortem interval. A regression formula was reported with a correlation coefficient r of 0.538. These authors commented that the shift in hypostasis was marked during the first 12 hours and decreased thereafter. They also claimed that hypostasis could be a useful means for determining the postmortem period up to 48 hours.

REFERENCES

1 Mallach HJ. Zur Frage der Todeszeitbestimmung. *Berlin Med.* 1964; **18**: 577–82.

2 Suzutani T, Ishibashi H, Takatori T. Studies on the estimation of the post-mortem interval. 2 The post-mortem lividity. *Hokkaido Zasshi* 1978; **52**: 259–67.

3 Fechner G, Koops E, Henssge C. Cessation of livor in defined pressure conditions. *Z. Rechtsmed.* 1984; **93**: 238–87.

4 Schuller E, Pankratz H, Liebhardt E. Farbortmessungen an Totenflecken. *Beitr. Gerichtl. Med* 1987; **45**: 169–73.

5 Vanezis P. Assessing hypostasis by colorimetry. *Forensic Sci. Int.* 1991; **52**: 1–3.

6 Vanezis P, Trujillo O. Evaluation of hypostasis using a colorimeter measuring system and its application to the assessment of the post-mortem interval (time of death). *Forensic Sci. Int.* 1996; **78**: 19–28.

Changes after death

LEONARD NOKES AND BURKHARD MADEA

The use of gastric contents in estimating time since death

BERNARD KNIGHT

A GENERAL ASSESSMENT OF THE RELIABILITY OF THE PROCEDURE

For very many years, examination of the contents of the stomach at autopsy has been used as an aid to determine the time since death, though claims as to its usefulness as probative evidence must be viewed with the greatest caution if potential miscarriages of justice are to be avoided. Opinions on the topic vary from author to author, but the following random extracts from standard English language textbooks indicate that strong evidential value can rarely be placed upon the use of gastric contents in timing death.

'The state of digestion of the stomach contents and bowel may be used as an additional means of fixing the hour of death in relation to the last meal. Most elaborate tables have been prepared of the time taken by the stomach to digest certain articles of diet, but these are wholly unreliable. The rate of digestion varies in different persons and gastric and intestinal activity is much retarded in cases of trauma and insensibility. Even without the paralysis of movement that is common to grave injury or deep insensibility, the process of emptying of the stomach may be much delayed.' (Simpson[1]).

'If undigested food is found in the stomach at a postmortem examination, it is often claimed that the deceased must have died within 3–4 hours of his last meal. This claim is of limited value as there are great individual variations in the emptying time of the stomach. As the rate of digestion is variable and as it is not possible to determine the degree of digestion of various foods from a naked-eye examination of the stomach contents, little reliance can be placed upon estimates of the post-mortem interval which are based upon the apparent state of digestion. Gastric digestion may continue post-mortem, this creating further difficulties.' (Gordon et al.[2]).

'Attempts to fix this time (of death) based solely on examination of the stomach contents are unsatisfactory even when allowance is made for the factors which either hasten or retard digestion; allowance must always be made for individual variation. …the foregoing (purported times of emptying), however, cannot be relied upon nor should it be relied upon, as crucial evidence which purports to fix the time of death within narrow limits.' (Polson et al.[3]).

'The rate of emptying of the stomach is so variable that it cannot be used to give any certain indication of the time that has elapsed between the last meal and the death. The state of the stomach and its contents might, however, help in making a decision when, for example, death could have taken place at two or more times. When a person dies in bed after taking supper, an empty stomach would point to death having occurred towards the end of the night, rather than earlier. If there is food in the stomach of a person found dead one morning on the kitchen floor, it might point to death after breakfast, rather than before it.' (Camps[4]).

'Never to be disregarded are the variations which exist in the speed with which food normally passes through the gastrointestinal tract of different persons Moreover, emotional upsets can produce changes in gastrointestinal motility. Thus psychogenic pylorospasm can prevent normal departure of a meal from the stomach for several hours. At the opposite extreme, hypermotility caused by emotional disturbance can result in hurried transit of food and chyme through the gut with resultant diarrhoea.

The physical and chemical facets of digestion are beset by so many imponderable and uncontrollable variables in vivo, that one cannot rely on the extent of mechanical dissolution and chemical breakdown of the gastric content, to help reach a reasonable estimate as to how long food was present in the stomach. Careful consideration of these factors indicates that one must be extremely wary about making statements about the time since death in relation to the last known meal on the basis of the "amount of digestion" of the gastric contents.' (Adelson[5]).

'In conclusion, the emptying of the stomach is a complex multifactorial process and its evaluation for determining the time of death requires caution and careful review of all limiting factors. Consideration must also be given to the possibility of one or more close consecutive meals.' (Spitz[6]).

'For many years, pathologists have argued over the reliability of the state of digestion of gastric contents as an indicator of the time between the last meal and death, the leading case in modern times being that of Truscott in Canada. There is now almost a consensus that with extremely circumscribed exceptions, the method is too uncertain to have much validity.' (Knight[7]).

'Thus this study demonstrates that the gastric emptying of either liquids or solids is subject to relatively wide differences in the same and different individuals, even if the same meal is ingested. If in addition to this we add differences in the weight, caloric content and composition of the meal we would see even greater differences in half-emptying time.' (Di Maio and Di Maio[8]).

This last quotation comes at the end of an excellent summary of many publications on the physiology of digestion and gastric emptying, which emphasizes succinctly the uncertainty provided by many variable factors.

These will be further discussed below, but some general aspects should be addressed. First, there are two ways in which gastric contents have been used to estimate the time of death:

1. By identifying the *nature* of the food in the stomach, and correlating this with a known type of meal eaten before death.
2. By attempting to assess the *quantity* and *state of digestion* as an index of the time elapsed since the last meal.

THE NATURE OF THE FOOD MATERIAL

The first method is certainly the most reliable, though circumstances rarely make it applicable. The rationale is that if the nature of the last meal that the deceased ate can definitely be determined by the investigating authorities, then positive identification of that same type of food in the stomach will almost certainly mean that death occurred after that known meal, and before the next scheduled meal. It certainly does not offer an absolute time-interval since the last meal

The method may be of most use where there has been a considerable delay after death before the body was discovered, when knowledge of a unique meal taken on a particular day might narrow down the time of death. For example, a homicide dealt with by the author involved a woman's body found in a submerged car. The stomach contained a considerable quantity of relatively undigested rice, chicken and vegetables, consistent with a Chinese meal, which was known to have been consumed at lunchtime several days previously, so that it was reasonable to infer that *given normal circumstances* death had probably occurred later that day.

Unfortunately, even this method suffers from several problems.

First, the 'normal circumstances' may not apply, especially in a criminal or other unnatural death. Fear, anger, pain, stress, trauma, coma, etc., may so have slowed digestion and gastric emptying, that the last recognizable meal may have sat unchanged in the stomach for a long period before death, thus misleading the investigators as to the true time of the demise. As mentioned again later, the author recollects an autopsy on the victim of a motorcycle accident, who survived in coma for a week before dying. The stomach contained a full meal, in a virtually fresh, undigested state. Similar cases have been quoted both in the literature and in court testimony, such as Truscott (see below). As quoted by Madea in the next

section, Puschel[9] published a series of cases in which he recorded delayed stomach emptying after trauma for up to 5 to 14 days.

Second, the identification of definitely recognizable food substances may be difficult or impossible, especially if digestion has already proceeded. Especially in these days of processed food of homogeneous consistency, to be able to allocate fairly non-specific animal or vegetable products to a particular meal would be an uncommon happening.

The amount of such recognizable, unique food product must be significant, as it is not legitimate to claim that some minute scrap of meat or cabbage is evidence of a particular specific meal, as particles from a previous meal may be retained in folds of gastric mucosa. Furthermore, eliminating the possibility of two similar meals being taken at different times may not always be practicable. Although it may have been known that a person had eaten a curry on Tuesday, it may not be known that they also had the same dish on Thursday; hence, when the body is found on the following Sunday, a substantial timing error might be made.

THE QUANTITY AND STATE OF DIGESTION OF FOOD MATERIAL

The second and most frequent – as well as dangerous – use of gastric contents is to attempt to interpret its quantity and digestive quality. This is where a whole range of variable factors conspire against the investigators to make firm conclusions extremely elusive. Although tentative estimates of the time of death may be offered, they should only be used as an aid to investigation and at best to reduce the margins of a wide range of possible times of death. They can never be used as free-standing probative evidence, and where they conflict with either good circumstantial evidence or reasoned calculations by other more accurate methods described in this book, the alternative estimates must always take precedence. To explore the reasoning behind attempts to use stomach contents as a timing mechanism, the physiology of gastric emptying and digestion must be studied.

Gastric transit

Food and fluid enter the stomach via the oesophagus and exit through the pylorus into the duodenum. The transit time has been the subject of extensive research over many decades, using a variety of investigative techniques – but the results vary very greatly.

The older, more simplistic opinion was that a 'typical meal' (whatever that is, given the enormous personal, cultural, geographic and ethnic variations in food availability and preference) spends about 2 to 3 hours in the stomach. Many of these publications were based on experiments using a meal of semi-liquid gruel (hardly 'typical food'), and the subjects were healthy and presumably free from trauma and stress – unlike many victims who come to the attention of forensic pathologists.

The medicolegal textbooks themselves give wide ranges for emptying times; for example, Spitz[6] says that a 'small' meal resides in the stomach for 1 to 2 hours, and a large meal for 3 to 5 hours.

Modi[10] claimed a residence time of 4 to 6 hours for a meat and vegetable meal, and 6 to 7 hours for a farinaceous meal.

Adelson[5] states that a light meal leaves the stomach in 2 hours, a medium meal in 3 to 4 hours, and a 'heavy' meal in 4 to 6 hours.

As in retrospect, it is often unknown what meal was last eaten by the subject (both in nature and quantity) and especially how much diluting fluid may have been taken before, with or after the meal, such inexact descriptions of the food taken further reduce the reliability of these assertions.

Experiments by Moore[11–14] on more realistic types of food than the usual experimental sludge, used the 'half' emptying time, as a measure which is more accurate than trying to determine when all food has passed. There was great variability in these times between different subjects, even when approximately the same volume and calorific value was used. These half-times ranged from 124 to 195 minutes, even in calm experimental conditions when no emotional factors were present. When the meal sizes and nature was more random, great variation in half-emptying times was noted, from 60 to 338 minutes. It was noted that some people had a long tag period, where the pylorus remained closed for an extended period.

The use of radioisotopes has greatly improved the technology of gastric investigations, but has only confirmed the range of variable factors. Brophy et al.[12] have been pioneers in such radionuclide techniques. From such investigations, it is known that fluids have a rapid transit time and that watery fluid may pass almost unhindered through an empty stomach. Where a meal is mixed with fluid, then the liquid component escapes more rapidly, leaving the solids behind. However, this provides another complicating factor, in that added fluids may emulsify a variable part of the previously solid food material and thus alter the solid/fluid ratio of the gastric contents, the fluid component then leaving the stomach rapidly. The transit of the fluid element does not seem to be dependent upon the amount and nature of the solid component, though Moore et al.[9–11] have shown that delayed passage of fluid may occur in aged males.

However, even fluids have different transit times according to their content. Those of high calorific value are markedly delayed, according to Brophy et al.,[12] who showed that carbohydrate-containing fluids, such as 150 g orange juice, have a half-emptying time ranging from 12 to 37 minutes. Strong alcoholic fluids, such as undiluted spirits and liqueurs may also be delayed, due to their irritant effect causing closure of the pylorus.

The calorific content of both fluids and solids affects the rate of transit, with an increasing nutrient value (especially from starch and fat) increasing the time the food stays in the stomach. A larger meal passes into the duodenum at a faster rate, in terms of unit volume per minute – though a large meal may still stay longer in the stomach than a smaller one, because of the sheer quantity present.

It is thus apparent that the factors affecting gastric emptying are multiple and complex. Brophy et al.[12] tested the same subjects on different days with identical meals and liquids. They showed that there was marked variation even in the same individual at different times; the half-emptying times of solids ranged between 29 and 92 minutes, whilst for orange juice the times varied between 12 and 30 minutes.

Attempting to use the *state of digestion*, rather than the quantity of food, as a measure of time since ingestion, is even more fraught with uncertainty. Assessing the stage of digestion in terms of time is subjective and almost impossible, as virtually no one has any standardized, control data for matching – and the original nature of the meal is usually unknown, so the appearance of the stage of digestion of say, porridge and bread would be utterly different, at 1 hour from swallowing, from meat and raw root vegetables.

In summary, the quantity and digestive appearance of gastric contents is modified by the following factors:

- The total quantity of food taken at a meal.
- Additional 'snacks' taken between meals, especially from the modern habit of 'grazing',

frequently upon quick 'convenience' foods. Where frequent snacking occurs, then food may still be in the stomach when the meal under consideration arrives.

- The ratio of solid to liquid in the meal and later 'top-ups' of liquid or solids.
- The carbohydrate/fat content compared with more inert fibre, etc.
- Marked variations between individuals.
- Variation in the same individual from day to day (Brophy et al.[12]).
- Dramatic variations due to the psychogenic and endocrine factors of emotion, fear, pain, anger, shock and trauma – with or without unconsciousness.

CONCLUSIONS

From the foregoing discussion, it is readily apparent that there are a whole range of variable factors which make it impossible to use stomach contents as definitive evidence in estimating the time since death.

Even the generalizations so often used by pathologists and other medical witnesses, can be wildly incorrect, sometimes to the detriment of justice. However eminent a pathologist might be, his or her expertise on this matter is of necessity limited. They may have conducted thousands of postmortem examinations, in every one of which the stomach contents have been noted. However, in the vast majority of cases, the issue of time since death need not be considered. Also in the vast majority, the time of and nature of the last meal is unknown, and is usually of no interest. So, where does the medical witness obtain the sometimes dogmatic evidence which he or she delivers in court with such pontifical gravitas?

It may be true that in the majority of persons, the 'average meal' passes from the stomach in something between 30 minutes and 3 hours. However, these persons are not the subjects of a forensic examination, necessitated by a violent crime which may have all the connotations of emotion, fear, injury, etc. that is well known to disrupt the digestive process. In addition, the 'majority of persons' leaves a very sizeable minority, whose gastric emptying may lie well outside the so-called 'normal' parameters. As proof in a criminal case must be 'beyond reasonable doubt', this leaves little scope for firm testimony based on such shifting sands as gastric physiology.

Unfortunately for defence counsel, the value of

such evidence tends to be one-sided – in other words, the unreliability of timing of death from stomach contents allows it to be legitimately claimed in almost all situations, that death *could* have occurred during the period alleged by the prosecution – whereas the same evidence can virtually never be used to claim that it *could not*, and thus remove the time of death into a period of alibi. This negative trend may be persuasive when added to other evidence, even though it has no probative value. A prime example of this is the Truscott case, described below.

A CASE HISTORY: STEVEN TRUSCOTT

The best-known instance where the estimation of time since death based on the postmortem evaluation of stomach contents became a matter of international controversy, is that of Stephen Truscott.

In 1959 in Ontario, Canada, this 14-year-old boy was accused of sexually assaulting and strangling a 12-year-old girl, Lynne Harper. He was found guilty and sentenced to be hanged, though on Appeal several months later, this was reduced to life imprisonment. Disquiet about his conviction led an investigative journalist, Isobel Lebourdais, to write a book on what was claimed to be an injustice; subsequently, a considerable political furore developed.

In 1966, the case was re-heard at the Supreme Court and many forensic experts from Canada, USA and Britain gave evidence, mainly on the reliability of estimating the time of death from gastric contents. These included Professor Milton Helpern from New York, Professor Francis Camps and Professor Keith Simpson from Britain, Dr Charles Petty (Baltimore, USA), Dr Frederick Jaffe (Toronto, Canada) Dr Sam Gerber (Cleveland), Mr John Funk (Toronto, Canada) and Dr Noble Sharpe (Toronto, Canada). The Supreme Court upheld the conviction, and Truscott served about 10 years in prison and on release, assumed a new identity. The case remained in the public eye, with television and press coverage at intervals and now (2001), Stephen Truscott has declared his intention of clearing his name, claiming that he is innocent of the crime for which he was convicted more than 40 years ago, and further expert medical opinion is being sought. The circumstances indicated that Truscott had only a period of 45 minutes in which he could have committed the crime, Lynne Harper being seen alive at 7.15 pm and Truscott being back home with numerous witnesses at 8.00 pm on the evening in question. The body was not discovered until 41 hours later, and a postmortem was carried out 48 hours later, two days after the girl was last seen alive. The pathologist was Dr John Penistan, a hospital histopathologist who also performed medicolegal autopsies. He gave evidence to the effect that, based on rigor mortis, hypostasis and stomach contents, the time of death lay within a 30-minute interval, two days previous to the autopsy.

The facts relating to the gastric contents were that the girl ate a meal of turkey, cranberry sauce, peas, potatoes and pineapple pudding between 5.30 and 5.45 that evening. There were other foods also on the table, but it is not known whether she took those, nor any knowledge of what fluids were taken.

The pathologist recorded that the stomach contents consisted of 'approximately one pint (568 ml)', though the evidence of two other doctors who examined the material in the forensic laboratory was that the volume was about 300 ml.

The material was described by Dr Penistan in his autopsy report as 'poorly masticated, only slightly digested food, including peas, onion, corn and a few shreds of apparent meat'. The forensic scientist, Mr Funk, described it as being of the consistency of 'a thick stew'. Dr Noble Share, a medically qualified forensic scientist, said it was like 'a lumpy porridge'.

Dr Penistan's actual words in his autopsy report, to which he adhered during the trial, were:

> 'Note on time of death; this opinion, which would place the time of death between 7.15 and 7.45 pm on 9 June 1959, is based on the following observations and assumptions:
>
> The extent of decomposition which is entirely compatible with death approximately 45 hours prior to identification, having regard to the environmental and climatic conditions.
>
> The extent of rigor mortis. This had almost passed off – a finding again compatible with death at the suggested time.
>
> The limited degree of digestion and the large quantity of food in the stomach. I find it difficult to believe that this food could have been in the stomach for as long as 2 hours unless some complicating factor was present, of which I have no information. If the last meal was finished at 5.45 pm, I would therefore conclude that death occurred prior to 7.45 pm. The finding would be comparable (sic) with death as early as 7.15 pm'.

Although Dr Penistan actually concludes with an opinion that death was *consistent* (though he uses the word 'comparable') with occurring as early as 7.15 pm, his earlier phraseology was that the findings were *indicative* of death occurring between 7.15 and 7.45 pm. This opinion was repeated throughout the trial and the later Supreme Court hearing, both by Dr Penistan and those expert witnesses who supported his view – in spite of the defence witnesses and lawyers forcibly indicating that the medical evidence also allowed death to have taken place well outside those unreasonably narrow limits.

Though there was considerable other non-medical evidence involved in this case, there is no doubt that a dogmatic adherence to unreliable pathological findings, which retrospectively placed the time of death within a 30-minute bracket from an autopsy two days later, contributed to the death sentence being passed on a 14-year-old boy.

REFERENCES

1 Simpson CK (ed.). *Taylor's Principles and Practice of Medical Jurisprudence.* 12th edition. J & A Churchill, London, 1965: 210.
2 Gordon I, Shapiro HA, Berson SD. *Forensic Medicine – A Guide to Principles*, 3rd edition. Churchill Livingstone, Edinburgh, 1988: 56.
3 Polson CJ, Gee DJ, Knight B. *The Essentials of Forensic Medicine.* 4th edition. Pergamon Press, Oxford, 1985: 32–3.
4 Camps FE (ed.). *Gradwohl's Legal Medicine*, 3rd edition. John Wright, Bristol, 1976: 98.
5 Adelson L. *The Pathology of Homicide.* Thomas, Springfield, Ill, 1974.
6 Spitz WU. *Spitz & Fisher's Medicolegal Investigation of Death.* 3rd edition. Thomas, Springfield, Ill, 19XX: 28–31.
7 Knight B. *Forensic Pathology*, 2nd edition. Edward Arnold, London, 1996: 89–90.
8 DiMaio D, DiMaio VJM. *Forensic Pathology.* Elsevier, New York, 1989: 36–42.
9 Püschel K. Nüchternheitsgebot und Aspirationprophylaxe aus rechtsmedizinischer Sicht. *AINS* 1996; **31**: 248–50.
10 Modi JP. *Medical Jurisprudence and Toxicology.* Tripathi, Bombay, 1957.
11 Moore JG, Christian PE, Brown JA. Influence of meal weight and caloric content on gastric emptying of meals in man. *Dig. Dis. Sci.* 1984; **29**: 513–19.
12 Moore JG, Christian PE, Coleman RE. Gastric emptying of varying meal weight and composition in man. *Dig. Dis. Sci.* 1981; **26**: 16–22.
13 Moore JG, Tweedy C, Christian PE *et al.* Effects of age on

gastric emptying of liquid-solid meals in man. *Dig. Dis. Sci.* 1983; **28**: 340.

14 Brophy CM, Moore JG, Christian PE *et al*. Variability of gastric emptying measurements in man employing standardized radiolabeled meals. *Dig. Dis. Sci.* 1986; **31**: 799–806.

Gastric contents and time since death

BURKHARD MADEA

The state of digestion and distribution of the last meal in the stomach and upper intestine have long been proposed as a method for estimating the time since death.[1–3] The volume of stomach content compared with the volume of the last meal and transportation distance into the small intestine must be known. Even if the volume of the last meal is not known from the kind of meal (breakfast, lunch), rough estimations of the daytime when death occurred may be possible.

Estimations of the time since death based on the stomach content are often also required however, as the police did not call for a forensic pathologist at the scene of crime.[4]

The state of digestion and transportation rate of food from the stomach into the duodenum depend on several antemortem (anatomical, physiological, psychological, pathological, agonal, kind of food) factors, which contribute to the great intra- and interindividual variability of gastric emptying. Therefore, it is not astonishing that diverging estimates on the time of death in relation to the last meal were made by different pathologists in the same case. Estimations considering all circumstances should be made only with great reservation. Digestion itself does not cease at death but progresses after death; the state of digestion is therefore only of little value estimating the time.

IS THERE POSTMORTEM TRANSPORT OF GASTRIC CONTENTS?

Previously published reports have claimed that postmortem transport of gastric contents into the duodenum occurs, these being based on animal experimental observations of postmortem electrical and pharmacological excitability of gastric smooth muscle and volume-dependent peristalsis of the gastric wall.[5,6] When pressure was applied to the gastric wall with high filling volumes of the stomach, contractions of the wall were observed.[5]

Our own animal experiments were carried out under the following questions and circumstances (Tables 6.1–6.4):

Table 6.1 *Postmortem gastric emptying. Observation of stomach and small bowel under direct view*

Material	Method
10 rats (HAN-SPRD, body weight about 100 g) No feeding 2 days prior to death Anaesthesia with ether Death due to KCl i.v. (5×) or ether/O_2-deficiency (5×)	Immediately after circulatory arrest: • opening of the abdomen • pinching off the pylorus • positioning of a stomach sound • instillation of blue-coloured gelatine into the stomach • removing the clamp In no case postmortem was there peristaltic transport of gastric content into the duodenum

Table 6.2 *Observing the stomach and small bowel under direct view. The dependence of antemortem transport on survival time*

Material	Method

4 rats (HAN-SPRD, body weight about 100 g) Anaesthesia with ether	During anaesthesia:
	
	• positioning of a stomach sound
	• instillation of blue-coloured gelatine into the stomach
	• survival time 2, 5, 10, 20 min, then
	• death due to KCl i.v.
	• opening of the abdomen
	
	Transport distance into the small bowel depending on the survival time:
	    2 min – 2 cm
	    20 min – 15 cm
	
	No postmortem gastric emptying, but postmortem transport of small bowel content did occur

Table 6.3 *Observing stomach and small bowel under direct view. The effect of prostigmin on postmortem transport*

Material	Method
4 rats (HAN-SPRD, body weight 200 g) No feeding 2 days prior to death Anaesthesia with ether Death due to KCl i.v. (2×) and exsanguination	• 4 min prior to death, 0.28 ml prostigmine given i.v. • opening of the abdomen immediately after circulatory arrest • pinching off the pylorus • Positioning of a stomach sound • instillation into the stomach • removing the clamp No postmortem transport of gastric content

Table 6.4 *Postmortem gastric emptying. Radiological control of gastric transport*

Material	Method
10 rats (HAN-SPRD), body weight 150–180 g No feeding for 1 day prior to death (7×) Feeding immediately prior to death (3×) Prostigmine i.v. 5 min prior to circulatory arrest (2×) Death by ether/O_2-deficiency	• Immediately after circulatory arrest, instillation of barium sulphate into the stomach by a stomach sound (3–5 ml, 10°C) • Radiological control taken anteriorly–posteriorly and laterally) of the abdomen immediately after circulatory arrest, 10–15 min postmortem, 30 min postmortem (Fig. 6.1a and b; Fig. 6.2a, b and c) • 2 hours postmortem: preparation of stomach and small bowel (Fig. 6.1c and d; Fig. 6.2d) No postmortem transport of gastric content (neither barium sulphate nor solid stomach content)

1. Is there any postmortem transport of stomach content which is applied immediately after circulatory arrest to the stomach?
2. Is there any transport of stomach content (gelatine) applied before death depending on the survival time?
3. Is there any effect of prostigmine on postmortem peristalsis?
4. Is there any effect of feeding prior to death?

The stomach and small bowel were either observed under direct vision after opening the abdomen, or the

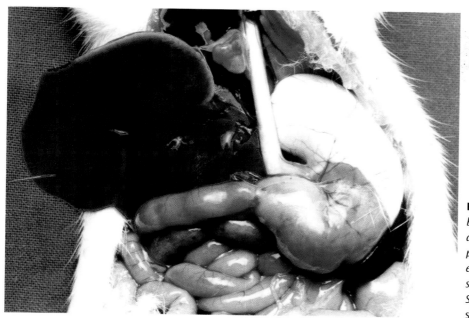

Plate 1 *Stomach filled with barium-sulphate, in the distal stomach solid food fed prior to death. No transport either of food or of barium-sulphate into the duodenum. Stomach and small bowel* in situ.

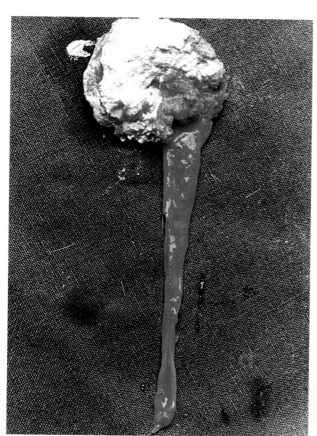

Plate 2 *Stomach filled with barium-sulphate, in the distal stomach solid food fed prior to death. No transport either of food or of barium-sulphate into the duodenum. Stomach and duodenum after preparation.*

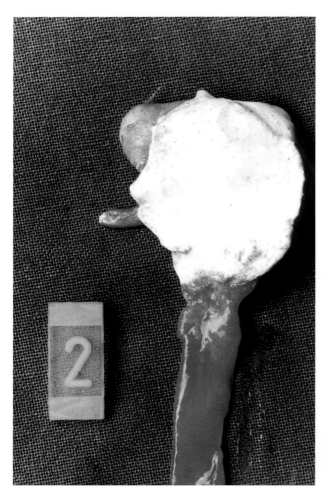

Plate 3 *Whole stomach filled with barium-sulphate. No transport into the duodenum. Stomach and duodenum after preparation.*

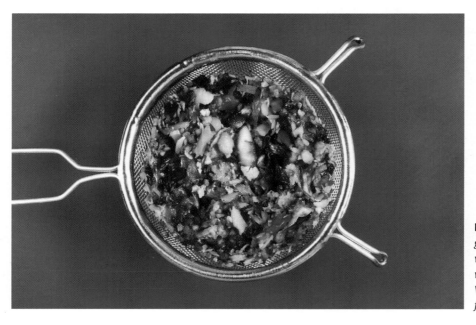

Plate 4 *Solid phase of gastric content consisting of vegetables (mixed salad) with only slight digestion. Victim stabbed soon after food intake (1–2 hours).*

stomach content (barium sulphate) by means of radiological control. In all cases, a preparation of the stomach and small bowel was carried out 2 hours postmortem.

Although peristaltic twitchings of the stomach were visible under direct view, there was in no case any peristaltic emptying of the gastric content after death.

Even in the cases with feeding immediately prior to death, there was no transport of food to the duodenum (Fig. 6.1a–c). Correspondingly, when the whole stomach was filled with barium sulphate, no transport into the duodenum occurred (Fig. 6.2a,b). Postmortem peristaltic transport of the small bowel

content may occur during the first minutes after death.

Under intravenous prostigmine, there is also no peristaltic gastric emptying, though the peristaltic twitchings may be stronger. Depending on the survival time, liquid stomach content (coloured gelatine) applied 2 to 20 minutes prior to death may be transported into the duodenum. Overall, there is no evidence of any functionally relevant postmortem gastric peristalsis with postmortem transport of the gastric contents.

The 'fastener' function of the pylorus clearly remains stable after death. These findings correlate with those

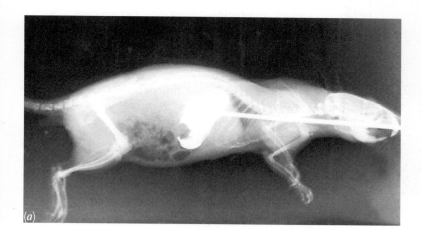

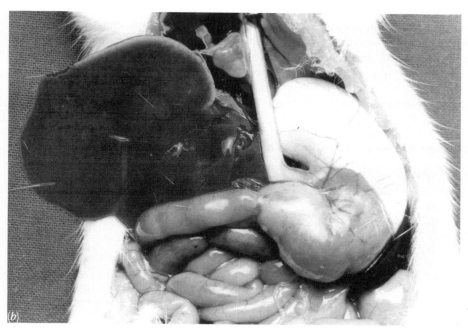

Figure 6.1 *Stomach filled with barium-sulphate, in the distal stomach solid food fed prior to death. No transport either of food or of barium-sulphate into the duodenum. (a) radiographical control (b) stomach and small bowel in situ. Pylorus fastened (c) stomach and duodenum after preparation. (See Plates 1 and 2.)*

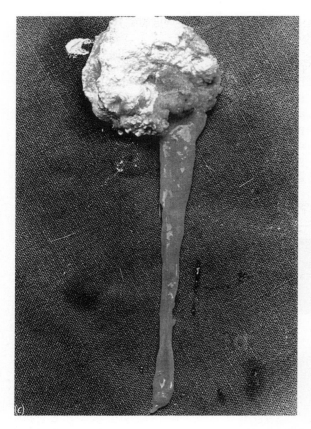

Figure 6.1 continued

found at autopsy by the German pathologist, Ludwig Aschoff (1921), who was able to perform autopsies at about 30 minutes after death during the first world war. Aschoff always found the pylorus fastened, while the supravital contraction of the pylorus was without relaxation followed by rigor mortis.[7]

Another argument for the postmortem stable fastener-function of the pylorus, and against post-mortem gastric emptying, is that in cases of newborn infants who survived only a few minutes, air may be found in the stomach but not in the small bowel. Furthermore, in the above-mentioned investigations which claimed postmortem peristaltic emptying of gastric content,[7,10] this could only be observed when high pressures were applied to the stomach wall.

GASTRIC EMPTYING PATTERN

Gastric emptying has been studied and quantified within the last decade using different methods (radio-logical, intubation-aspiration, radioisotopic, ultra-sound, absorption kinetics of orally administered solutes, ferromagnetic traces).[8]

Liquids leave the stomach much more rapidly than do solids. For liquids, gastric emptying clearly follows an exponential function, but solids show a linear emptying pattern. A mixed meal shows an exponential emptying pattern, with the emptying time itself depending on the volume and composition of the last meal(s), and carbohydrates, proteins and lipids leaving the stomach in that order. The following gastric emptying times have been cited in the literature:

- 1–3 hours for a light, small-volume meal;
- 3–5 hours for a medium-sized meal; and
- 5–8 hours for a large meal.

Data relating to the gastric emptying pattern of solids and liquids are based on radionuclide studies (Table 6.5), but in the older German literature tables were provided which indicated how rapidly different liquids, vegetables and mixed meals leave the stomach (Table 6.6).

Table 6.5 *Solid and liquid gastric emptying in normal subjects assessed by dual isotopic radionuclide methods*

Authors	No. of subjects	Meal size (g)	Solid 50% emptying time (min)	Liquid 50% emptying time (min)
Fischer *et al.* (1982)	20	380	100 ± 4	30 ± 3
Heading *et al.* (1976)	10	185	120 ± 6	45 ± 4
Horowitz *et al.* (1984)	22	250	78 ± 4	19 ± 1
Moon *et al.* (1981)	8	300	77 ± 5	38 ± 4
	8	900	146 ± 26	81 ± 12
	10	1692	277 ± 44	178 ± 22
Wright *et al.* (1993)	31	410	87 ± 9	63 ± 6

Modified according to Horowitz and Pounder.[8]

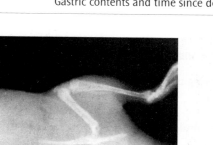

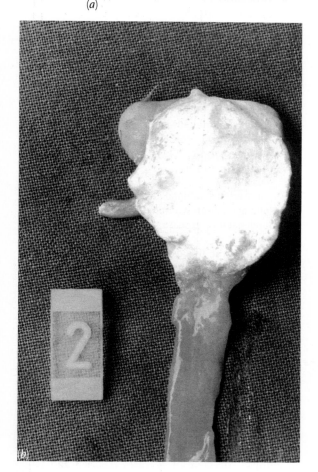

Figure 6.2 *Whole stomach filled with barium-sulphate. No transport into the duodenum (a) radiographical control (b) stomach and duodenum after preparation. (See Plate 3.)*

It should be borne in mind that different anatomical and functional disorders cause either delayed or rapid gastric emptying (Table 6.7). For example, in cases of raised intracranial pressure, gastric emptying may cease for several days. Püschel[10] recently reported data relating to solid stomach content found at autopsy 10 days after scalding, at 5 days after subdural haematoma, 9 days after scalding, 11 days after polytrauma, and even a bolus death 14 days after subdural haematoma with entirely parenteral nutrition.

Horowitz and Pounder[8] summarized their review on gastric emptying as follows:

1. Simultaneously ingested liquid, digestible solid and non-digestible solid foods leave the stomach at different rates.
2. The emptying pattern of low-calorie liquids approximates a monoexponential (volume-dependent) process that results primarily from the motoric activity of the proximal stomach.
3. The emptying of digestible solids usually occurs much more slowly than liquids, and approximates a linear pattern following an initial lag period. It is primarily dependent on the motoric activity of the distal stomach.
4. The emptying of larger, non-digestible particles chiefly occurs during the interdigestive periods, as a specific result of gastric motor activity.
5. Meals of higher osmotic and caloric content are emptied more slowly.
6. There is a substantial variation in emptying rates in normal subjects, and this variation may even be altered by diseases.

Table 6.6 *Solid and liquid (g) gastric emptying according to Pensold and Stinzing (in Tröger et al.[9])*

Food leaving stomach	Quantity (g)
1–2 hours	
Water	100–200
Carbon dioxide, water	220
Tea	200
Coffee	200
Cocoa	200
Beer	200
Light wines	200
Milk (boiled)	100–200
Beef tea	200
2–3 hours	
Coffee with cream	200
Cocoa with milk	200
Open wine	200
Water or beer or boiled milk	300–500
Egg (uncooked), scrambled or boiled	100
Beef/sausage	100
Boiled fish	200
Cauliflower	150
Potatoes	150
Cherries	150
White bread	70
Asparagus	150
3–4 hours	
Date	100
Bread	40
Boiled chicken	220–230
Beef, boiled or uncooked	250
Ham	160
Roast veal	100
Rice	150
Apple	150
Bean/spinach	150
4–5 hours	
Fat ham	120
5 eggs	5 eggs
Beefsteak, roasted	250
Hare, roasted	150
Goose, roasted	250
Herring, salted	200
Lentils (porridge)	150
Peas (porridge)	200

ESTIMATION OF TIME OF DEATH FROM GASTRIC CONTENTS

From the examination of the stomach content, only a rough estimation can be derived, and this may extend

Table 6.7 *Aetiology of delayed and rapid gastric emptying*

Transient delayed gastric emptying
- postoperative illness
- acute viral gastroenteritis
- hyperglycaemia
- drugs: morphine, anticholinergics, levodopa, beta-adrenergic agonists, nicotine
- stress: labyrinthine stimulation, cold, pain, pectin supplementation

Chronic gastric stasis
- diabetes mellitus
- postsurgical – truncal vagotomy with pyloroplasty and antrectomy
- gastro-oesophageal reflux
- anorexia nervosa
- progressive systemic sclerosis
- chronic idiopathic intestinal pseudo-obstruction
- amyloidosis
- myotonia dystrophica
- familial dysautonomia
- dermatomyositis
- tachygastria
- paraplegia
- idiopathic myocardial infarction
- acute abdomen
- laparotomia
- physiological: liquids, acid, lipids, left-side position

Rapid gastric emptying
- after gastric surgery
    - vagotomy
    - antrectomy/subtotal gastrectomy
- Zollinger–Ellison syndrome
- duodenal ulcer disease
- reserpine
- physiological: liquids, hunger

Modified according to Horowitz and Pounder[8] and Tröger et al.[9]

over a few hours. According to Horowitz and Pounder,[8] only the solid components of a mixed solid and liquid meal should be considered, and the weight of the stomach contents should be compared with the estimated weight of the last meal and reference made to the known 50% emptying times for the solid components of meals of various sizes (see Table 6.5).

Tröger et al.[9] compared the gastric content (volume) found at autopsy to time and volume of last meals on an autopsy collective of 47 cases (sudden and unexpected death, exclusion of brain tumours, gastrointestinal tract surgery, intoxication, alcoholism). The gastric content (as per cent volume of the last meal) was plotted against the survival time. Only a gastric contents weight over 10 g was considered, and a regression line and 90% and 98% confidence limits were calculated (Fig. 6.3a, b).

The following conclusions were derived from the graph obtained:

- If 90% of the last meal is still found in the stomach, the last food intake was probably within the last hour before death, with 98% confidence limits of 3 to 4 hours.

- At autopsy, if 50% of the volume of the last meal is found in the stomach, the last food intake was about 3 to 4 hours before death, with 98% confidence limits of not less than 1 hour and not more than 10 hours.

- If only 30% of the last meal is found, the last food intake was about 4 to 5 hours before death, with

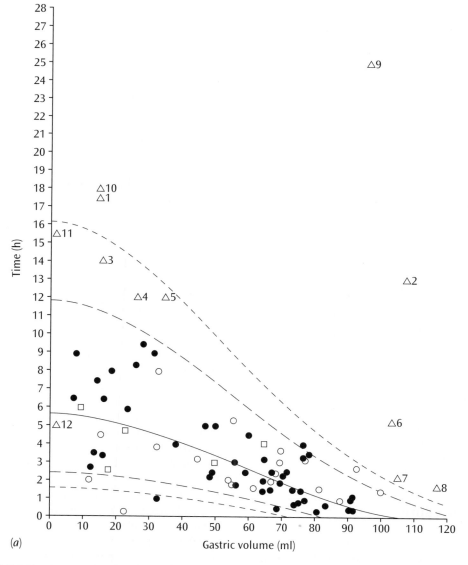

(a)

Figure 6.3 (a) Relation between gastric volume of a mixed meal in per cent of ingested volume and time after food intake with regression line, 90 and 98% limits of confidence. Whole samples consists of 48 cases. ● normal cases; ○ alcohol concentration between 0.3‰ and 3.18‰ (n = 17); □ death after hospitalization (n = 8); ▲ special cases (intoxication, trauma to the head).

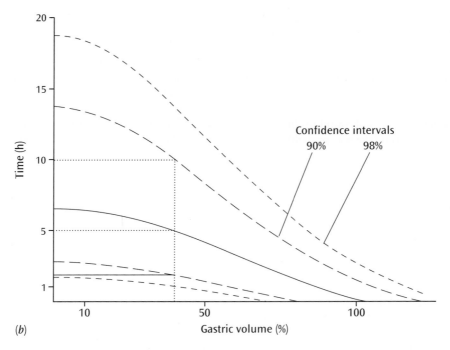

Figure 6.3 *(b) Procedure in practice. From the stomach content in per cent of the ingested volume and estimation of the survival period can be made (from Moore* et al., *1984[19]).*

98% confidence limits not less than 1 to 2 hours and not more than 10 to 11 hours.

It must be borne in mind that the data shown in Fig. 6.3 is valid only for mixed food. If the volume of the last meal is not known exactly, tables for the calculation of restaurant portions have been published by Tröger *et al.*[9]

Pure carbohydrate food leaves the stomach earlier than mixed food. Therefore, a specialized graph was also derived for pure carbohydrate food (gastric content in relation to the volume of the last meal) as well (Fig. 6.4), while for baby food a graph is also available (Fig. 6.5). Due to the small sample size, confidence limits could not be calculated, and in the practical case only mean values could be estimated.

Practical procedure

In practical terms, the stomach content at autopsy (mixed food with proof of meat, carbohydrates, vegetables) is weighed and compared with the volume of the last meal. If the volume of the last meal is not known exactly, the gastric content can be compared to typical restaurant portions. The remaining volume, expressed as percent-

age of the ingested volume, provides the mean survival time after food intake, with the corresponding confidence limits. The practical case must be comparable with the case from which the graph was calculated.

For mixed food, these graphs are advantageous when estimating time since death, as the confidence limits derived from casework material can be used, and subjective rough estimations can be avoided. For the identification of food ingredients in stomach contents, the use of microscopical and/or immunological identification methods may be necessary, and these have been described in detail in a monograph.[9] For special identification methods, experts must be consulted.

In order to examine gastric contents, an additional sieve analysis is recommended,[11] using a sieve tower. This consists of a collecting basin and four sieves, each of 20 cm diameter, which can be fitted together. The mesh diameters of the four sieves are 6.3, 4, 2 and 1 mm, respectively.

After weighing the gastric content, the whole volume is placed into the upper sieve (6.3-mm mesh). If the content is viscous, water will be added; this permits the content to be separated into one liquid and up to four solid phases, and these can be further analysed as appropriate (Figs. 6.6 and 6.7).

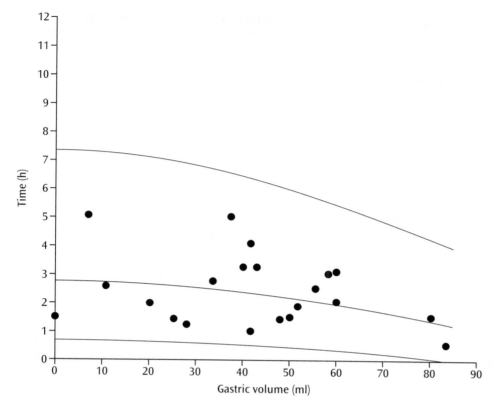

Figure 6.4 *Pure carbohydrate food: rest volume in per cent of ingested volume plotted against the survival period after food intake. Regression line and 90% limits of confidence (from Moore* et al., *1984[19]).*

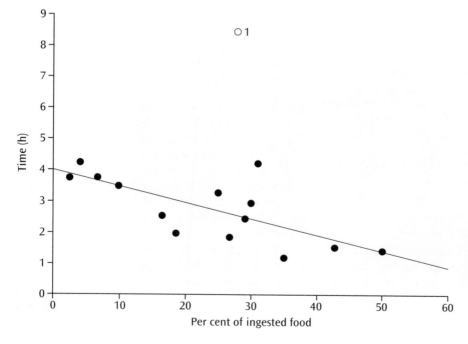

Figure 6.5 *Babies up to 10 months – rest volume in per cent of ingested volume in relation to the time since food intake. One case of fatal intoxication (from Moore* et al., *1984[19]).*

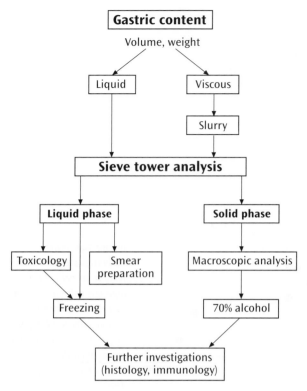

Figure 6.6 *Sieve tower analysis of gastric content allowing further preparation and investigation of the various phases of gastric content (from Holczabek, 1961[16]).*

REFERENCES AND BIBLIOGRAPHY

1 Merkel H. Über Mageninhalt und Todeszeit. *Dtsch. Z. Gerichtl. Med.* 1922; **1**: 346–58.

2 Sonderegger W. Zeitbestimmungen nach biologisch-medizinischen Methoden in dem Gebiete der Rechtsmedizin. Med Diss, Zürich, 1916.

3 Sorge A. Die Verwertung des Mageninhaltes zur Bestimmung der Todeszeit und der Zeit der letzten Nahrungsaufnahme. *Z. Medizinal Beamte* 1904; **17**: 373–90.

4 Berg S. Der Beweiswert der Todeszeitbestimmung (Über-lebenszeit). *Beitr. Gerichtl. Med.* 1969; **25**: 61–5.

5 Forster B, Hummelsheim G, Döring G. Tierexperimentelle Untersuchungen über die postmortale Magenperistaltik bei Leuchtgas- und Parathion-Vergiftung. *Dtsch. Z. Gerichtl. Med.* 1965; **56**: 148–59.

6 Joachim H. Probleme der frühen Todeszeitbestimmung und die sogenannten supravitalen Reaktionen im Tierversuch. Habil. Schrift, Freiburg.

7 Aschoff L. Diskussionsbemerkung zu Mangold E: Über Automatie, Erregbarkeit und Totenstarre in verschiede-nen Teilen des Froschmagens. *Dtsch. Med. Wochenschr.* 1920; **16**: 447–8.

8 Horowitz M, Pounder DJ. Gastric emptying – forensic implications of current concepts. *Med. Sci. Law* 1985; **25**: 201–14.

9 Tröger HD, Baur C, Spann KW. Mageninhalt und Todeszeitbestimmung. Schmidt-Römhild, 1987.

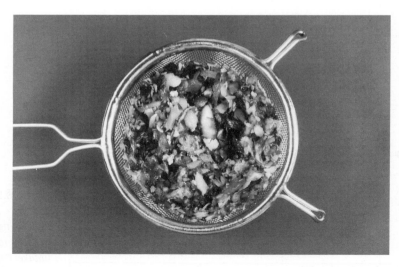

Figure 6.7 *Solid phase of gastric content consisting of vegetables (mixed salad) with only slight digestion. Victim stabbed soon after food intake (1–2 hours). (See Plate 4.)*

10 Püschel K. Nüchternheitsgebot und Aspirations prophylaxe aus rechtsmedizinischer Sicht. *AINS* 1996; **31**: 248–50.

11 Rabl W, Sigrist Th. Auftrennung des Mageninhaltes mittels Siebturm-Technik. *Arch. Kriminol.* 1992; **189**: 164–8.

12 Baur C, Spann KW, Tröger HD, Schuller E. Magenfüllung und Todeszeitpunkt. *Beitr. Gerichtl. Med.* 1980; **38**: 193–7.

13 Brophy CM, Moore JG, Christian PE, Egger MJ, Taylor AT. Variability of gastric emptying measurements in man employing standardized radiolabeled meals. *Dig. Dis. Sci.* 1986; **31**: 799–806.

14 Camps FE. Establishment of the time of death – a critical assessment. *J. Forensic Sci.* 1959; **4**: 73–82.

15 Camps FE. *Gradwohl's Legal Medicine*, 3rd edition. John Wright & Sons Ltd, Bristol.

16 Holczabek W. Zur Untersuchung des Magen-Darmtraktes für die Todeszeitbestimmung. *Beitr. Gerichtl. Med.* 1961; **21**: 23–7.

17 Madea B, Oehmichen M, Henssge C. Postmortaler Transport von Mageninhalt. *Z. Rechtsmed.* 1986; **97**: 201–6.

18 Madea B, Oehmichen M, Henssge C. Postmortale Magenperistaltik? Festschrift Prof Spann. Springer, Berlin, Heidelberg, New York, 1986: 200–5.

19 Moore JG, Christian PE, Brown JA, Brophy C, Datz F, Taylor A, Alazraki N. Influence of meal weight and caloric content on gastric emptying of meals in man. *Dig. Dis. Sci.* 1984; **29**: 513–19.

Blood changes and time since death

LEONARD NOKES

A wealth of data on biochemical material in the blood after death is available. Some of these indices remain relatively stable during the early postmortem period, whilst others show varying degrees of change. One of the most detailed reviews of postmortem blood chemistry was carried out by Coe in 1974.[1] Below are listed the various postmortem blood biochemical markers and how their analysis may help in determining the time since death.

CARBOHYDRATES

Glucose

Early work by Hampden *et al.* (cited in Coe[1]) demonstrated that glycolysis varied after death, and that blood from the right atrium commonly had high glucose values as a result of glycogenolysis. Diabetics tended to have high peripheral glucose due to slower glycolysis. Since 1940, numerous investigators have reported their analysis of glucose after death, though to the author's knowledge none has attempted to estimate the postmortem period from these data. Hill reported that glycolysis occurred at the rate of 12.8 mg/dl per hour, but no attempt has been made to utilize this information as a means to calculate the time of death.

Lactic acid

Jetter (cited in Coe[1]) reported that during life there are very small amounts of lactic acid in both plasma and erythrocytes. There is a progressive increase (relationship not stated) so that at 12 to 24 hours after death, the lactic acid values were 50- to 75-fold the normal antemortem concentrations.

NITROGENOUS COMPOUNDS

Blood urea, nitrogen and creatinine

Numerous investigators reported very little variation in the concentration of urea, nitrogen and creatinine in postmortem blood, compared with antemortem levels.

Non-protein nitrogen, amino acid nitrogen, ammonia and uric acid

For all four markers, it was found that a sharp increase in concentration occurred during the early postmortem period. Unfortunately, for all except amino acid nitrogen, no rates of increase are given. For amino acid nitrogen, values less than 14 mg/dl were usually found under 10 hours postmortem, but by 48 hours after death the concentration had risen to 30 mg/dl.[1]

OTHER ORGANIC COMPOUNDS

It is generally agreed among investigators that blood concentrations of cholesterol, lipids and protein vary little between postmortem and antemortem levels.

ENZYMES

Acid and alkaline phosphatase

Enticknap (cited in Coe[1]) demonstrated that the concentrations of acid phosphatase increased to a value 20 times the normal antemortem level by 48 hours after death. Similarly, the levels of alkaline phosphatase were found to rise after death from 1.15 to 5.3 Vodansky units at 10.5 hours postmortem.

Phosphoglucomutase (PGM)

Gupta et al.[2] reported that the ratio of postmortem to antemortem levels of PGM varied according to the mode of death. These authors also concluded that the estimation of the time since death by analysing PGM activity depends upon many factors, including the environmental conditions.

Amylase, glutamate-oxalate transaminase (AST4) and lactate dehydrogenase (LDH)

Concentrations of all three enzymes increased postmortem. Amylase reached its highest level in the second day postmortem (three to four times normal antemortem levels), whilst AST and LDH increased linearly over the first 60 hours after death. Enticknap (cited in Coe[1]) concluded that, due to the linear relationship between AST (LDH) and the time since death, it may be possible to calculate the postmortem period.

ELECTROLYTES

Sodium

Jetter (cited in Coe[1]) demonstrated that, up to 12 hours postmortem, the concentration of sodium in serum remained constant, but after 12 hours there was a decrease. Coe[1] reported that there was an immediate decrease in the sodium concentration after death, but that the rate of decrease shows considerable variation between investigations. The average rate of decrease was found to be 0.9 mEq/l per hour.

Chloride

Several investigators reported various rates of decrease in plasma chloride through intracellular shift after death. Jetter (cited in Coe[1]) quotes 80–90 mEq/l per day, whilst Schleyer (cited in Coe[1]) reported rates between 0.25 and 1 mEq/l per hour. Querido[3,4] found the rate to be approximately 0.95 mEq/l per hour.

Potassium

Numerous investigators have reported an initial rapid increase in serum potassium concentration over the first 1 to 2 hours after death, but after this period the rate declined steadily. The rapid release of potassium from cells immediately after death makes its evaluation impossible as a means of investigating the postmortem period.

Sodium/potassium ratio

Querido[3,4] demonstrated that there was a strong relationship between the ratio of the postmortem concentration of sodium and potassium to the time since death (Fig. 6.8). He concluded that, although the work was carried out on rats, the results could be transferred to the human model due to the similarities between rat and human blood.

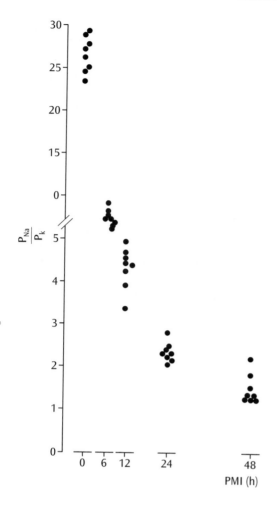

Figure 6.8 *Plasma sodium/ potassium concentration ratio (P_{Na}/P_K) plotted as a function of the postmortem interval (PMI).*

Calcium

A number of investigators have found that the concentration of serum calcium is approximately the same between post- and antemortem samples.

Phosphorus

Jetter (cited in Coe[1]) found a postmortem increase in the concentration of organic phosphorus in serum, reaching levels of 20 mEq/l at 18 hours after death. Schleyer (cited in Coe[1]) also found similar results.

Magnesium

After death, haemolysis results in large amounts of magnesium being released into the plasma. Due to the uncertainty over the mechanism of the release of magnesium and the highly variable rate of release between individuals, no attempt has been made to determine the time of death using this technique.

WHITE BLOOD CELLS

In an unusual approach, Laiho and Penttila[5] investigated the viability of white blood cells, spermatozoa of the epididymis cells from minced spleen, lymph node, lung and cells aspirated from the bone marrow of the sternum. The analysis was carried out using the vital dye exclusion test, which involves the cellular uptake of trypan blue.

The loss of viability of white blood cells showed a moderate correlation ($r = -0.78$) with the postmortem period. The results for other tissues were not significant.

HORMONES

Cortisol, adrenaline and noradrenaline

No literature could be found to correlate these hormones with the time since death.

Thyroxine (T4) and thyroid-stimulating hormone (TSH)

Coe[1] found that T4 levels tended to fall after death. The rate of the fall was inconsistent and was not a valid method of determining time since death. TSH showed very little variation between postmortem and antemortem values.

Insulin

No reports have been found that attempt to correlate the time since death with the changes in insulin concentration in serum.

BLOOD GASES: OXYGEN TENSION

Patrick (cited in Coe[1]) reported that the oxygen tension PO_2 increased after death from approximately 21–25 mmHg at 6 hours after death to 45 mmHg at 24 hours postmortem. No attempts were made to determine the time of death using this information.

CASCADE SYSTEM

In an unusual approach to the estimation of the postmortem period, Komintato et al.[6] reported the analysis of the third component of complement (C3) and its breakdown in relation to the time since death. After complex measurement procedures involving immunoelectrophoresis, they reported a strong correlation between the percentage of C3 cleavage (breakdown products of C3) and the postmortem interval (Fig. 6.9).

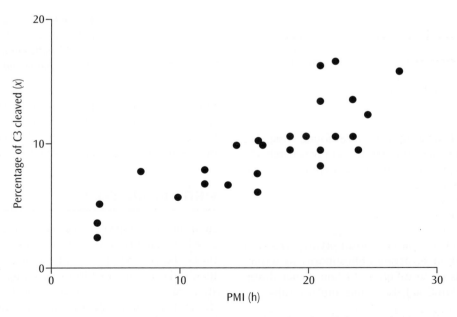

Figure 6.9 *Measured percentage of C3 cleavage (x) in cadaver blood plotted against their respective PMIs. Regression analysis of the points creates a line with the equation:*

$$PMI\ (hours) = 1.64 + 1.56x$$

The correlation coefficient is r = 0.832.

BLOOD CELLS

Penttila and Laiho[5,7] analysed the morphology of various types of cell in the peripheral blood of human cadavers. The results suggest that various cellular elements of the postmortem blood appear quite resistant to autolysis and, as such, are of little use in determining the time since death.

FLUIDITY OF BLOOD

Takeichi et al.[8] investigated the fluidity of blood after death. Although a number of biochemical processes are altered, i.e. fibrinolytic activity and acidosis increase, no indices could be found that would enable the accurate estimation of the postmortem period.

REFERENCES

1 Coe JI. Post-mortem chemistry: practical considerations and a review of the literature. *J. Forensic Sci.* 1974; **19**: 13.
2 Gupta H, Dixit PC, Jaydish C. Relationship of phosphoglu-comutase in post-mortem blood with time and cause of death. *Indian J. Med. Ves.* 1983; **77**: 159–62.
3 Querido D. Double logarithmic, linear relationship between plasma sodium/potassium concentration ratio and post-mortem interval during the 6 to 96 hour post-mortem period in rats. *Forensic Sci. Int.* 1990; **44**: 125–34.
4 Querido D. Linearization of the relationship between post-mortem plasma chloride concentration and post-mortem interval in rats. *Forensic Sci. Int.* 1990; **45**: 117–28.
5 Laiho K, Penttila A. Autolytic changes in blood cells and other tissues of human cadavers viability and ion studies. *Forensic Sci. Int.* 1981; **17**: 109–20.
6 Komintato Y, Horada S, Yamazaki K, Misava J. Estimation of post-mortem interval based on the third component of complement (C3) cleavage. *J. Forensic Sci.* 1988; **33**: 404–9.
7 Penttila A, Laiho K. Autolytic changes in blood cells of human cadavers II, morphology studies. *Forensic Sci. Int.* 1981; **17**: 121–32.
8 Takeichi S, Tokunaga I, Hayakumo K, Maeiva M. Fluidity of cadaveric blood after sudden death, Part III. *Am. J. Forens. Med. Path.* 1986; **7**: 35–8.

Cerebrospinal fluid chemistry

BURKHARD MADEA

Postmortem changes of cerebrospinal fluid (CSF) electrolytes are due to autolytic changes of cell membranes with resultant greater permeability, so that intracellular ions of higher concentrations will diffuse out into the extracellular fluid, while ions with a higher extracellular concentration will decrease due to the increased volume of distribution.[2] Postmortem changes of CSF electrolytes are based mainly on hypoxic damage of the choroid plexus.

The investigations of Schleyer[2] on chloride and magnesium concentrations in CSF, of Schleyer and Janitzki[3] on inorganic phosphorus in CSF, and of Dotzauer and Naeve[4] on sodium and calcium concentrations in CSF revealed that determination of these parameters is of no use in estimating the time since death – not even in the early postmortem interval (PMI). Calcium showed a tendency to increase in the later PMI, and sodium to decrease with increasing PMI.[4] Mason et al.[5] were the first to report on a relationship between time since death (t) and $[K^+]$ (in mmol/l) in cisternal fluid with the regression:

$$[K^+] = 48.56 + 61.45 \lg t$$

and a standard deviation of ± 9.4 mg K^+/100 ml.

This standard deviation is equivalent to a halving or doubling of the time since death calculated from the cisternal fluid potassium. Neither Mason et al.[5] nor Dotzauer and Naeve[4] recommended cisternal fluid electrolyte determination for estimating the PMI.

A postmortem increase of K^+ was also reported by Naumann[1], and Murray and Hordynsky.[6] The latter authors drew the following conclusions from their investigations on 46 bodies in the time interval from 2 to 24 hours postmortem:

1. Spinal fluid cannot be compared with cisternal fluid due to the obvious divergent gradients of diffusion.
2. The concentrations of sodium, magnesium and calcium have no obvious relationship to time since death.
3. The amount of K^+ increased at a constant rate in relation to the temperature of the body.
4. Severe infections or toxic processes which exist for an extended period prior to death influence the subsequent rate of diffusion.

Schleyer's results[7] show, in addition to the previous studies on cisternal fluid K^+, a great scatter of values over the PMI. According to Schleyer[7], bloody cisternal fluid shows no excessively high K^+ values. Further studies on CSF K^+ concentration, with similar results, were published by Fraschini et al.[8], Paulson and Stickney[9] and Weischer.[10]

In spite of these disappointing results, Urban et al.[11–16] carried out extensive investigations on CSF electrolytes. The results were obtained from cases of sudden death. On 147 bodies, cisternal fluid was withdrawn repeatedly at half-hourly intervals; on 143 bodies, only one sample was taken. Rectal temperature was taken simultaneously. As expected from the literature, the concentrations of calcium and magnesium showed no correlation with the time since

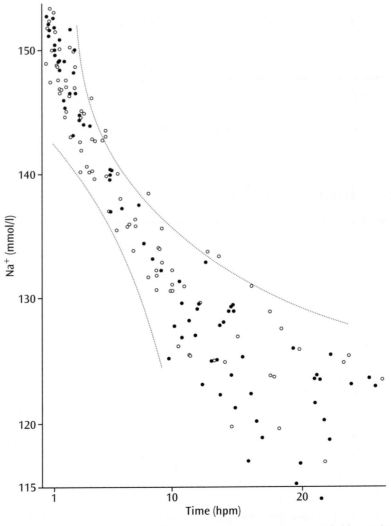

Figure 6.10 *Temperature dependence of the decrease of sodium concentration in cisternal fluid over the PMI.* ○ *Ambient temperature = 5°C;* ● *ambient temperature = 20°C. There is no temperature dependence.*

death. Sodium concentrations decrease exponentially during the first 20 hours postmortem; two subgroups which were kept at ambient temperatures of 5 and 20°C showed no difference (Fig. 6.10).

The exponential rise of cisternal fluid K^+ during the first 20 hours postmortem showed a stronger relationship with the time since death (Fig. 6.11). This rise of potassium was also not influenced by environmental temperature. In Fig. 6.11, the single values are plotted with 98% confidence limits. During the first 10 hours the variation was ± 1 hour with the exception of four cases dying from liver failure or uraemia. All the other cases were sudden deaths. Fig. 6.11b appears to indicate that the rise of cisternal potassium is not influenced by environmental temperature. Urban and Tröger[13] could reduce the deviations between real and extrapolated time since death from ± 1.5 hours in the first 15 hours postmortem to −0.75 to +1 hour by taking the actual rectal temperature and the cooling velocity into consideration. In 1987, the authors presented a 'Potassium – time since death nomogram' claiming 95% confidence limits of ± 1.4 hours, which is wider than the published variations of ± 1 hour up to 10 hours postmortem.

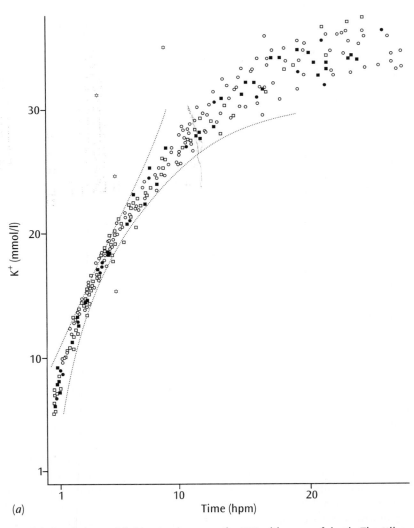

Figure 6.11 (a) Exponential rise of cisternal fluid potassium over the PMI with cause of death. Throttling, manual strangulation ■; asphyxiation, drowning ●; cardiac failure: pulmonary thromboembolism, myocardial infarction ○; cardiac failure: shooting, stabbing □; liver failure, uraemia ☆; four cases with liver failure/uraemia had a marked deviation.

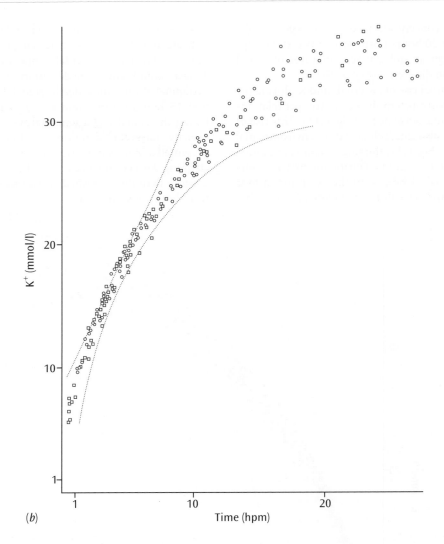

Figure 6.11 *(b) Rise of potassium for two different environmental temperatures: 5°C □; 20°C ○.*

In 1987, 95% confidence limits of death-time estimation from cisternal fluid potassium of ± 2.36 hours up to 15 hours postmortem were reported.[16] By taking temperature into consideration, these could be reduced to ± 1.4 hours in the interval up to 15 hours postmortem; during the interval up to 10 hours postmortem, the 95% limits were ± 1.03 hours.[16] The author found a strong linear correlation between estimated time since death from cisternal potassium and estimated time since death from rectal temperature using the nomogram method of Henssge (see Chapter

3) (Fig. 6.12). The author assessed cisternal K⁺ to be the most precise method of death-time estimation in the early PMI, because the 95% confidence limits are only ± 1.4 hours compared with ± 2.8 hours using Henssge's nomogram method. The high correlation between death-time estimation from cisternal potassium and body temperature strengthens the value of combining different methods for a reliable statement on the time since death.

Urban[12,16] recommends the application of his method for all cases except the following:

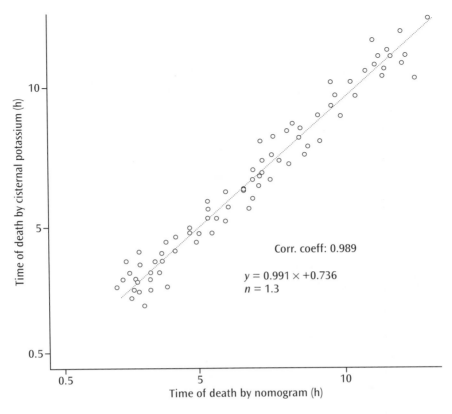

Figure 6.12 *Correlation between estimated time since death from K⁺ in cisternal fluid and rectal temperature (using the nomogram method of Henssge).*

- Intracranial/intracerebral bleeding with haemorrhage into ventricles or cisterns.
- Chronic lingering disease with electrolyte imbalances.
- Death from hypothermia.

The value of these recent investigations on the increase of cisternal potassium are without any doubt, since Urban has, unlike other authors, studied the cisternal potassium concentration during its steepest rise, and not during the interval where the equilibrium has already been achieved.

However, succeeding authors (Madea *et al.*[17], Fig. 6.13a; Wiesböck *et al.*[18], Fig. 6.13b) found a much wider range of scatter even in sudden deaths. Comparing the raw data of Mason *et al.*[5] with Urban's results (Fig. 6.14), Mason's 19 values taken serially from eight bodies have a greater scatter of values, although Mason *et al.*[5] claim to have eliminated all cases with diseases that might influence serum potassium.

In the 46 cases of Murray and Hordynsky[6] (Fig. 6.15), as well as in Schleyer's cases, there is a much wider range of scatter than was found by Urban. However, the random sample of the latter authors included cases with causes of death such as encephalitis, glomerulonephritis, chronic hepatitis, stroke and bronchopneumonia, which may cause antemortem dysregulation of electrolyte homeostasis.

The discrepancies between our results[17,19] and those of Urban cannot be explained by differences in the random samples, because we studied exclusively cases of sudden death. Our sample consisted mostly of natural deaths, while Urban's group consisted of traumatic deaths such as strangulation, throttling, shooting and stabbing, which he was in part able to investigate within 1 hour of death.

According to Urban, the differences in taking the samples (single sample-taking–repeated sample-taking) cannot be taken into consideration as a cause of the different scatter: he found no systematic difference

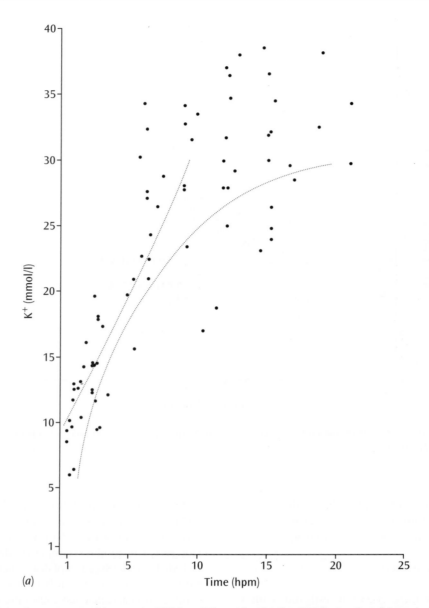

(a)

Figure 6.13 *(a) Potassium concentration over the PMI (n = 76); sudden deaths. 98% limits of confidence by Urban. Although the sample consists only of sudden deaths, the range of scatter is much wider than in Urban's sample.*

in the scatter of potassium values between single sample-taking and repeated sample-taking (unlike Schourup[20]).

The cause of the discrepancies regarding the scatter of values remains unclear, and further studies are necessary to clarify this situation. At present, we cannot recommend use of the method of Urban and his narrow 98% confidence limits.

REFERENCES

1 Naumann HN. Cerebrospinal fluid electrolytes after death. *Proc. Soc. Biol. Med.* 1958; **98**: 16–18.
2 Schleyer F. Untersuchungen über die Beziehungen der postmortalen Chlor- und Magnesiumkonzentration in Liquor und Plasma zu Leichenalter und Todesursache. *Frankfurter Z. Pathol.* 1959; **69**: 644–8.

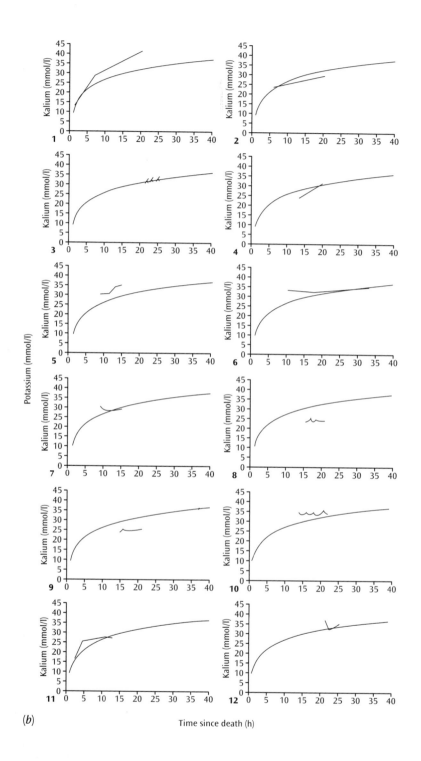

(b)

Time since death (h)

Figure 6.13 (b) Individual courses of cisternal potassium in 12 cases of sudden death after repeated sample taking (ambient temperature 5°C) over the time since death. The regression curve was calculated on 76 independent potassium values (single sample taking). The 'rise' of cisternal potassium is irregular; in some cases there is a drop of the potassium concentration (cases 7, 8, 10, 12) even in the early PMI (case 7). From Wiesbock et al.[18].

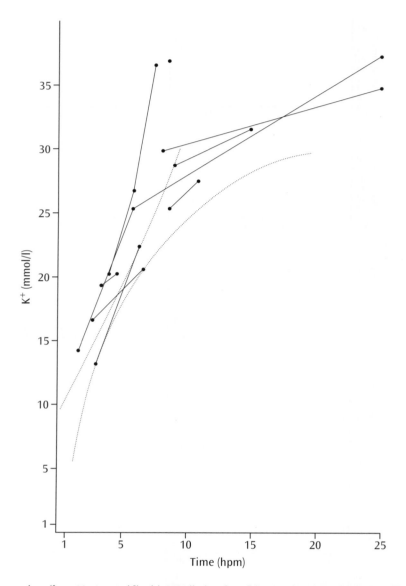

Figure 6.14 *Potassium values (from Mason* et al.[5]*) with 98% limits of confidence. Nineteen values were taken from eight bodies.*

3 Schleyer F, Janitzki U. Untersuchungen über den post-
mortalen Phosphatgehalt von Liquor und Serum in
Beziehung zum Leichenalter. *Deutsch. Z. ges. Gerichtl.
Med.* 1959; **49**: 229–34.

4 Dotzauer G, Naeve W. Vergleichende Untersuchungen
über den Natrium- und Kaliumgehalt im Serum wie im
Liquor post mortem. *Dtsch. Z. Gerichtl. Med.* 1960; **49**:
406–19.

5 Mason JK, Klyne W, Lennox B. Potassium levels in the
cerebrospinal fluid after death. *J. Clin. Path.* 1951; **4**:
231–3.

6 Murray EF, Hordynsky W. Potassium levels in the cerebrospinal fluid and their relation to duration of death.
J. Forensic Sci. 1958; **3**: 480–5.

7 Schleyer F. *Postmortale klinisch-chemische Diagnostik und
Todeszeitbestimmung mit chemischen und physikalischen
Methoden.* Stuttgart: Thieme Verlag, 1958.

8 Fraschini F, Muller E, Zanoboni A. Postmortem increase
of potassium in human cerebrospinal fluid. *Nature* 1963;
98: 1208.

9 Paulson G, Stickney D. Cerebrospinal fluid after death.
Confinea Neurol. 1971; **33**: 149–62.

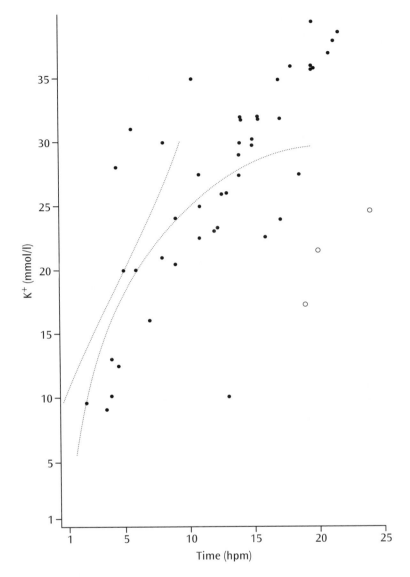

Figure 6.15 *Forty-six potassium values (from Murray and hHordynsky[6]) with 98% limits of confidence by Urban. In three cases only spinal fluid was available; this has systematically lower potassium values than cisternal fluid.*

10 Weischer K. *Biochemische Liquoruntersuchungen an Leichen.* Münster University: MD Thesis, 1982.

11 Urban R, Tröger HD, Krüger HJ. Todeszeitbestimmung im früh-postmortalen Intervall durch Elektrolytbestimmung im Zisternenliquor. Vortrag 64. Jahrestagg. *Dtsch. Ges. Rechtsmed.* 1985: 7–11 September, Hamburg.

12 Urban R, Tröger HD. Einfluss der Todesursache auf die Leichenliegezeitbestimmung im Zisternenliquor. Vortrag 17. Jahrestreffen der Arbeitsgemeinschaft Nord- und Westdtsch. *Rechtsmed.* 1986.

13 Urban R, Tröger HD. Todeszeitbestimmung Möglichkeiten und Grenzen der Elektrolytbestimmung im Leichenliquor. *Beitr. Gerichtl. Med.* 1987; **45**: 157–61.

14 Urban R, Tröger HD. Todeszeitbestimmung im frühpostmortalen Intervall – Kalium–Todeszeit-Bezugsnomogramm. Vortrag 66. Jahrestagg. *Dtsch. Ges. Rechtsmed.*, 1987: 8.

15 Urban R. Persönliche Mitteilung zur Methodik der Kaliumbestimmung (1987).

16 Urban R. Elektrolytbestimmung im Liquor cere-

brospinalis – mathematische Analyse experimenteller Befunde unter Berücksichtigung forensisch relevanter Einflussfaktoren zur Todeszeitbestimmung im frühpostmortalen Intervall. Habil. Schrift, Hanover, 1987.

17 Madea B, Henssge C, Püschel K, Honig W. Wie zuverlässig ist die Todeszeitbestimmung aus der Kaliumkonzentration in Zisternenliquor? Beitr. Gerichtl. Med. 1988; 46: 375–81.

18 Wiesböck J, Josephi E, Liebhart E. Intraindividuelle Kaliumverschiebungen im Liquor cerebrospinalis nach dem Tod. Beitr. Gerichtl. Med. 1989; 47: 403–5.

19 Madea B, Henssge C. Informationswert der Kaliumkonzentration in Glaskörperflüssigkeit für die Todeszeit – Präzisionsgewinn durch Erfassung antemortaler Dysregulationen? Beitr. Gerichtl. Med. 1987; 45: 151–5.

20 Schourup K. Dodstidsbestemmelse pa grunlag af postmortelle cisternevaedskevorandringer og det postmortelle axiltemperaturfald. Summary: Determination of the time since death. Med. Diss, Kopenhagen, 1950, Dansk Vindenskabs, Kobenhavn.

Pericardial fluid and miscellaneous methods

LEONARD NOKES

PERICARDIAL FLUID CONSTITUENTS

Aoki[1] was one of the few investigators to attempt to estimate the time since death by chemical analysis of the pericardial fluid. A negative correlation was found between the concentrations of glucose, lactic acid and cholesterol in the pericardial fluid and the postmortem period.

Some correlation (though this was not specified) was found between concentrations of non-protein nitrogen, amino acid nitrogen and certain enzymes, i.e. glutamate-oxaloacetate transaminase (GOT), glutamate-pyruvate transaminase (GPT), and the time since death. Similarly, ultraviolet analysis failed to find a clear relationship between various pericardial fluids and the postmortem period.

Aoki selected pericardial fluid as a test medium due to the absence of blood cells which might give rise to spurious results. However, the various detailed biochemical analyses failed to provide a single accurate method of determining the time since death. He concluded by stating: '… we are obliged to estimate time since death by various methods collectively'. This method of approach is now, after many years, slowly being accepted as perhaps the optimum technique to adopt when determining the time since death with any degree of confidence.

MUSCLE ENZYMES

Mayer and Neufeld[2] measured the postmortem activity of two enzymes found in rat skeletal muscle. Myofibrillar protease activity at room temperature was found to increase linearly against time since death. In contrast, the activity of creatinine phosphokinase (CPK) declined linearly after death. Exceptions occurred when the environmental temperature was around 4°C, when very little activity occurred for either enzyme. Although the activity of these two enzymes is temperature-dependent, Mayer and Neufeld speculated that by comparing the ratio between protease and CPK against time (Fig. 6.16) it might be possible to determine accurately the time since death.

Over a similar postmortem period, Gallois-Montbrun et al.[3] recorded other muscle biochemical components from hen pectoral muscle. These authors found that there was a strong positive correlation between:

- the ratio of non-protein nitrogen and total soluble protein and the time since death; and
- creatinine concentration and time since death.

A negative correlation was found between aspartic aminotransferase activity and time since death. The relationships are illustrated in Figs 6.17–6.19.

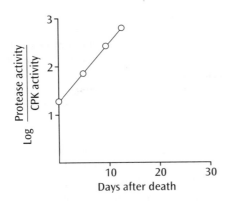

Figure 6.16 *Changes in the protease/creatinine phosphokinase (CPK) activities during muscle storage after death.*[2]

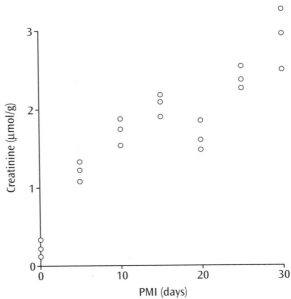

Figure 6.18 *Scatterplot of creatinine concentration in muscle versus PMI.*[3]

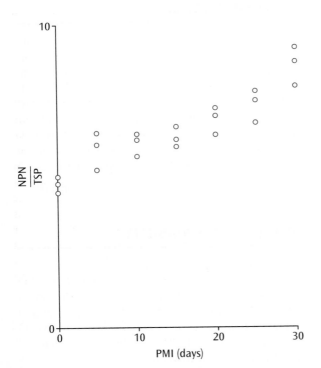

Figure 6.17 *Scatterplot of NPN/TSP ratio versus PMI.*[3]

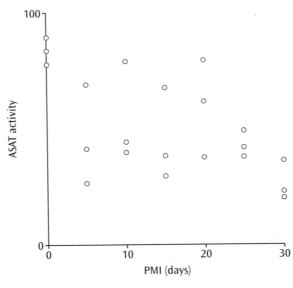

Figure 6.19 *Scatterplot of ASAT activity in muscle versus PMI.*[3]

ULTRASOUND VELOCITY IN MUSCLE

In a novel application of ultrasound, Webb *et al.*[4] reported the velocity of ultrasound waves passing through the calf muscle of cadavers. These authors found that, although the velocity varies from case to case, the rate at which the velocity changes at a given postmortem interval is similar in each case. Taking nine cases of known time since death, a standard gradient curve was constructed (Fig. 6.20). The time since death can be calculated by measuring two velocities at a known time interval and comparing the gradient over this time with the standard curve.

For example, if the first velocity reading was 1545 m/s and the second velocity reading was 1541 m/s, with a time interval of 2 hours, the gradient will be 2. From Fig. 6.20 the time since death is approximately between 7.5 and 8 hours prior to the first velocity reading.

The physical factors affecting the ultrasound velocity in muscle are density, bulk and water content. Webb *et al.* suggest that the observed changes in velocity over time are not directly related to rigor but are due to either fluid or blood loss.

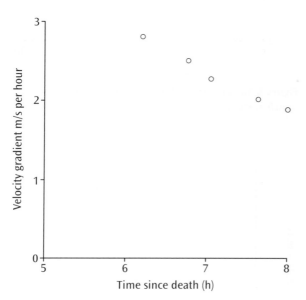

Figure 6.20 *Graph of velocity through calf muscle against time since death.*[4]

BONE MARROW CYTOLOGY

It has been known for at least 30 years that human bone marrow cells still exhibit some physical characteristics after death, including motility.

In 1960, Perry *et al.*[5] examined the motility of bone marrow cells in order to assess their viability in marrow transplantation. Mobile cells were present up to 50 hours after death of the donor.

Similar results were reported by Porteous,[6] who presented the data shown in Table 6.8. Again, the aim of the paper was to assess the viability of cells in transplantation.

Table 6.8 *Mobility of bone marrow cells after death*[6]

	Hours after death	
	0–20	> 20
Motile cells	18	3
Non-motile cells	0	5

In 1964, in a detailed paper, Hoffman *et al.*[7] reported observations on the morphological changes in ante- and postmortem bone marrow cells. Again, the summary was based on the possible use of postmortem cells in haematological disorders.

No reference is made in any of the reviewed papers to the use of bone marrow cell viability after death as a means of determining the time since death.

NERVE CONDUCTION

A study was conducted by McDowal *et al.*[8] to investigate the feasibility of using the absolute refractory period of nervous function as a tool for estimating the postmortem interval. These authors found a strong correlation between the duration of the absolute refractory period and postmortem interval. This relationship appears to be linear, with a correlation coefficient (r) of 0.86. In order to calculate the time of death, a linear regression formula was devised which stated:

$$\text{Time of death} = 164.61 - (4.17 \times \text{rectal temperature}).$$

SPERMATOZOAN VIABILITY

In a unique approach, Lorenzen and Lawson[9] reported their observations on sperm viability after death, and its possible use in determining the postmortem interval. The experiments involved the removal and storage of bull testes over a period ranging from 2 to 168 hours after death. The results showed that the spermatozoa remained viable in the epididymis for a considerable period postmortem. On removal from the epididymis, the spermatozoa die at various rates depending on the length of storage and the environmental temperature. An increase in temperature shortens the life-span of the spermatozoa by increasing their metabolic rate. The authors concluded that further work is required to analyse postmortem changes in motility, morphology and histochemical appearance of spermatozoa.

DNA DEGRADATION

In a novel approach, Cina,[10] in 1994, quantified the amount of DNA within the cells of human corpses against time, using flow cytometry. The report was a preliminary investigation, and at the time of going to press a graphical means of plotting the DNA fragmentation with respect to the postmortem time was being undertaken.

REFERENCES

1 Aoki T. Studies on the estimation of time after death. *Jikei Med. J.* 1965; **12**: 164–77.

2 Mayer M, Neufeld B. Post-mortem changes in skeletal muscle protease and creatinine phosphokinase activity – a possible marker for determination of time of death. *Forensic Sci. Int.* 1980; **15**: 197–203.

3 Gallois-Montbrun FG, Barres DR, Durigon M. Post-mortem estimation by biomechanical determination in bird muscle. *Forensic Sci. Int.* 1988; **37**: 189–92.

4 Webb PA, Terry HJ, Gee DJ. A method for time of death determination using ultrasound: a preliminary report. *J. Forensic Sci. Soc.* 1986; **26**: 393–9.

5 Perry VP, Stevenson RE, McFarland W, Zink GA. Motility studies of human post-mortem bone matter. *Blood* 1960; **16**: 1020–8.

6 Porteous LB. Persistence of motility in bone marrow cells form the cadaver. *Nature* 1961; **11**: 569–70.

7 Hoffman SB, Morrow GW, Pease GL, Stoebel CF. Rate of cellular autolysis in post-mortem bone marrow. *Am. J. Clin. Path.* 1964; **41**: 281–6.

8 McDowal KL, Lenihan DV, Busuttil A, Glasby MA. The use of absolute refractory period in the estimation of the early post-mortem interval. *Forensic Sci. Int.* 1998; **91**: 163–70.

9 Lorenzen GA, Lawson RL. A possible new approach for determining the post-mortem interval. *J. Criminal Law, Criminology Police Sci.* 1971; **62**: 560–3.

10 Cina ST. Flow cytometric evaluation of DNA degradation. A predictor of post-mortem interval? *Am. J. Forens. Med. Path.* 1994; **15**: 30–2.

Synovial fluid

BURKHARD MADEA

Synovial fluid is a well-investigated fluid compartment in rheumatology,[1-14] and handbooks of joint fluid analysis are available.[15] However only a few studies of medicolegal interest on synovial fluid have been published, dealing with alcohol concentration of, and drug distribution into synovial fluid, as well as postmortem chemistry regarding cause of death.[16-19] One study dealt with the estimation of postmortem interval according to time course of potassium ion activity in cadaveric synovial fluid.[20] The potassium ion activity increased more than two-fold within the first two days postmortem. A precision of death time estimation of ± 50 minutes in the postmortem interval from 6 to 36 hours and within ± 55–60 minutes in 36 to 48 hours was claimed.

Our own investigations[21] on potassium concentration in synovial fluid compared with vitreous humour revealed an almost linear rise of the synovial fluid potassium (knee-joints), the slope being flatter than in vitreous humour (Fig. 6.21).

The range of scatter of potassium values in synovial fluid is as great as in vitreous humour. In cases where vitreous humour cannot be obtained, synovial fluid may be used for death time estimation with all precautions known from vitreous humour.

IMPEDANCE

Querido[22-24] has produced three papers examining the viability of electrical impedance of animal tissues, such as abdominal wall and scalp, as a means of estimating the early postmortem period. All of the papers have reported the work carried out in rats, each describing the various resistance patterns over postmortem periods of up to 504 hours. The application of this to

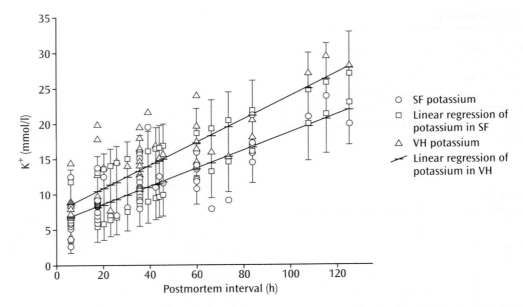

Figure 6.21 *Rise of potassium in synovial fluid (SF) (knee joint) compared to potassium in vitreous humour (VH). The rise is steeper in vitreous humour. The range of scatter in both fluid compartments is comparable.*[21]

the human model has, to the author's knowledge, not been reported.

REFERENCES

1 Arthur E, Stern M, Galeazzi M, Baldassare AR, Weiss TD, Gorgers JR, Zuckner J. Synovial fluid lactic acid in septic and nonseptic arthritis. *Arthritis Rheum.* 1983; **26**: 1499–505.

2 Binzus G. Substrate, Enzyme und Metaboliten in der Synovialflüssigkeit verschiedener Genese. 1979. In: *Synovialflüssigkeit und synoviales Milieu* (Thumb N, Kellner G, Klein G, Zeidler H, eds.). Georg Thieme Verlag Stuttgart, S54–S63.

3 Brook I, Reza MJ, Bricknell KS, Bluestone R, Finegold SM. Synovial fluid lactic acid. *Arthritis Rheum.* 1978; **21**: 774–9.

4 Cummings NA, Nordby GL. Measurement of synovial fluid pH in normal and arthritic knees. *Arthritis Rheum.* 1966; **9**: 47–56.

5 Duncan S, Owen J. Aspiration and injection of joints and soft tissues. In: *Textbook of Rheumatology*, 3rd edition (Kelley WN, Harris E, Ruddy S, Sledge CB, eds.). WB Saunders Co., Philadelphia, London, Toronto, Montreal, Sydney, Tokyo, 1989.

6 Fehr K, Meihle W, Schattenkirchner M, Tillmann K. *Rheumatologie in Praxis und Klinik*, Georg Thieme Verlag Stuttgart, 1989, New York.

7 Greiling H, Kleesiek K, Stuhlsatz HW. Zur klinischen Biochemie der Synovialflüssigkeit. In: *Synovialflüssigkeit und synoviales Milieu* (Thumb N, Kellner G, Klein G, Zeidler H, eds.). Georg Thieme Verlag Stuttgart, 1979: S43–S54.

8 Kellner G. Zytologie und Zytochemie der Synovial-flüssigkeit. In: *Synovialflüssigkeit und synoviales Milieu* (Thumb N, Kellner G, Klein G, Zeidler H, eds.). Georg Thieme Verlag Stuttgart, 1979: S84–S91.

9 Kushner I, Somerville JA. Permeability of human synovial membrane to plasma proteins. *Arthritis Rheum.* 1971; **14**: 560–70

10 Müller W. Die Untersuchung der Synovialflüssigkeit. *Laborblätter* 1976; **26**: 25–35.

11 Schumacher HR. Synovial fluid analysis and synovial biopsy. In: *Textbook of Rheumatology*, 3rd edition (Kelley WN, Harris E, Ruddy S, Sledge CB, eds.). WB Saunders Co., Philadelphia, London, Toronto, Montreal, Sydney, Tokyo, 1989.

12 Singer F, Kolarz G, Thumb N, Schieler K. Zur differential-diagnostischen Wertigkeit von nephelometrisch be-stimmten Proteinfraktionen in der Synovialflüssigkeit. *Z. Rheumatologie* 1987, **46**: 245–9.

13 Sita F, Krizala JF, Dite P, Krupar V. Nachweis einiger Heilmittel in der Kniegelenksynovialflüssigkeit. *Arch. Toxikol.* 1971; **27**: 242–7.

14 Tillmann K, Binzus G. Spezielle gasanalytische Befunde in der Synovialflüssigkeit. In: *Synovialflüssigkeit und syn-*

oviales Milieu (Thumb N, Kellner G, Klein G, Zeidler H, eds.). Georg Thieme Verlag Stuttgart, 1979: S79–S84.

15 Gatter RA. *A Practical Handbook of Joint Fluid Analysis.* Lea & Febiger, Philadelphia, 1984.

16 Audrilicky I, Pribilla O. Über die Alkoholkonzentrationsbestimmung in der Kniegelenksynovialflüssigkeit lebender Menschen. *Blutalkohol* 1965/66; **3**: 503–11.

17 Gastmeier G, Lehmann K. Bedeutung von glaskörperflüssigkeit und Kniegelenksynovialflüssigkeit für die Begutachtung von Intoxikationsfällen. *Kriminal. Forens. Wiss.* 1982; **47**: 41–6.

18 More DS, Castellano Arroyo M. Technical note. Biochemical changes of the synovial liquid in corpses with regard to the cause of death. 1: Calcium, urea nitrogen, uric acid, proteins and albumin. *J. Forensic Sci.* 1985; **30**: 541–6.

19 More DS, Castellano Arroyo M. Technical note. Biochemical changes of the synovial liquid in corpses with regard to the cause of death. 2: Alkaline phosphatase, lactic acid dehydrogenase (LDH), and glutamic oxaloacetic transaminase (GOT) *J. Forensic Sci.* 1985; **30**: 547–51.

20 Madea B, Kreuser C, Banaschak S. Postmortem biochemical examination of synovial fluid – a preliminary study. *Forensic Sci. Int.* 2001; **118**: 29–35.

21 Alybaeva KN. Estimation of postmortem interval according to time course of potassium ion activity in cadaveric synovial fluid. *Sud. Med. Ekxert.* 1987; **30**: 18–20.

22 Querido D. Time-dependent changes in electrical resistance of the intact abdomen during the 1–504 hours postmortem period in rats. *Forensic Sci. Int.* 1994; **67**: 17–25.

23 Querido D, Phillips MRP. Changes in the resistance of reactive components of the abdominal impedance during the 1–21 days post-mortem period in rats. *Forensic Sci. Int.* 1997; **85**: 163–75.

24 Querido D. A preliminary study of changes in scalp impedance during the early post-mortem period in rats. *Forensic Sci. Int.* 1999; **101**: 123–30.

Vitreous potassium

LEONARD NOKES

Lange *et al.*[1] investigated the use of vitreous potassium as a means of estimating the early postmortem interval by analysing the data from six different studies. In this way, and by performing some simple linear regression calculations, these authors concluded that the postmortem interval estimates based on vitreous potassium are more accurate when the curves are combined. Caution was expressed regarding the use of vitreous potassium beyond 100 hours postmortem, however.

REFERENCE

1 Lange N, Swearer S, Sturner WQ. Human post-mortem interval estimation from vitreous potassium. An analysis of original data from six different studies. *Forensic Sci. Int.* 1994; **66**: 159–74.

7

Practical casework

CLAUS HENSSGE, BURKHARD MADEA AND BERNARD KNIGHT

Integration of different methods in casework

CLAUS HENSSGE AND BURKHARD MADEA

INTRODUCTION

The great interindividual variability of the postmortal changes as a consequence of many influencing factors restricts the accuracy of death-time estimation and, if the limits of confidence of a method are not exactly known, impairs the reliability. As no single method allows a sufficiently exact and reliable estimation of the interval of death in any particular case, it is recommended that several different methods are used. The selection of methods requires some consideration of the level of investigation and the consequent expenditure of effort.

The following scheme of integration of different methods is recommended for estimating the time of death in casework at the scene. The guidelines are:

1. Whenever possible, use measurements instead of subjective evaluations.

2. Avoid a 'mean value' for the resulting time of death, instead always offer a 'range', i.e. the minimum and maximum limits.
3. Take into account important influencing factors upon each criterion.
4. Use no more methods in a particular case than are potentially useful.
5. Give a preliminary statement of the interval of death at the scene.
6. The reliability of a stated range of time since death is more important than attempting to give an unrealistically narrow range.

The examination of the body at the scene usually begins with the use of the temperature-based method by using the nomogram as described in Chapter 3. The margins of error of this method can be reduced in many cases by using the following methods, though they themselves have wider margins of error. In a few cases, where the temperature-based method must not be used because of contrary circumstances, those methods should still be used.

THE TIME-RELEVANT CRITERIA OF DIFFERENT METHODS

Development of rigor

For more detailed information, see Chapter 5.

Hitherto, the grade of rigor has generally been evaluated subjectively for estimating the time of death in casework of human bodies. Measurement with a special device[1] is uncommon for a variety of reasons.[2,3] The description of the stages of the subjectively evaluated rigor differs from author to author.[4–6] For our purposes, only those stages of rigor which are relevant to the time of death are of interest. According to the statistical analysis by Mallach[5,6] of the data in the literature, this is given only for the following stages: 'beginning', 'full development', 'duration' and 'complete resolution' of rigor. The latter two stages are not relevant, because of their late postmortal onset of 57 ($\pm$ 14) hours postmortem and 76 ($\pm$ 32) hours postmortem, respectively. The stages of rigor are not exactly described either by Mallach,[5,6] or in the only other experimental reports of Von Hofmann in 1876 and 1877.[7] (All the other data of Mallach's statistical analyses are figures from textbooks without any experimental basis.) 'Beginning' may mean 'you can observe slight rigor in the joints'. 'Full development' or 'complete development' (shortened to 'maximum' in the following tables) may mean 'rigor is strongly developed in all joints'. There is a third useful marker – the re-establishment of rigor after breaking it. The re-established rigor is less strong than it was before breaking. To avoid a false-positive result, it is necessary to ensure that rigor was broken completely by fully moving the elbow joint several times. A negative result should be stated only if the examined joint had not been manipulated (e.g. by transport or removal of clothing) between breaking the rigor and examination for re-establishment.

The death-time relationship of these three suitable marks of rigor can be seen in Table 7.1.

Lividity

For more detailed information, see Chapter 5.

Subjective methods are also employed for the evaluation of lividity. Attempts to make the evaluation of lividity objective[8,9] have not been generally accepted in practical work until now. Data in the literature – exceptionally figures from textbooks without experimental basis – were analysed statistically by Mallach[5,6] for the following degrees of lividity (Tables 7.2 and 7.3): 'beginning', 'confluence', 'maximum of expansion and intensity' (shortened as 'maximum'), 'complete displacement by slight pressure' (using the thumb; shortened to 'thumb pressure'), 'complete shifting' and 'incomplete shifting' after turning the body over. Complete shifting means that lividity disappears completely in the upward facing parts of the body after turning it over, and then appears in the downward parts; this is apparently dependent on the death-time and may take from a few minutes to up to 1 hour. Incomplete shifting means that lividity fades only in the upward facing parts and appears only slightly in the downward facing parts after turning the body over. The maximum stage of lividity should be stated only after a second examination carried out later, especially in cases where bleeding had occurred. The criterion 'complete shifting' can be observed at the scene frequently when the body, or even parts of it, had been moved to a new position in the course of the investigative procedure. 'Incomplete shifting' is found to be more likely at autopsy if the body had been transported in another position than that examined at

Table 7.1 *Rigor related to the time of death (hpm)*

Stage	Mean	Standard deviation	Limits	
			Lower	Upper
Beginning	3	2	0.5	7
Maximum	8	1	2.0	20
Re-establishment			2.0	8

Lower and upper limits of variance computed from literature data (1811 to 1960).[5]

Table 7.2 *Hypostasis related to the time of death (hpm)*

Stage	Mean	Standard deviation	Limits	
			Lower	Upper
Beginning	0.75	0.5	0.25	3
Confluence	2.50	1.0	1.00	4
Maximum	9.50	4.5	3.00	16
Thumb pressure	5.50	6.0	1.00	20
Complete shifting	3.75	1.0	2.00	6
Incomplete shifting	11.00	4.5	4.00	24

Lower and upper limits of variance computed from literature data (1905 to 1963).[5]

Table 7.3 *Probability of a time interval of ± 0.1 hour around the mean value of the time since death (examples) related to the standard deviation*

Criterion stage	Mean	Standard deviation	Probability
Hypostasis			
Complete shifting	3.75	1.0	0.08
Thumb pressure	5.50	6.0	0.01
Maximum	9.50	4.5	0.02
Incomplete shifting	11.00	4.5	0.02

The probabilities were computed according to eqn 7.1 for a time interval of ± 0.1 hour (12 min) around the mean.

the scene. Two other criteria – 'incomplete displacement after strong pressure' and 'only small fading after turning the body' – were not taken into account because they do not bring further information to the early death-time interval in which we are interested.

The reason for non-displacement and non-shifting of lividity is not the early diffusion of haemoglobin, as supposed formerly, but the haemoconcentration by loss of fluid which penetrates the wall of those vessels related to the hydrostatic pressure, as shown by Hilgermann.[10]

Mechanical excitability of skeletal muscle

For more detailed information, see Chapter 5.

Sufficient data are given in the literature on the two phenomena of postmortal mechanical excitability:

1. Tendon reaction, or Zsako's phenomenon, described first by Zsako[11] and examined as follows[12]: striking at the lower third of the quadriceps femoris muscle about 10 cm above the patella with a reflex hammer causes an upward movement of the patella because of a contraction of the whole muscle.

2. Idiomuscular contraction (bulge) tested as described by Dotzauer[13] and Prokop[12]: striking at the biceps brachii muscle with the back of a knife causes a muscular bulge at the point of contact due to local contraction of the muscle. The related times of death listed in Table 7.4 are taken from Popwassilew and Palm.[14] The muscular bulge is maintained for some hours if the examination takes place several hours postmortem, as is usually the case, when ATP levels are low. Nevertheless, in order to avoid a false-negative result, it should be carefully checked whether a local contracture appears after striking the muscle, but immediately disappears again, as may happen in the very early postmortem period due to high levels of ATP.

The electrical excitability of skeletal muscle

For more detailed information, see Chapter 5.

There is an extensive literature on this subject since the 'second' start of the investigations in this field by Prokop.[15] We refer here only to the results of the extensive experimental material of Klein and Klein[16] on 447 bodies. As the type of electrical stimulus used influences the muscle reaction, the following data of death-time are related to stimulation by 'rectangular-like' impulses of a duration of a 'few milliseconds' in a repetition rate of 30 to 70 per second and an amplitude of 50 volts (resistance 1 kOhm).[16] A small battery-operated generator with constant-current rectangular impulses of 30 mA, 10 ms duration and a frequency of 50 per second is now available commercially (for details: contact Peschke J; http://home.t-online.de/home/j-peschke/rzg1.htm). The time data of Table 7.4. can be transferred when using this device.

Needle electrodes are inserted 5 to 7 mm deep into the nasal part of the upper eyelid at a distance of 15 to 20 mm (Fig. 7.1). The grade of reaction is divided into six degrees according to the spread of the reaction of the mimic muscles. The strongest reaction (degree VI) is obtained if the reaction includes the upper and lower eyelids, forehead and cheek. In the minimal

Table 7.4 *Chronological arrangement of the lower and upper limits of the time since death related to the different stages of the cited methods according to literature data*[18]

Parameter checked	Answer ↓ Result reduction of the lower limit ($t \geq hpm$)		Answer ↓ Result reduction of the upper limit ($t \leq hpm$)	
Lividity				
Beginning?	Yes	0.0	No	3.0
Confluence?	Yes	1.0	No	4.0
Thumb pressure?	No	1.0	Yes	20.0
Complete shifting?	No	2.0	Yes	6.0
Maximum?	Yes	3.0	No	16.0
Incomplete shifting?	No	4.0	Yes	24.0
Rigor mortis				
Beginning?	Yes	0.5	No	
Re-establishment?	No	2.0	Yes	8.0
Maximum?	Yes	2.0	No	20.0
Mechanical excitability				
Zsako's phenomenon?	No	0.0	Yes	2.5
Idiomuscular contraction?	No	1.5	Yes	13.0
Electrical excitability				
Eye VI?	No	1.0	Yes	6.0
Eye V	No	2.0	Yes	7.0
Eye IV?	No	3.0	Yes	8.0
Eye III?	No	3.5	Yes	13.0
Eye II?	No	5.0	Yes	16.0
Eye I?	No	5.0	Yes	22.0
Orbicularis oris muscle?	No	3.0	Yes	11.0
Chemical excitability Iris				
Atropine/Cyclopent?	No	3.0	Yes	10.0
Mydriaticum Roche?	No	5.0	Yes	30.0
Acetylcholine?	No	14.0	Yes	46.0

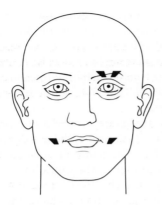

Figure 7.1 *Position of insertion of electrodes for facial stimulation.*

reaction (degree I), only a small local fascicular contraction of the nasal angle of the upper eyelid appears (Fig. 7.2). In addition, the electrodes can also be inserted 10 mm from each corner of the mouth.

We extracted the data of Table 7.4 from the original data produced by Klein and Klein,[16] and computed the permissible variation of 95%.[17] In cases with haematoma or emphysema of the eyelid, the time figures are much greater; in cases of long terminal episode the time figures are much smaller than those given in Table 7.4.[16] At present, and regardless of the criticisms,[17,18] this method seems to be the most suitable of all the reported 'electrical' methods for casework. Apart from the nomogram method it is more useful than any of the other methods reviewed in this volume (see Table 7.7).

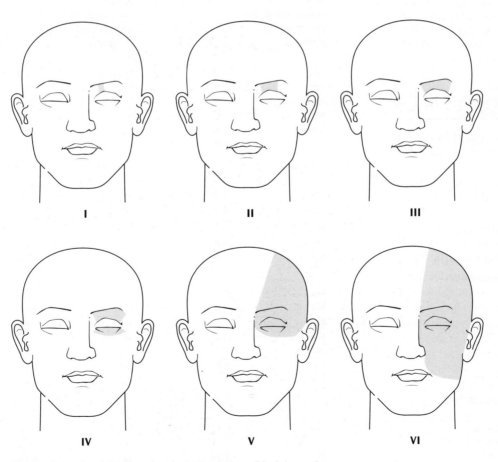

Figure 7.2 *Degrees of reaction following electrical stimulation of facial muscles.*

The chemical excitability of the iris

For more detailed information, see Chapter 5.

From the extensive literature in this field we refer only to the systematic investigations of Klein and Klein[16] on 5765 eyes of 3979 bodies. From these results, we utilized the data listed in Table 7.4. To examine this reaction, about 0.5 ml of the solution is injected subconjunctivally at the limbus corneae[15]; the concentration used is not important (e.g. 5%). The onset of the reaction begins between 5 and 30 minutes after the injection, and lasts at least 1 hour. Acetylcholine (miosis) and noradrenaline (mydriasis) have the same time interval of postmortem reaction. However, the effect of acetylcholine is more reliable and the application of noradrenaline is preferable only if the starting width of the pupil is small. The so-called double reaction, firstly miosis (e.g. acetylcholine), followed by mydriasis (e.g. atropine) on the same eye, or vice versa, gives no further time information than each reaction separately (using both eyes) (all according to Klein and Klein[16]). In order to avoid mistakes, it is recommended that the starting diameter of the pupil is measured with a slide caliper to determine whether there was a reaction, or not.

ARRANGEMENT OF DATA

As we concluded in the introduction to this section, there is no statistical evidence for the use of *mean* values of the time since death in a special case. Remembering the mathematical relationship between the probability of a short time interval ($X < X_k$) around the mean (x) and the standard deviation (SD):

$$\text{Prob } (X < X_k) = X - x/\text{SD} \tag{7.1}$$

there is only a very small probability of the mean values being accurate because of the great standard deviations (examples in Table 7.3). In compliance with this, the mean value of the idiomuscular contraction (6.9 hours postmortem) occurred in only 6% of the cases of an experimental study.[13] To avoid great errors in our statements of the time since death, we have to avoid the use of mean values. Therefore, we recommend only the use of the upper and lower time limits of any criterion as the basis of statements. In the example of the idiomuscular contraction sought by striking the biceps muscle, no case was reported as having had idiomuscular contraction after the 13th hour postmortem. In no case was this reaction missed

before 1.5 hours postmortem. This means that, if the reaction occurs, we can say only that the time since death must be less than 13 hours. If there is no reaction, we can state only that the time since death must be greater than 1.5 hours. Integrating the results of all examinations in the same manner, the greatest figure of any lower limit and the smallest figure of any upper limit reduces the interval within which the death occurred – with a high probability of at least 95%.

From this point of view, and for practical purposes, data will be best arranged chronologically, according to the lower and the upper limits (Table 7.4).

PRINCIPLE OF USING A SPECIAL CHART

For casework, we rearranged the data of Table 7.4 into a special chart (Fig. 7.3), which facilitates the choice of the subsequently helpful criteria in an actual case. In the example of Fig. 7.3 the examination began with measurement of the rectal temperature, followed by use of the nomogram method. The result was 4.5 hours postmortem (lower limit) and 10.1 hours postmortem (upper limit). The lower limit can be confirmed or improved only by a criterion with a higher figure for its lower limit. Looking at the chart in the left-hand column we can quickly find only two criteria that could improve the lower limit: the electrical excitability if there is a negative result; and the chemical excitability of the iris by Mydriaticum Roche®, also if there is a negative result. The upper limit (10.1 hours postmortem) can be confirmed or improved only by a criterion with a lower figure for its upper limit. We can quickly find the possibly helpful criteria on the chart, in the right-hand column: the electrical excitability again if there is a reaction of degree IV (or V or VI); or the chemical excitability of the iris by atropine or Cyclopent® if there is a reaction and the re-establishment of the rigor after breaking if it occurs. We examined the electrical excitability of the mimic muscles, the chemical excitability of the iris by atropine (one side) and by Mydriaticum Roche® (other side), and we broke the rigor of one elbow joint. The other criteria need not be examined because they could not help in this case. (As a routine we always examine the stages of rigor and hypostasis.)

The results of the examined criteria are put into the chart (Fig. 7. 3) Only the electrical excitability (degree IV) and the re-established rigor were helpful: they reduced the upper time limit of the temperature-based

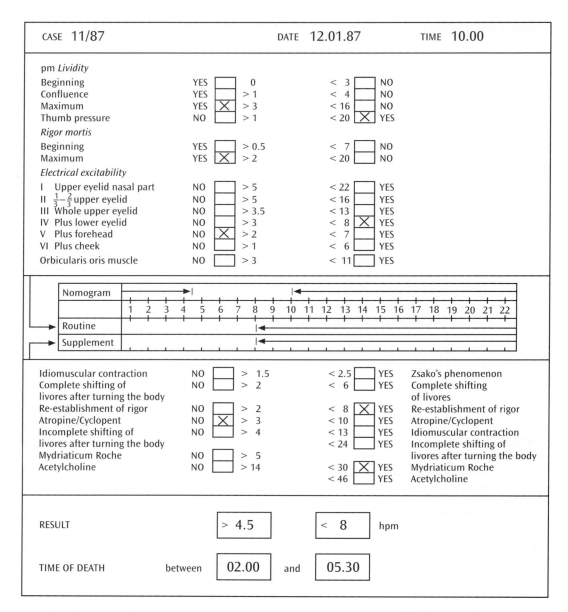

Figure 7.3 *Integrating chart for casework at a scene of crime with an example.*[18]

nomogram result from 10 to 8 hours postmortem. The chemical examinations did not provide an improvement in this case. In so far as this example is a typical one, the electrical examination gives rather more of an improvement than the other criteria (see Table 7.7). The final result in this case is: with a high probability (95%), the death occurred between 4.5 and 8 hours before the examination. Meanwhile, a computer program for a note-book computer was developed which leads the procedure of examining the body at the scene according to this logistic; additionally, it automatically performs all mathematical operations including those of the nomogram method (for details, contact Henssge CA; http://home.t-online.de/home/Christoph.Henssge/t-zeit.htm). The computer program was evaluated in a field study.[21,22]

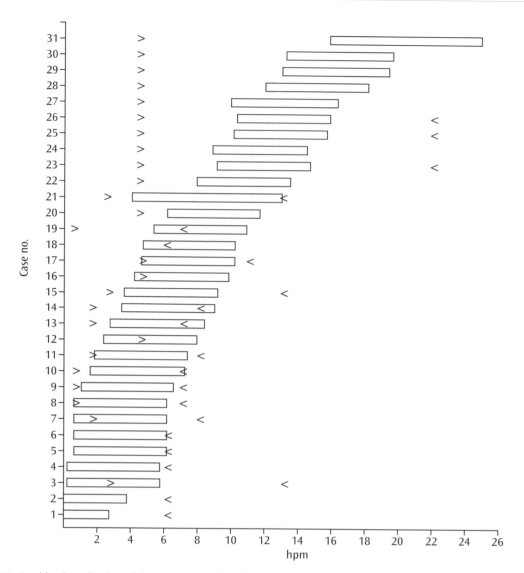

Figure 7.4 *Combined application of the temperature-based nomogram and the electrical excitability for determining the time since death.*[19] *Case numbers according to* Table 7.5. *Boxes: death-time estimation by the nomogram method (lower and upper 95% limits of confidence; see* Table 7.5*).> < Death-time information based on the degree of electrical excitability. For instance, degree III positive (case 15) not only reveals the information that the time since death is < 13 hpm but also means degree IV negative and therefore that the time since death is 3 hpm. Especially during the time period from 3 to 8 hpm, combining electrical excitability with the nomogram method reveals a more precise death-time estimation than using one method alone. The real time since death was always within the calculated time since death.*

EXPERIENCES IN CASEWORK

In 32 cases with investigated death-times between 2 and 13 hours, both the nomogram and the electrical excitability of mimic muscles were used (Fig. 7.4; Table 7.5).[19] The results provide evidence that the range of death-times resulting from the temperature nomogram becomes smaller in some cases by application of the method of electrical excitability of facial muscles according to Fig. 7.2. Nevertheless, in the other cases the self-confidence of the investigator in his opinion on the time since death, increases by

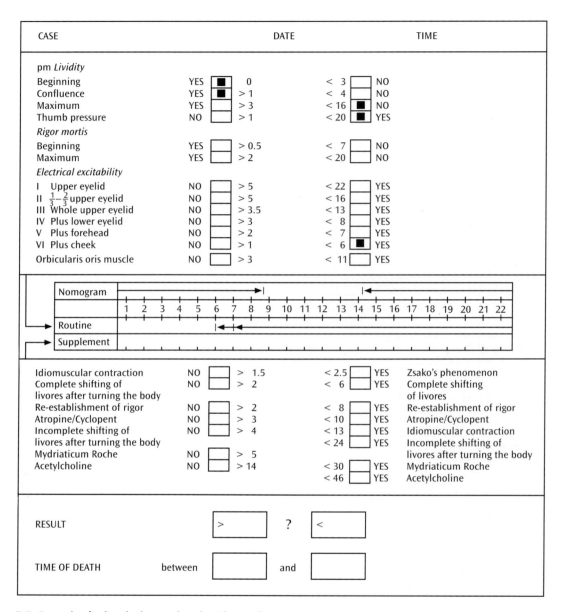

Figure 7.5 *Example of using the integrating chart (see text).*

using two independent methods with a common result. In addition, the 32 investigated cases confirmed the results of Klein and Klein.[16]

Two special cases[20] may demonstrate that factors which influence the time course of electrical excitability in a contrary direction to body cooling may mislead or confuse the investigator when not taken into account (Figs. 7.5 and 7.6).

In the case of Fig. 7.5, the temperature-based nomogram method showed the death-time interval to be from 8.8 to 14.3 hours, corresponding to 26.6°C rectal temperature, 10°C ambient temperature and 72 kg body weight. Rigor mortis had not begun, and electrical excitability showed a full reaction (degree VI) resulting in a death-time of less than 7 and 6 hours, respectively. These results excluded each other. The

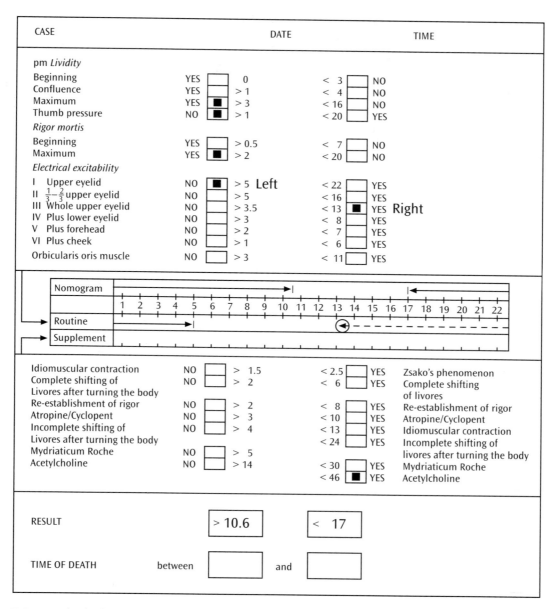

Figure 7.6 *Example of using the integrating chart (see text).*

suspicion of fatal hypothermia, as a result of purple-red patches of discoloration of the skin on and around the elbow and knee joints, was confirmed by autopsy findings such as haemorrhagic erosions of the stomach, haemorrhage of the pancreas and its ductus. The fatal hypothermia explains the contrary results of death-time estimation between the temperature-based nomogram method and the electrical excitability

method: the hypothermia simulated a long time since death because of the fall in central body temperature during life. The nomogram method must not be used in such a case (see page 77). Electrical excitability is not influenced by hypothermia. The investigated time of death was really 2.5 hours.

In the other special case (Fig. 7.6), there was a large difference in the electrical excitability of the right (re)

Table 7.5 *Death-time estimation from body temperature (using the nomogram) and the degree of electrical excitability*[19]

No.	Cause of death	Time of investigation	T_R	T_A	Body weight	f	Death-time estimation (nomogram)	Degree of electrical excitability	Death-time estimation (hours)
1	Female, 44 years, 3 homicidal shotgun wounds of the neck	13.20	37.2	35.5	60	0.5	0–2.8	VI	<6
2	45 years, male, suicidal shotgun wound of the head	13.30	37.1	17	70	1.2	0–3.8	VI	<6
3	30 years, female stab wounds of the heart	16.10	35.6	14.5	54	1.1	0.2–5.8	III	>3<13
4	53 years, female, stab wounds of the neck and chest	15.55	36.5	18.5	74.3	1.2	0.2–5.8	VI	<6
5	Male suicidal shotgun injury of heart and lung	03.15	36	20.9	56	1.2	0.6–6.2	VI	<6
6	48 years, male, homicidal stab wounds of the chest	01.45	36.1	24.8	80	1	0.6–6.2	VI	<6
7	6 years, female, blunt force injury to the skull	06.15	26.4	2.3	19.8	1	0.6–6.2	IV	>2<8
8	80 years, female, coronary artery disease	16.20	36.7	23.6	71	1.9	0.6–6.2	V	>1<7
9	42 years, male, stab wounds of the neck	19.30	36.5	17.7	62.5	1.9	1–6.6	V	>1<7
10	20 years, female, fatal heroin intoxication	20.45	33.2	20.7	36.3	1	1.6–7.2	V	>1<7
11	35 years, female, stab wounds of chest and neck	04.25	33.3	9.5	60	1	1.8–7.4	IV	>2<8
12	72 years, female, homicidal strangulation	19.00	34.8	19.7	60.1	1.2	2.4–8	I neg.	>5
13	29 years, male, homicidal gunshot wound of the heart	10.25	34.7	18	75	1.05	2.8–8.4	V	>1<7
14	39 years, female, homicidal gunshot wound of the skull	09.20	34.9	21.5	75.5	1.1	3.4–9	V	>1<7
15	14 years, male, homicidal gunshot wound of the skull	09.00	33.4	20	61.2	1	3.6–9.2	III	>3<13
16	22 years, female, blunt force injury to skull and neck	04.45	32.1	20.6	50	1	4.2–9.8	I neg.	>5
17	45 years, female, alcoholic bleeding from gastric erosions	08.00	30.2	21.5	35.4	1	4.6–10.2	I orb. oris +	>5<11
18	44 years, male, homicidal shotgun wound of the heart	03.15	34.4	22.8	80	1	4.6–10.2	VI	<6
19	58 years, male, homicidal blunt force injury of the skull	13.15	28.3	6	65	1	5.4–11	V	>1<7
20	Homicidal stab wounds of the neck	11.15	32.9	24	71.5	1.1	6.2–11.8	I neg.	>5
21	3 years, female, drawing	00.30	26.2	22.9	16	1	4.1–13.1	III orb. oris +	>3<11
22	56 years, male, homicidal blunt force injury of the skull	10.45	33.2	22.5	90	1	8–13.6	I neg.	>5
23	Female, homicidal stab wounds of the neck	11.00	30.6	23.5	59.8	1.1	9–14.6	I	>5<22
24	Male, homicidal stab wounds of the neck	11.30	33.6	22.9	97.5	1.1	9.2–14.8	I neg.	>5
25	Male, homicidal stab wounds of the chest	12.10	32.7	21.5	87	1.2	10.2–15.8	I neg.	>5
26	79 years, female, throttling	04.00	31	21.8	65	1.2	10.4–16	I	>5<22
27	Female accidental traumatic asphyxia	12.30	25.9	19.6	42	1	10–16.4	I neg.	>5

Table 7.5 *– continued*

No.	Cause of death	Time of investigation	T_R	T_A	Body weight	f	Death-time estimation (nomogram)	Degree of electrical excitability	Death-time estimation (hours)
28	Female, throttling	19.10	25.7	16.1	64	1	12–18.2	I neg.	>5
29	39 years, male, stab wounds of the neck	10.10	27.5	18	75.5	1	13–19.4	I neg.	>5
30	22 years, female, homicidal gunshot wound of the chest	23.20	26.5	19.1	62.6	1–1.2	13.2–19.6	I neg.	>5
31	73 years, female, homicidal strangulation	13.00	27.5	18	74	1.3	15.9–24.9	I neg.	>5
32	41 years, male, chronic alcoholic, pneumonia	12.05	38.9	24	72	1	—	IV orb. oris + thenar+++	>2<8

T_R = rectal temperature (°C)
T_A = ambient temperature (°C)
f = corrective factor.

and left (li) eyelids. The right upper eyelid had emphysema due to an incised wound in the glabella region. Because of the higher figure obtained for death-times with regard to the degree of electrical excitability in cases with emphysema or fresh haemorrhage,[16] the reaction of the right eyelid (degree III) cannot be used as an upper limit of death-time (13 hours). The investigated time since death was really 15 hours.

Recently, the experiences with the complete 'integrated method' used in a field study of 72 consecutive cases at the scene were published.[21,22] Subsequent to the use of the temperature nomogram as primary method (see Tables 3.15 and 3.18), the non-temperature-based methods (Table 7.4; Fig. 7.3) were selectively used to improve (or at least confirm) the range of death-times resulting from the temperature nomogram. The case-oriented selection of the additional methods followed the principle discussed above (Fig. 7.3), and was supported by the interactive note-book program discussed above (see p. 251). The program defines the term confirmation of the range of death-time resulting from the temperature nomogram as follows: Henssge CA, http://home.t-online.de/home/Christoph.Henssge/t-zeit.htm.

To confirm the upper and lower time-limits obtained by the primary nomogram method, an additional criterion is only requested if its time-limit is 20% or at least 1 hour higher, or 20% or at least 1 h lower, respectively (Fig. 7.7).

Using this logistic, only those criteria were used that could be potentially helpful in the actual cases

examined. In three cases, none of the required examinations could be performed due to the particular situation at the scene. In several cases the required additional examinations could only be performed incompletely. Nevertheless, the range of death-time as estimated by the nomogram method became smaller by application of additional methods in 49 cases (examples in Table 7.6). In a further six cases the additional methods confirmed the time-limits obtained by the temperature method. In three of four cases where the temperature method should not be used, the period since death was estimated by the non-temperature-based methods exclusively (Table 7.6). As expected, the electrical examination gave rather more of an improvement, but the other criteria also contributed to improvement in many cases (Table 7.7). As can be seen from the examples in Table 7.6, the developing cascade of stepwise limitation of the period since death by examination of each further criterion contributes to the self-confidence of the investigator in his or her opinion on the period since death. The application of the integrated method including the nomogram method and the additional non-temperature-based criteria led to total spans of the period since death in the order of 1.5 hours in five cases, and up to 3.5 hours in a further 15 cases. In only one of the 72 cases (case number 23 in Table 7.6) did the upper limit of the estimated period since death concluded from the re-establishment of rigor (8 hours postmortem) contradict the time of death investigated by the crime police (9.4 hours postmortem). However, the upper limits of the period since death concluded from the nomogram method (11.7 hours post-

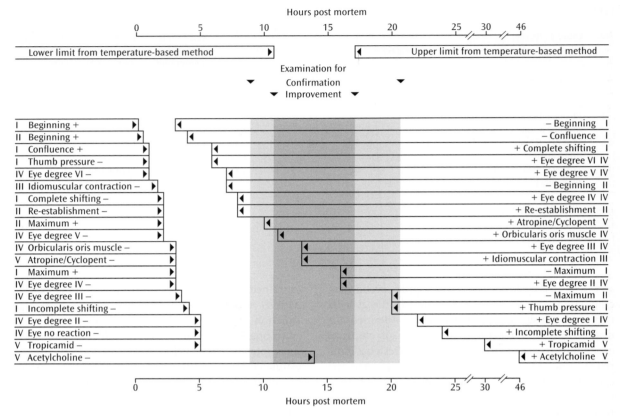

Figure 7.7 *Logistic of the 'integrated method' (see* Table 7.4). *Only those criteria should be checked which can improve or confirm the time limits from the nomogram method should be used in an actual case.*

mortem) and from the criterion mydriasis of iris to atropine (10 hours postmortem) were not in contradiction.

The field study clearly demonstrates the usefulness of estimating the period since death in the early postmortem period by application of the 'integrated method' described in this volume.

DISCUSSION

It must be emphasized that the proposed system is not the result of simultaneous measurements of experimental investigations, but rather is based only on separate data from the literature. Most of the data are again not the result of experimental investigations, but figures taken from textbooks. Therefore, not all cited limits will be the last word. For example, case number 23 in Table 7.6 points to a higher upper time limit of the criterion re-establishment of rigor (9.5 hpm) than

the literature-based 8 hpm (Tables 7.1 and 7.4).

Nevertheless, these data chosen and arranged from statistical and practical points of view are now evaluated in two field studies with simultaneous examination of the combined temperature-based nomogram method and the electrical excitability,[19] as well as of combination of all the parts of the integrated method.[20,21]

Using the proposed combined method in casework at the scene, in several cases we were able to assist the criminal investigation in its earliest stage. In other cases the additional examination of the listed criteria did not provide reduced limits for the nomogram reading. The overall result is an estimation of a time interval within which the death occurred – longer or shorter – but reliable within at least 95% limits if the instructions about using the nomogram and the other methods are followed. We feel that this is the best we can do at present, when giving a statement concerning the time of death.

Table 7.6 *Examples of cases in which the non-temperature-based methods provided a reduction and/or a confirmation of the lower and/or upper limit of the period since death obtained by the nomogram method*

Case number	Estimation — lower limit (hpm)	Method/criterion	Upper limit (hpm)	Ascertainment — lower limit (hpm)	upper limit (hpm)	Method/criterion	Comments
4	2.0	Cooling by nomogram method		5.8	6.3	Cooling by nomogram method	
	3.0	Lividity maximum					
	4.0	Lividity no incomplete shifting					
	5.0	**No electr. excit. eye**	7.6				
15	0.3	Cooling by nomogram method	11.0			Electr. excit. orbic. oris m.	
	1.0	Electr. excit. eye NO VI	10.0			Mydriasis to atropine	
	1.0	Lividity confluence	8.0			Rigor re-establishment	
	2.0	Rigor maximum+	7.0			Electr. excit. eye V	
	3.0	**Lividity maximum+**	6.0			Lividity complete shifting +	+After repeated examination at autopsy two hours later
			5.9	4.3	4.5	**Cooling by nomogram method**	
20	3.5	Electr. excit. eye NO III	10.0			Idiomuscular contraction	
	5.6	**Cooling by nomogram method**	8.0			Cooling by nomogram method	
						Electr. excit. orbic. oris m.	
						Mydriasis to atropine	
						Electr. excit. eye IV	
21	5.0	No electr. excit. eye	30.0		9.8*	Mydriasis of iris to Mydriaticum^R	*Missing for 9.8 h
			29.9	2.8*		Cooling by nomogram method	*Finding the body 2.8 h before examination
	18.1+	**Cooling by nomogram method**	24.0+	?	?	**Lividity incomplete shifting***	*The body found lying prone was transported lying back; the incomplete shifting of lividity was observed at autopsy. +Survival of the fatal pressure on the neck for 'at least 30 minutes up to 3 h': some contravascular emigration of polymorphic leucocytes in the subcutaneous fat of the ligature mark
23	3.0	Lividity maximum	13.0			Electr. excit. eye III	
	3.0	Electr. excit. eye NO IV	11.7			Cooling by nomogram method	
			10.0			Mydriasis of iris to atropine	
	6.1	**Cooling by nomogram method**	8.0	9.3	9.4	**Rigor re-establishment+**	+Being inconsistent with the time of investigation
26	2.0	Electr. excit. eye NO V	11.9			Cooling by nomogram method	
	2.0	Rigor no re-establishment		7.4	7.4	**Electr. excit. eye IV**	
	6.3	**Cooling by nomogram method**	8.0				
28	3.0	No electr. excit. orbic. oris m.	16.0			Electr. excit. eye II	
	3.5	Electr. excit. eye NO I	10.0			Mydriasis of iris to atropine	
	3.5	Cooling by nomogram method	9.1			Cooling by nomogram method	
	5.0	**No mydriasis of iris to Mydriaticum^R**	8.0	6.6	6.9	**Rigor re-establishment**	
34	1.0	Lividity confluence	8.9			Cooling by nomogram method	
	2.0	Electr. excit. eye NO V	8.0			Electr. excit. eye IV	
	3.3	**Cooling by nomogram method**	6.0	4.8	5.5	**Lividity complete shifting**	

Table 7.6 – continued

Case number	Estimation lower limit (hpm)	Method/criterion	Upper limit (hpm)	Method/criterion	Ascertainment lower limit (hpm)	Ascertainment upper limit (hpm)	Comments
40	3.0 5.0 **8.9**	No electr. excit. orbic. oris m No electr. excit. eye **Cooling by nomogram method**	14.5 **10.0**	Cooling by nomogram method **Mydriasis of iris to atropine**	7.5*	12.3+	*Finding the body +Infliction of the stab wounds
44	0.5 1.0 1.1 **3.0**	Rigor beginning Lividity confluence Cooling by nomogram method **Electr. excit. eye NO IV**	13.0 11.0 8.0 **6.7**	Electr. excit. eye III Electr. excit. orbic. oris m. Rigor re-establishment **Cooling by nomogram method**	3.6	4.3	
46	3.0 3.0 3.0 4.9 **5.0**	No mydriasis of iris to atropine Electr. excit. eye NO IV No electr. excit. orbic. oris m. Cooling by nomogram method **No mydriasis of iris to Mydriaticum®**	13.0 13.0 10.5 8.0 **6.0**	Idiomuscular contraction Electr. excit. eye III Cooling by nomogram method Rigor re-establishment **Lividity complete shifting**	5.8	6.1	Same scene as 47
47	2.0 3.0 3.5 **5.0**	Rigor maximum Lividity maximum Cooling by nomogram method **Electr. excit. eye NO II**	10.0 **9.1**	Mydriasis of iris to atropine **Cooling by nomogram method**	7.3	7.6	Same scene as 46; examination 1.5 hours later than 46 The man shot first the woman and then himself in the presence of witnesses: 'Contemporarily' proved
48	3.0 5.0 **8.8** 14.0+	Lividity maximum No electr. excit. eye **Cooling** No miosis of iris to acetycholine	**14.4**	**Cooling**	11.0	14.0	*This finding would provide an extraordinarily small range of the period since death. As a precaution, the statement at the scene did not take this criterion into account The upper limit of the time since death investigated later on (14.0 hpm) was identical to the lower limit of the estimated period since death based on this criterion
52	1.4 2.0 2.0 **3.0**	Cooling by nomogram method Rigor maximum Electr. excit. eye NO V **Lividity maximum**	11.0 8.0 8.0 **7.0**	Electr. excit. orbic. oris m. Electr. excit. eye IV Rigor re-establishment **Cooling by nomogram method**	3.6	4.8	
57	5.0 5.0 11.6 **14.0**	No electr. excit. eye No mydriasis of iris to Mydriaticum® Cooling by nomogram method **No miosis of iris to acetylcholine**	20.0 **17.2**	Cooling by nomogram method **No miosis of iris to acetylcholine**	3.2	18.7	
58	5.0 **13.7**	Electr. excit. eye NO II **Cooling by nomogram method**	24.0 20.1 **20.0**	Lividity incomplete shifting+ Cooling by nomogram method **Lividity positive thumb pressure**	14.3	16.1	+The body found lying prone was transported lying back; the incomplete shifting of lividity was observed at autopsy
59	1.8 1.5 2.0 **3.0**	Cooling by nomogram method No idiomuscular contraction Electr. excit. eye NO V **No mydriasis of iris to atropine**	8.0 8.0 **7.4**	Electr. excit. eye IV Rigor re-establishment **Cooling by nomogram method**	2.4	4.5	

Table 7.6 – *continued*

Case number	Estimation lower limit (hpm)	Method/criterion	Upper limit (hpm)	Method/criterion	Ascertainment lower limit (hpm)	upper limit (hpm)	Comments
63		Idiomuscular contraction	13.0				
		Lividity maximum	11.2				
	3.0	Rigor re-establishment	8.0	Cooling by nomogram method			
	5.6	**Cooling by nomogram method**	**7.0**	**Electr. excit. eye V**	**6.7**	**7.1**	
67	3.0	No mydriasis of iris to atropine					
	3.0	No electr. excit. orbic. oris m.					
	3.5	Electr. excit. eye NO III					
	4.9	Cooling by nomogram method	16.0	Electr. excit. eye II			
	5.0	**No mydriasis of iris to Mydriaticum®**	**10.5**	**Cooling by nomogram method**	**9.3**	**10.3**	
68	2.0	Electr. excit. eye NO V					
	3.0	Lividity maximum	15.9	Cooling by nomogram method			
	6.9	**Cooling by nomogram method**	**8.0**	**Electr. excit. eye IV**	**5.7**	**11.2**	
69		Electr. excit. orbic. oris m.	11.0				
		Mydriasis of iris to atropine	10.0				
	1.7	Cooling by nomogram method	7.3	Cooling by nomogram method			
	3.0	**Lividity maximum**	**6.0**	**Electr. excit. eye VI**	**3.1**	**3.4**	
71	5.0	No electr. excit. eye	23.4	Cooling by nomogram method			
	14.4	**Cooling by nomogram method**	**20.0**	**Lividity positive thumb pressure**	**17.2**	**17.7**	
72		Cooling by nomogram method	9.5				
		Electr. excit. eye IV	8.0				
	2.0	Electr. excit. eye NO V	8.0	Cooling by nomogram method			*Observed at the scene after turning the body from lying prone to lying back
	3.9	**Cooling by nomogram method**	**6.0+**	**Lividity complete shifting+**	**5.1**	**5.4**	

Cases where the nomogram method must not be used

Case number	Estimation lower limit (hpm)	Method/criterion	Upper limit (hpm)	Method/criterion	Ascertainment lower limit (hpm)	upper limit (hpm)	Comments
31	1.0	Lividity confluence	10.0	Mydriasis of iris to atropine			Because of the particular circumstances the temperature-based nomogram method could not be used
	3.0	**Electr. excit. eye NO IV**	**8.0**	**Rigor re-establishment**	**4.8**	**5.3**	
38	0.5	Rigor beginning	11.0				The temperature-based method was not used because of heat exposure by a room-fire
		Lividity confluence	10.0	Mydriasis of iris to atropine			
	1.0	**Electr. excit. eye NO VI**	**7.0**	**Electr. excit. eye V**	**3.0**	**?**	
45	1.0	Lividity confluence	10.0				The temperature method was not used because of the particular cooling conditions
	2.0	Rigor maximum					
	3.0	No electr. excit. orbic. oris m.		Mydriasis of iris to atropine			
	5.0	**Electr. excit. eye NO II**	**8.0**	**Rigor re-establishment**	**4.5**	**7.5**	

Table 7.7 *Number of instances where a criterion of a non-temperature-based method led to improvement or confirmation of the upper or lower limit of the period since death estimated from body cooling*

Method/criterion	Improvement	Confirmation
Electrical excitability eye	33	18
Electrical excitability orbicularis oris muscle	6	5
Mydriasis of iris to atropine	9	3
Mydriasis of iris to Mydriaticum Roche	4	1
Miosis of iris to acetylcholine	1	2
Rigor beginning	5	4
Rigor maximum	3	0
Rigor re-establishment	6	7
Idiomuscular contraction	1	1
Lividity beginning	0	0
Lividity confluence	6	3
Lividity maximum	9	3
Lividity complete displacement by thumb pressure	3	0
Lividity complete shifting after turning over	5	5

REFERENCES

1 Forster B, Ropohl D, Raule P. A new formula for the measurement of rigor mortis: the determination of the FFR-Index (German, English summary). *Z. Rechtsmed.* 1977; **80**: 51–4.

2 Beier G, Liebhardt E, Schuck M, Spann M. Measurement of rigor mortis on human skeletal muscles in situ (German, English summary). *Z. Rechtsmed.* 1977; **79**: 277–83.

3 Schuck M, Beier G, Liebhardt E, Spann W. On the estimation of lay-time by measurements of rigor mortis. *Forensic Sci. Int.* 1979; **14**: 171–6.

4 Berg S. *Grundriss der Rechtsmedizin* (German). München: Müller und Steinicke, 1984.

5 Mallach HJ. Zur Frage der Todeszeitbestimmung. (German). *Berl. Med.* 1964; **18**: 577–82.

6 Mallach HJ, Mittmeyer HJ. Rigor mortis and livores. (German, English summary). *Z. Rechtsmed.* 1971; **69**: 70–8.

7 Hofmann EV. Die forensisch wichtigsten Leichenerscheinungen (German). *Vierteljahresschr. Gerichtl. Med.* 1876; **25**: 229–61 and 1877; **26**: 17–40.

8 Hunnius PV. *Das Verhalten der Totenflecken bei quantitativen Druckmessungen in Abhängigkeit vom Leichenalter* (German). Dissertation, Tübingen, 1973.

9 Hunnius PV, Mallach HJ, Mittmeyer HJ. Quantitative pressure measurements of livores mortis relative to the determination of the time of death (German, English summary). *Z. Rechtsmed.* 1973; **73**: 235–44.

10 Hilgermann R. *Histochemische Untersuchungen zur Frage der Diffusions-Totenflecke* (German). Marburg University: MD Thesis, 1973.

11 Zsako S. Die Bestimmung der Todeszeit durch die muskelmechanischen Erscheinungen (German). *Münch. Med. Wochenschr.* 1916; **3**: 82.

12 Prokop O. Supravitale Erscheinungen (German). In: *Forensische Medizin* (Prokop O, Göhler W, eds.). Berlin: Verlag Volk und Gesundheit, 1975: 1, 27.

13 Dotzauer G. Idiomuskulärer Wulst und postmortale Blutung (German). *Dtsch. Z. Gerichtl. Med.* 1958; **46**: 761–71.

14 Popwassilew J, Palm W. Über die Todeszeitbestimmung in den ersten 10 Stunden. *Z. Ärztl. Fortbildung* 1960; **54**: 73–7.

15 Prokop O. *Lehrbuch der gerichtlichen Medizin* (German). Berlin: VEB Verlag Volk und Gesundheit, 1960.

16 Klein A, Klein S. *Die Todeszeitbestimmung am menschlichen Auge* (German). Dresden, Med. Akademie: MD Thesis, 1978.

17 Henssge C. *Methoden zur Bestimmung der Todeszeit.* Berlin, Humboldt-Universität: MD Thesis, 1982.

18 Madea B, Henssge C. *Estimation of the Time since Death – Integration of Different Methods.* Digest of the International Meeting of P.A.A.F.S. & Police Medical Officers, Wichita, USA, August 10–14, 1987.

19 Madea B, Henssge C. Electrical excitability of skeletal muscle postmortem on casework. *Forensic Sci. Int.* 1990; **47**: 207–27.

20 Henssge C, Madea B. Determination of the time since death. Body heat loss and classical signs of death – an integrated approach. *Acta. Med. Leg. Soc.* 1988; **I**: 9.

21 Henssge C, Althaus L, Bolt J, Freislederer A, Haffner H-T, Henssge CA, Hoppe B, Schneider V. Experiences with a compound method for estimating the time since death. I. Rectal temperature time of death nomogram. *Int. J. Legal Med.* 2000; **113**: 303–19.

22 Henssge C, Althaus L, Bolt J, Freislederer A, Haffner H-T, Henssge CA, Hoppe B, Schneider V. Experiences with a compound method for estimating the time since death. II. Integration of non-temperature-based methods. *Int. J. Legal Med.* 2000; **113**: 320–31.

Summary and practical scheme for casework

BERNARD KNIGHT

In spite of the great amount of theoretical and experimental work that has been carried out for more than a century on the estimation of the time since death, it is obvious that the great accuracy portrayed in innumerable detective novels and television fiction is unattainable.

Using temperature methods alone, Henssge claims a maximum precision within 95% confidence limits, of ± 2.8 hours either side of the actual time of death. This accords well with the opinion of Simonsen[1] that, where the body temperature was still above 25°C, the errors were of the order of 2.5 hours each side of the true time – and greater where the body temperature had declined below 25°C.

Madea and Henssge recommend that, wherever required, the best obtainable time range from temperature calculations be further refined by integrating other methods, such as electrical stimulation of muscle, pupillary changes, vitreous potassium, etc., as described in Chapter 6. These authors emphasize that this is not to obtain a mean time, which might be fallacious, but as a means of attrition to narrow the ranges obtained by other techniques, leaving a tighter time bracket, which still fulfils a 95% confidence criterion.

After the mass of highly technical material put forward in the preceding chapters, the reader – and especially those in the front line of law enforcement and the administration of justice, such as pathologists, detectives, prosecutors and defence lawyers – may feel bewildered by the mass of detail and arcane mathematics, etc. which have been offered – some of it apparently contradictory – with little consensus as to the 'best method'.

There is no 'best method', as different situations, the availability of equipment, the experience or otherwise of the investigator and the nature of the circumstances of the death and its environment dictate what can be done in any specific circumstance.

The methodology employed by highly experienced staff from a large European forensic institute in a suspicious death in a closed apartment with constant central heating, investigated by a police department trained in scientific methods, will of necessity be quite different from a hospital medical officer in a remote country obliged to undertake the 'occasional' forensic case, equipped only with a mercury thermometer, dealing with a body found in a forest during a day of highly variable weather.

Familiarity with the method(s) is also a potent factor in obtaining accuracy, or the lack of it. For example, the nomogram method of Henssge was checked in a large-scale collaborative exercise between a number of forensic institutes in Germany and adjacent countries, with general confirmatory results. Yet when the same method was used in a small number of cases by other authors of this book, considerable discrepancies were obtained. This was no doubt because they had insufficient experience in applying the 'correction factors', which are such an integral part of the nomogram method.

Thus, familiarity with a technique is essential, and a 'butterfly-like' dabbling with a range of methods is to be avoided. Better to stick to one possibly arbitrary method until practice and trial-and-error tactics bring the operator to the best available performance, than to flit between various techniques but fail to obtain the optimum results from any of them.

A PRACTICAL SCHEME

In the first part of this chapter, Henssge and Madea set out in considerable detail an integrated system for obtaining the narrowest possible time range within which death would have occurred in 95 out of every 100 cases. This scheme is commended for use where the investigator is familiar with the methods employed, where the equipment is available and where the importance of the case merits the effort expended.

However, in many deaths these criteria cannot be met and a compromise must be employed. It is suggested that the following is a reasonable scheme of procedure, modified again by expertise, equipment, time and opportunity. Some of the recommendations will require preplanning, such as a standing agreement between pathologist and detectives about the routines to be followed in all suspicious deaths, even before the arrival of the doctor at the locus of the body, whether that be the scene of death or a mortuary.

At the earliest possible moment, the environmental temperature at the scene of the discovery of the body should be taken. Ideally, this should be carried out as routine by the police, as soon as is practicable. The calling of more senior detectives by juniors often precedes the arrival of a pathologist, police surgeon or medical examiner and, by the time the latter arrive, the scene may have been greatly distorted by the early phases of the investigation. Doors will have been opened, even windows. People will have been passing in and out, causing draughts. Central heating or air-conditioning may have been turned on or off. Many police, scenes-of-crime officers, photographers, etc. may have crowded into a small room, their body heat altering the environmental temperature, and other variables may have been introduced by the bustle of an investigation.

In outdoor scenes, the weather – wind, rain, sun – or other conditions may have changed between the discovery of the body and the arrival of the pathologist or other doctor. It is therefore good practice for detectives to carry a thermometer to measure the environmental temperature, and even to check at intervals the direction and rate of change of that temperature. In a number of countries, including Britain and Germany, specially trained police, such as scenes-of-crime officers, are responsible for scientific matters such as trace evidence collection; some have been equipped with thermometers and are instructed to take scene temperatures as soon as possible in the investigative process. The cautions of Henssge about taking these temperatures as close as possible to the body should be remembered, as different areas of a scene may have significantly different temperatures.

As well as the actual scene temperatures, notes should be made, either by the medical examiner on arrival or by the scene investigators at an earlier time, of general and special conditions at the scene. These include details of any changes in heating or air-conditioning in internal locations, and weather changes in outdoor situations. These details are to assist in any adjustments or corrections to the actual recorded scene temperatures, as best as can be made in a retrospective fashion. Enquiries may have to be made of local weather stations or the meteorological service to learn of prior air temperatures, rain, frost, etc. in the area of the discovery.

The pathologist or other medical examiner examines the body on his or her arrival at the scene. If the body is already at a mortuary, as sometimes happens, then the whole process of estimating the time of death is rendered more inaccurate. As mentioned below, it may be impossible to take temperatures, etc. at the scene, even if the pathologist attends, but then at least he or she has been able to assess the conditions there; removal to the mortuary usually occurs relatively soon after this.

At the scene, the pathologist assesses the environment and is almost always able to test rigor by manipulating the limbs, jaw, etc. The pupils can be examined, and there would rarely be any objection to the use of drugs to test their residual reactivity.

The major problem at the scene is taking a rectal temperature. Because of the ever-present possibility of sexual or homosexual activity – which may have profound relevance to the criminal investigation – it is an almost invariable rule to take vaginal and anal swabs, and perhaps fluid samples, usually during the first stages of the autopsy at the mortuary, before any disturbance of the perianal areas. It is also common practice for the scenes-of-crime officers or forensic scientists, if called, to take 'adhesive tapings' of the clothing and to retain all clothing, inner and outer, for detailed forensic examination. For example, female pants may have seminal drainage which needs chemical and biological examination.

Gaining access to the anus requires removal of clothing or cutting or splitting of seams in the clothing, and this may be viewed with disfavour by the investigating or scientific officers. The act of introducing a thermometer into the anus runs the risk of transferring seminal traces from the perineal skin, as from vaginal drainage or direct ejaculation on to the perineum, to the margins or inside of the anal canal. The manipulation of clothing, or splitting clothing, may transfer semen or blood to other parts of skin or clothing and move, or even lose, extraneous pubic hairs or other trace material.

As an example, a body wearing tight jeans, especially in a confined space in a passageway, automobile or behind furniture, may present a very difficult problem in the removal of clothing without considerable disturbance of the body. Removal to a mortuary, with cautious, organized removal of garments one by one, in good lighting, with proper facilities for examination and packing for laboratory transit, is obviously better than a struggle in dimly lit, cramped conditions at some scenes, or wet and windy weather at an outdoor location.

However, it is for the pathologist and detective and scientific officers to come to some prearranged scheme of procedure. If the investigative team can either dispense with examinations for semen, etc. at the scene, or the taping of skin and garments, then the pathologist may carry on with temperature measurements. Alternatively, it may be possible to carry these out at the scene, before the pathologist is allowed access to the perineum for measurements.

If the nomogram regime of Henssge is used, then only a single temperature recording is required; as Henssge has argued in Chapter 3, multiple records are actually counterproductive, because calculations derived from multiple readings may give information based only on that part of a quite variable temperature-decline curve.

Other researchers prefer multiple recordings, but as said earlier, each doctor must decide on his or her own calculation regime.

If access to the rectum is forbidden at the scene, because of the probability of sexual interference and the need for detailed forensic science investigation, a further line of procedure would be to take the temperature in one or both ears, nostrils and axillae. This makes the calculations intended for rectal temperatures invalid, especially the more complex ones such as the nomogram, but may be of assistance in a less accurate estimation and may be useful in assessing the value of later rectal temperatures taken when the body reaches the mortuary.

If the equipment is available, then electrical stimulation of muscle may be employed.

Whether or not the temperature is taken at the scene, it should always be repeated at the mortuary,

assuming that the autopsy is to be performed as soon as the body is transferred there from the locus of the death, as it usually is in Britain. Because of the radical change in environment and the changes inherent in transit, whatever algorithm is used is distorted to some extent. Naturally, the longer the transit and delay period and the greater the difference in environmental conditions between scene and mortuary, the greater will be the errors in calculation.

In methods using multiple sequential temperature measurements over a period of time, and those employing multiple measuring sites, such as rectum, ear, nose, etc., the body must be undisturbed for an appreciable period. This may be difficult (or even impossible) in operational conditions where the investigators are eager to proceed with scientific examinations and the autopsy. Where the environmental temperature is high, the body temperature decline is slow, and therefore an even longer time is needed to measure significant differences.

Chemical methods, such as vitreous humour chemistry, are really confined to the mortuary and, as they are more valuable in the later postmortem period, there is less urgency to perform them at the scene. Vitreous fluid can be withdrawn before the autopsy, except where some possible damage to the eye requires full examination before any interference.

In the usual situation of having obtained a single rectal temperature reading, either at the scene or soon after arrival at the mortuary (given a minimal delay between scene and mortuary), then the pathologist uses the algorithm of his or her choice, preferably decided by long usage and familiarity. (The Henssge nomogram or computation is explained in Chapters 3 and 5.) Full attention must be paid to the correction factors, and the body weight must also be known.

Other algorithms are set out in Chapter 2. Where no range of accuracy and confidence limits are stated, as with the Henssge programme, then the experience of the pathologist, with an assessment of rigor, clothing, body size and posture, environmental factors, etc., must be taken into account in adding a time bracket to the central point derived by calculation. Though Madea's electrical stimulation equipment is rarely available outside Germany, other methods such as pupillary response to drugs and vitreous potassium may be incorporated to attempt to refine further the bracket of death-times, though Madea's warning against the temptation to 'average them out' must be heeded.

The last word must go to John Davey[2], the pioneer of the estimation of the time of death, already quoted in Chapter 2:

'Much judgement, however, and nice discrimination may be requisite on the part of the medical man ... so as to enable him when called on for his opinion, to give one which will be satisfactory to the legal officers – and to himself, on reflection'.

REFERENCES

1 Simonsen A, Voigt J, Jeppesen N. Determination of the time of death by continuous post-mortem temperature measurement. *Med. Sci. Law* 1977; **17**: 112–21.
2 Davey J. *Researches, Physiological Anatomical*. London, 1839.

Index